COVID-19 and SARS-CoV-2

The Science and Clinical Application of Conventional and Complementary Treatments

Edited by
Srijan Goswami
Chiranjeeb Dey

CRC Press
Taylor & Francis Group
Boca Raton London New York

CRC Press is an imprint of the
Taylor & Francis Group, an **informa** business

First edition published 2022
by CRC Press
6000 Broken Sound Parkway NW, Suite 300, Boca Raton, FL 33487-2742

and by CRC Press
4 Park Square, Milton Park, Abingdon, Oxon, OX14 4RN
CRC Press is an imprint of Taylor & Francis Group, LLC

Library of Congress Cataloging-in-Publication Data

Names: Goswami, Srijan, editor.
Title: COVID-19 and SARS-CoV-2 : the science and clinical application of conventional and complementary treatments / edited by Srijan Goswami, Chiranjeeb Dey.
Description: First edition. | Boca Raton : CRC Press, 2022. | Includes bibliographical references and index.
Identifiers: LCCN 2021060936 (print) | LCCN 2021060937 (ebook) | ISBN 9781032011950 (hardback) | ISBN 9781032014135 (paperback) | ISBN 9781003178514 (ebook)
Subjects: LCSH: COVID-19 (Disease)--Treatment.
Classification: LCC RA644.C67 C683193 2022 (print) | LCC RA644.C67 (ebook) | DDC 614.5/92414--dc23/eng/20220211
LC record available at https://lccn.loc.gov/2021060936
LC ebook record available at https://lccn.loc.gov/2021060937

ISBN: 978-1-032-01195-0 (hbk)
ISBN: 978-1-032-01413-5 (pbk)
ISBN: 978-1-003-17851-4 (ebk)

DOI: 10.1201/9781003178514

Typeset in Kepler Std
by Deanta Global Publishing Services, Chennai, India

This book is dedicated to the scientists, doctors, academicians, medical and paramedic personnel, researchers, and all those persons who are working tirelessly day and night in silence to combat and defeat the ongoing COVID-19 pandemic, by sacrificing their own wellbeing.

Contents

Preface

Since the end of December 2019, the world has been battling with a global health emergency called COVID-19. The ongoing pandemic has claimed millions of lives worldwide and has made a serious impact on global healthcare. Information and facts about the virus and the pandemic are constantly evolving, expanding, and are available in a scattered manner. Above all, various rumors and false information have spread through word of mouth or social media in relation to the pandemic. In situations like this, it becomes hard for a common person as well as professionals to keep track of the fundamental concepts, ongoing scientific advancements and differentiate between the facts and myths.

Within a short period of time, COVID-19 has changed the landscape of healthcare systems, public health communications, and economic aspects worldwide. Globally, as of 4:51 pm CET, 13 December 2021, there have been 269,468,311 confirmed cases of COVID-19, including 5,304,248 deaths, reported to WHO. As of 13 December 2021, a total of 8,200,642,671 vaccine doses have been administered. Even after that, the COVID-19 pandemic keeps coming through the first wave, second wave, and a third wave, and each time acquiring an increased infection and transmission capability. We can clearly see the casualties because COVID-19 cases have increased to a disturbingly huge number in approximately two years. Because of the desperate need of the situation, the regulatory authorities introduced certain unproven experimental drugs (hydroxychloroquine, lopinavir-ritonavir, favipiravir, and remdesivir to name a few) for the treatment of COVID-19 patents under emergency use authorization (EUA) because the healthcare system did not have any proven medicines for the treatment of COVID-19. All of these experimental drugs failed to treat the condition and instead showed adverse drug reactions and thus their use was stopped from EUA. At the same period of time, physicians were successfully treating COVID-19 patients with Ayurveda, homoeopathy, the Siddha system, and holistic nutrition treatments. Unfortunately, because of the lack of basic understanding of holistic science of complementary and alternative systems of medicine, all these treatments were sidelined as non-evidence-based practices. In order to find a proper treatment for COVID-19, the knowledge gap and conceptual mismatch between conventional and complementary and alternative systems of treatment should be addressed first. The ongoing pandemic has proved that no single medicine system can address all aspects of a disease in totality. An integrated and multidisciplinary approach is required to establish effective prevention, treatment, and management protocol.

So, keeping the existing knowledge gap and conceptual mismatch in mind, the present textbook presents the COVID-19 situation from both a reductionistic and a holistic perspective. The experienced authors from diverse backgrounds have made a collective effort to present different aspects of COVID-19 treatment and management through conventional and complementary and alternative medical practices. The present book is grouped into three broad sections and 17 chapters illustrating coronavirus and SARS-CoV-2 molecular biology, conventional treatment regimens, and supportive, complementary, and alternative treatment strategies. This book will help researchers, medical students, and practitioners from diverse backgrounds to acquire basic knowledge about COVID-19. This book is an outcome of interactions and experiences shared by different practitioners and professionals in their respective domains.

Srijan Goswami and Chiranjeeb Dey

MATLAB® is a registered trademark of The MathWorks, Inc. For product information, please contact:

The MathWorks, Inc.
3 Apple Hill Drive
Natick, MA 01760-2098 USA
Tel: 508 647 7000
Fax: 508-647-7001
E-mail: info@mathworks.com
Web: www.mathworks.com

Editors

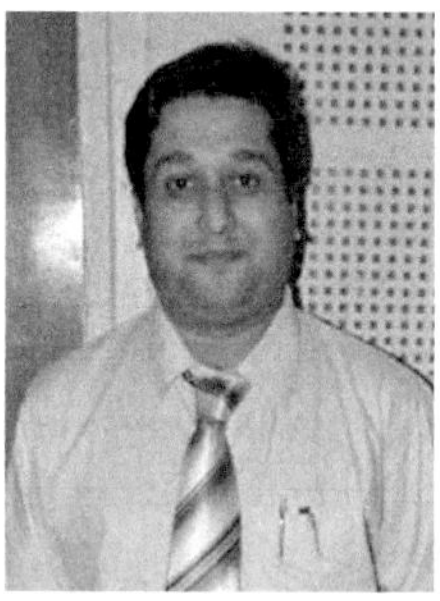

Srijan Goswami is the Founder Director of the Indian Council of Complementary Therapy and Allied Sciences, Kolkata, India (a non-government, non-profit, and ISO 9001:2015 Certified Organization). Presently, he is associated with the Guest Faculty of Immunology at the Department of Zoology (PG Courses), Serampore College, India. He is experienced in teaching at a diverse range of paramedical and Lifesciences departments of reputed colleges and institutions. Dr. Goswami is a Physician of Biochemic System of Medicine and also holds specializations in Medical Biotechnology and Clinical Nutrition. He received his professional training on Community Nutrition and Childcare, Medical Microbiology, and Medical Biochemistry from reputed medical colleges in Kolkata, India.

Dr. Goswami has around eight years of experience in the field of teaching and research and has around 30 research papers published in national and international journals and has medical books (of PG level) to his credit. He has independently and successfully guided around ten undergraduate and postgraduate students with their complete research work and publications in the past three years. Dr. Goswami has qualified the entrance test for Ph.D. in 2018.

Dr. Goswami has received four Letters of Commendation for Global Community Services and the Certificate of Honor for his contribution in the field of science and knowledge from the *International Journal of Agricultural Research, Sustainability and Food Sufficiency* (IJARSFS), the *International Journal of Advances in Medical Sciences and Biotechnology* (IJAMSB), and the *International Journal of Health, Safety and Environment* (IJHSE) in 2019, 2020, and 2021. *Current Research in Nutrition and Food Science* (Enviro Research Group) and Academia Scholarly Journals awarded him the Certificate of Excellence as a Reviewer in 2020. He is actively associated as an Editorial Review Board Member of 15 international journals and holds the post of Honorary Vice-Principal and Head of the Department of Physiology at Shree Krishna Biochemic College, Kolkata, India. His domain of interest includes molecular biology, medical-informatics, clinical nutrition, immunonutrition, mechanisms of drug action, nutraceuticals, and functional food.

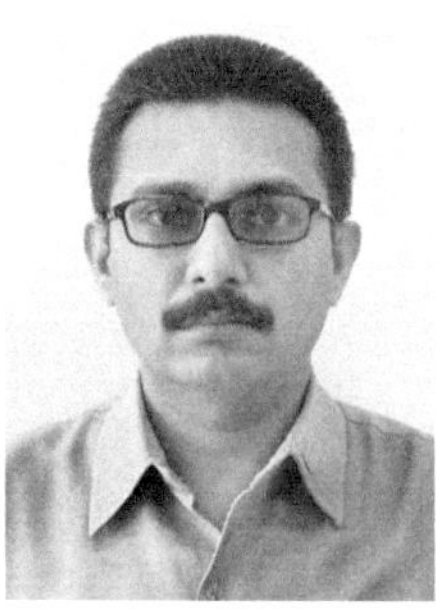

Chiranjeeb Dey graduated with an MSc in Zoology with specializations in parasitology and immunobiology from the University of Calcutta in 2001. He is a recipient of a national scholarship from CSIR-UGC, New Delhi, for his doctoral thesis and was awarded his Ph.D. degree in Zoology from the University of Calcutta in 2007 on the ultrastructure of an avian cestode tegument. Dr. Dey was a recipient of the Sudev Bhushan Ghosh Young Scientist award from the Zoological Society, Kolkata, in 2007. He was a post-doctoral fellow in a CSIR project at the Department of Biophysics, Bose Institute, Kolkata, India. He joined as an Assistant

Professor in Zoology, Serampore College (affiliated to the University of Calcutta) in 2008. Dr. Dey has published more than 25 research papers in peer-reviewed national and international journals. In addition, he has published a few textbooks for undergraduate students in Zoology from the University of Calcutta. His Ph.D. thesis was published by Scholars Press, Germany, in 2013. Apart from his research career, he has also taught zoology in undergraduate and postgraduate courses since 2002. Dr. Dey acted as examiner/evaluator and guest faculty in different undergraduate colleges and universities in India, and he has more than 19 years of research and teaching experience. His field of research interest is parasitology, especially on helminths, and their physiology, biochemistry, tegument biology (ultrastructural level), and ecology with respect to their host. Dr. Dey has collaborated in his research with a good number of institutes, namely Zoological Survey of India, Kolkata; Bose Institute, Kolkata; Department of Anatomy, All India Institute of Medical Sciences, New Delhi; USIC, Jadavpur University, Kolkata; Drug Research and Development Centre, Dum Dum, Kolkata; S. N. Bose National Centre for Basic Sciences, Salt Lake, Kolkata; and West Bengal University of Animal and Fishery Sciences, Kolkata. He has acted as a regular reviewer in international journals, notably *Experimental Parasitology* and the *Journal of Parasitic Diseases*. Dr. Dey has been supervising postgraduate students' project/dissertation works in the elective parasitology and immunobiology of the postgraduate course in zoology at Serampore College (affiliated to the University of Calcutta), Sikkim Manipal University, and Netaji Subhas Open University. Also, Dr. Dey supervises a number of students in their Ph.D. work (one of them was under DST, Govt. of WB, India MRP). He is a life member in the Zoological Society, Kolkata, Social Environmental and Biological Association (SEBA), a member of the Academy of Biodiversity Conservation (ABC), and a member of the Progressive Biochemic Practitioners Association, Ichapur, West Bengal, India. Dr. Dey participated and presented his research papers in a number of national and international level seminars and workshops. In the administrative domain, he has acted as the Head of the Department of Zoology and Convenor of the PG course in Zoology from 2010 to 2013, Co-ordinator in the PG course in Zoology from 2014 to 2016, and also acted as Chairperson (PGEC) in the PG course in Zoology from 2016 to 2019 at Serampore College, Serampore, India.

Contributors

Ushmita Gupta Bakshi
Indian Council of Complementary Therapy and Allied Sciences
Provaspally, India

Malay Banerjee
Department of Mathematics and Statistics
IIT Kanpur
Kanpur, India

Shreya Bhattacharya
Indian Council of Complementary Therapy and Allied Sciences
Provaspally, India

Subhra Bhattacharya
Department of Physiology
R. G. Kar Medical College and Hospital.
Kolkata, India

Biswaroop Roy Chowdhury
Hospital and Institute of Integrated Medical Sciences (HIIMS)
Dera Bassi
Mohali, India

Debdeep Dasgupta
Department of Physiology
Bankura Sammilani Medical College
Bankura, India

C. R. Desai
HPS Wellness
Pune, India

Soumyajit Dutta
Department of Oral Medicine and Radiology
Haldia Institute of Dental Sciences and Research
Banbishnupur, India

Shyamali Guha
Homoeopathic Practitioner
Amiya Homoeopathic Clinic
Uttarpara, India

Dona Khamaru
Indian Council of Complementary Therapy and Allied Sciences
Provaspally, India

Rehab A. Rayan
Department of Epidemiology, High Institute of Public Health
Alexandria University
Alexandria Governorate, Egypt

Sonali Sain
Department of Community Medicine
NRS Medical College and Hospital
Kolkata, India

Swarnali Sharma
Department of Mathematics
Vijaygarh Jyotish Ray College
Kolkata, India

Aikaterini Tata
Faculty of Medicine
University of Athens
Athina, Greece

Christos Tsagkaris
Faculty of Medicine
University of Crete
Heraklion, Greece

Imran Zafar
Department of Bioinformatics and Computational Biology
Virtual University of Pakistan
Punjab, Pakistan

Part I

The Molecular Biology of Coronaviruses and SARS-CoV-2

Chapter 1

Coronaviruses, History, Classification, and COVID-19

Ushmita Gupta Bakshi*, Srijan Goswami, and Chiranjeeb Dey

CONTENTS

INTRODUCTION

In December 2019, in the city of Wuhan in China, there were reports of a cluster of pneumonia cases of unknown etiology that were thought to have spread from the seafood and animal markets of the region (WHO, 2020a). Through subsequent investigation, it was confirmed that the cases of pneumonia were caused by a newly discovered member of the coronavirus family (Huang et al., 2020). The World Health Organization (WHO) named the disease COVID-19 (WHO, 2020a). The disease first spread within China and then to the rest of the world, encompassing 216 countries, areas, and territories. On January 30, 2020, the outbreak was declared a Public Health Emergency of International Concern by the World Health Organization. Globally, as of 5:05 pm CET, November 29, 2021, there have been 260,867,011 confirmed cases of COVID-19, including 5,200,267 deaths, reported to the WHO. As of November 25, 2021, a total of 7,702,859,718 vaccine doses have been administered (https://covid19.who.int/; Tables 1.1 and 1.2).

CORONAVIRUSES: DEFINITION, HISTORY, AND CLASSIFICATION

Coronaviruses belong to a family of viruses that have ribonucleic acid (RNA) as their genetic material and have the ability to cause diseases in birds and mammals. The viruses belonging to the

DOI: 10.1201/9781003178514-2

TABLE 1.1 CORONAVIRUS DISEASE (COVID–19) OUTBREAK REGIONS AROUND THE WORLD AS OF NOVEMBER 29, 2021

Region of the World	Total Cases	Total Recovered	Total Deaths
Europe	73,283,934	64,579,014	1,410,608
North America	58,957,922	47,478,076	1,191,694
South America	38,966,844	37,046,170	1,181,508
Asia	82,031,304	79,310,935	1,212,438
Africa	8,724,485	8,123,035	223,520
Oceania	366,421	191,722	4,201

Source: https://covid19.who.int/.

coronavirus family have been reported to have the largest RNA genome (Dimmock et al., 2007). Electron microscopic analysis revealed the morphological appearance of this virus family, and they were thus named coronavirus (WHO, 2020). The word "corona" in Latin means "crown like structure" (Etymonline, n.d.). Two scientists called June Almeida and David Tyrrell were the first to observe and study three previously uncharacterized human respiratory viruses (Almeida, 1967) and named the viruses "coronaviruses" based on their appearance (Tyrrell et al., 2002). The term "coronavirus" was first published (print form) in the journal *Nature* in November 1968 (Almeida et al., 1968). Figure 1.1 points out the major historical events related to the discovery and subsequent research on coronaviruses. A scientist named David Baltimore introduced the Baltimore classification system, which classifies viruses into seven different families depending on the type of genetic material they possess. The Baltimore classification system is represented in Figure 1.2. According to the Baltimore classification system, the members of the coronavirus family are grouped as class 4 because they possess positive-sense, single-stranded RNA (+ssRNA). The +ssRNA is converted to its antisense RNA, which is then reconverted to +ssRNA (Dimmock et al., 2007). In 1960, the International Committee on Taxonomy of Virus (ICTV) classified viruses depending on their taxonomic rank as order, family, subfamily, and genus. It does not emphasize the kingdoms, phyla, or class of viruses within this scheme (Dimmock et al., 2007). On the basis of taxonomy, the SARS-CoV-2 is classified under order – *Nidovirales*, family – *Coronaviridae*, and genera – *Betacoronavirus* (Rehman et al., 2020). Figure 1.3 represents the taxonomic classification of SARS-CoV-2.

TABLE 1.2 CORONAVIRUS DISEASE (COVID–19) TOP FIVE OUTBREAK COUNTRIES AS OF NOVEMBER 29, 2021

Region of the World	Total Cases	Total Recovered	Total Deaths
Worldwide	262,331,631	236,865,753	5,223,984
United States	49,267,877	39,001,529	801,049
India	34,583,597	34,008,183	468,790
Brazil	22,084,749	19,894,660	614,428
Russia	9,604,233	8,295,811	273,964
United Kingdom	10,189,059	9,025,773	144,810

Source: https://covid19.who.int/.

1930	Acute Respiratory Infections of Domesticated Chickens by Infectious Bronchitis Virus (IBV). Referenced in: Estola, T. (1970).
1931	New respiratory infections of chicken. First reported by Arthur Schalk and M.C. Hawn. Referenced in: Fabricant, J. (1998).
1937	Isolation and Cultivation of Infectious Bronchitis Virus (IBV). First isolated and cultivated by Fred Beaudette and Charles Hudson. Referenced in: Decaro, N. (2011).
1940s	Isolation of two animal coronaviruses Mouse Hepatitis Virus (MHV) Transmissible Gastroenteritis Virus (TGEV). Referenced in: McIntosh, K (1974).
1960s	Discovery of Human Coronaviruses. Referenced in: Kahn, JS, 2005; Mahase, E, 2020.
1960s	Isolation of novel common cold virus B814 at Common Cold Unit of the British Medical Research Council. E.C. Kendall, Malcom Byone, and David Tyrrell Referenced in: Kendall, et al (1962); Richmond, C, (2005).
1965	Successful cultivation of B814. Malcom Byone, and David Tyrrell Referenced in: Byone, et al. (1965).
1966	Isolation of novel common cold virus 229E at University of Chicago. Dorothy Hamre and John Procknow. Referenced in: Knapp, (n.d.); Dorothy et al. (1966).
1967	Imaging study of B814 and 229E under Electron Microscope by June Almeida (Scottish Virologist). Referenced in: Almeida J. (2008); Almeida, et al. (1967).
1968	Introduction of the term "Coronavirus" and nomenclature of the family. Referenced in: Almeida, et al. (1968).
2002	Detection of SARS-CoV. Referenced in: Su, et al. (2016); Zhu, et al. (2020).
2012	Detection of MERS-CoV. Referenced in: Su, et al. (2016); Zhu, et al. (2020).
2019	Detection of SARS-CoV-2. Referenced in: Su, et al. (2016); Zhu, et al. (2020).

Figure 1.1 The major historical events related to the discovery and subsequent research on coronaviruses.

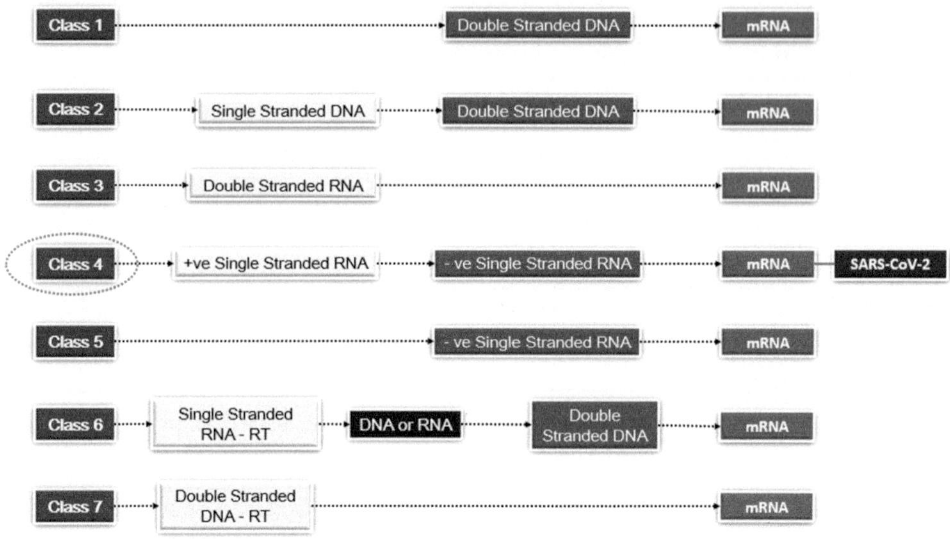

Figure 1.2 The Baltimore classification system of SARS-CoV-2.

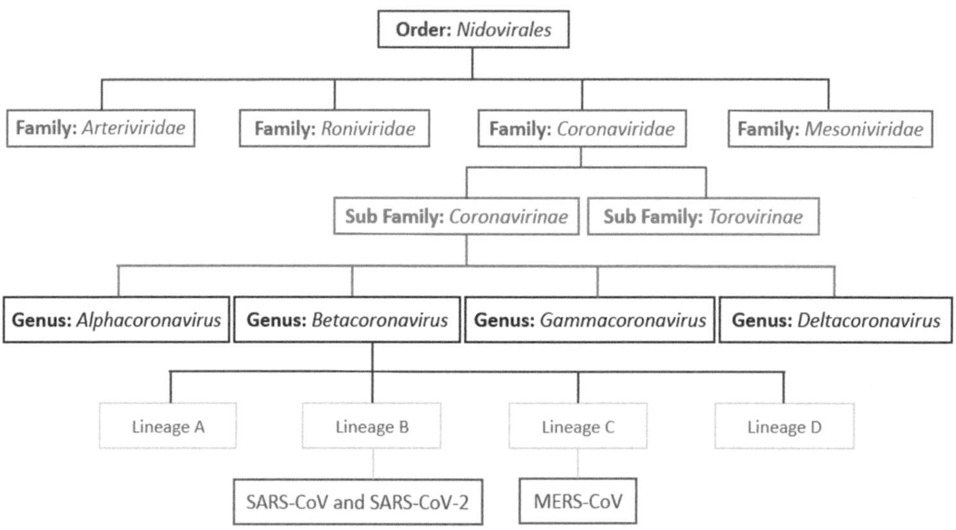

Figure 1.3 The taxonomic classification of SARS-CoV-2.

UNDERSTANDING THE WAY A VIRUS BEHAVES

SARS-CoV-2 is the causative organism for COVID-19. This correlation between the pathogen (in this case, the virus itself) and the disease (COVID-19) is based on the concept of the germ theory of disease introduced by Sir Louis Pasteur. According to this theory, diseases are caused by germs (or microorganisms). If this concept holds, then the obvious way to cure COVID-19 is to kill or eliminate the causative organism SARS-CoV-2. It is important to understand that it is not possible to kill viruses because they are neither living nor dead. The unique feature of viruses is that they only start functioning as living organisms when they infect a host cell. The general mechanisms of action of viruses are similar to the functioning of USB memory devices. For understanding the relationship between viruses and host cells, we will be using USB memory devices as an example. USB devices (like pen drives) are portable plug-in devices that can be attached to the USB port of a computer. Portable memory devices contain memory but they lack an operating system of their own, which means even if they have certain information stored in them, autonomous functioning is not possible. The program or information stored in the memory stick can only be transferred to the computer if the memory stick is connected to a computer (having a proper operating system) through the USB port (the receptor). The information or program stored in the memory stick becomes functional when it interacts with the operating system of the computer, present within the system. Viruses are comparable to memory sticks. Viruses are neither living nor do they have functional metabolism when present outside host cells. It is a capsule containing the information to overrule and control the genetics and metabolism of host cells. So, viruses, in general, can be thought of as invisible memory sticks existing in nature and one of these memory sticks has the ability to plug itself into a host cell that has the appropriate receptors. Following attachment with the appropriate receptor on the host cell, the information present inside the virus is passed into the host cell just like how files are transferred from memory sticks into a computer. The metabolic functions of the host cell are then taken over by viral genetic machinery which reprograms it accordingly to produce more virus particles. The gathering of newly synthesized viral particles inside the host cells after being replicated results in the spread of virus particles into the system which ultimately leads to cell death. These newly synthesized virus particles then infect other host cells and continue their lifecycle. This process goes on like a domino effect (Lipton, 2020; Dutta et al., 2021).

TRACING THE ORIGIN OF nCOV-19

Severe acute respiratory syndrome coronavirus 2 (SARS-CoV-2) belongs to the coronavirus family as it has remarkable similarity with the SARS virus, the virus that caused severe acute respiratory syndrome in 2002 (WHO, 2020: 36). Several studies have confirmed that the SARS virus of 2002 first originated in bats (initial host) where it mutated and achieved the ability to infect other hosts (intermediate host). Naturally, coronaviruses are benign but they might gain the ability to cause severe diseases in humans if they undergo appropriate mutations in primary and intermediate hosts. After severe acute respiratory syndrome caused by the SARS virus in 2002 and Middle East respiratory syndrome by the MERS virus in 2012, in 2019, SARS-CoV-2, a member of the same family, first mutated inside bats (primary host), then jumped to an intermediate host (the actual source of the intermediate host is still under investigation), and it further mutated and gained the ability to infect human beings, causing COVID-19 (WHO, 2020). Several studies have revealed that viruses (including coronaviruses) possess the tendency to undergo periodic mutations which provides them with the ability to cross the species barrier. This phenomenon is known as a zoonotic spillover event, a term used to indicate the situation when a virus overcomes the naturally occurring barriers necessary to "spillover" from one species to another. An accurate prediction of a viral-spill timeframe is not easy as it involves multiple factors (Figure 1.4).

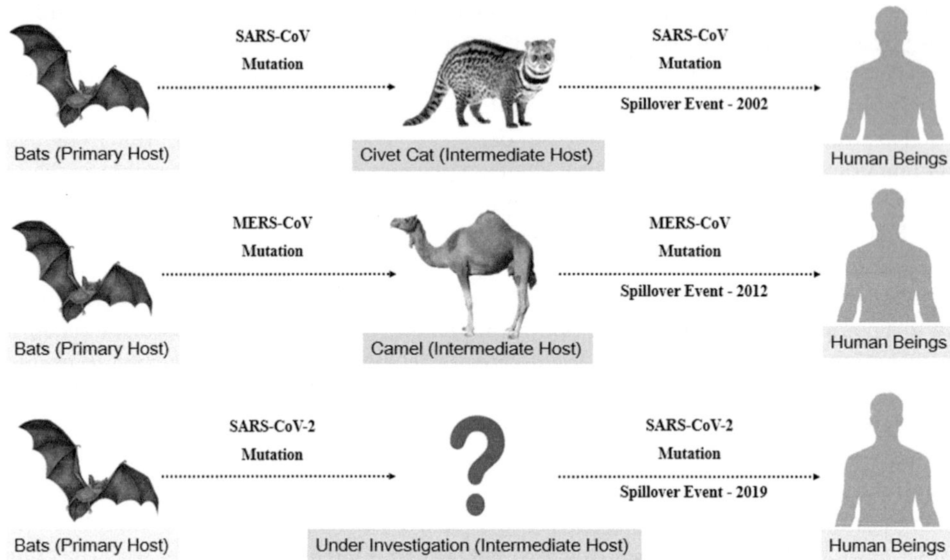

Figure 1.4 Three major spillover events.

NOMENCLATURE OF A NOVEL CORONAVIRUS AND THE DISEASE

In December 2019, a novel strain of coronavirus was found to be responsible for several cases of pneumonia. This newly identified coronavirus was named the novel coronavirus of December 2019 (nCoV-19) (WHO, 2020). The ICTV and the WHO are the two regulatory authorities responsible for naming a virus and the disease caused by it, respectively. The systematic naming of the virus as well as the disease caused by it helps in the development of diagnostic procedures, vaccines, and medications, enables scientific research, the designing of standard protocols for the understanding of transmissibility and severity, and strategize preventive measures, treatment, and management. Based on the nature of genetic the material, nCoV-19 was officially named "severe acute respiratory syndrome coronavirus 2 (SARS-CoV-2)" by ICTV on February 11, 2020. Also, on February 11, 2020, the WHO, the World Organization for Animal Health, formerly Office International des Epizooties (OIE), and the Food and Agriculture Organization of the United Nations (FAO) jointly named the disease caused by SARS-CoV-2 as COVID-19 (coronavirus disease of 2019) (WHO, 2020).

TRANSMISSION OF COVID-19

There are two basic ways by which an individual can become infected by SARS-CoV-2, one is through "respiratory droplets" and the other one is through "droplet nuclei" (WHO, 2020). Respiratory droplets are droplet particles that are >5–10 μm in diameter, whereas droplet particles with a size of <5 μm in diameter are called droplet nuclei (WHO, 2014). Several researchers have reported that respiratory droplets and contact routes are the primary modes of transmission between individuals (Liu et al., 2020; Chan et al., 2020; Li et al., 2020; Huang et al., 2020; Burke et al., 2020; WHO, 2020a). Transmission through droplets is possible when an individual is in close

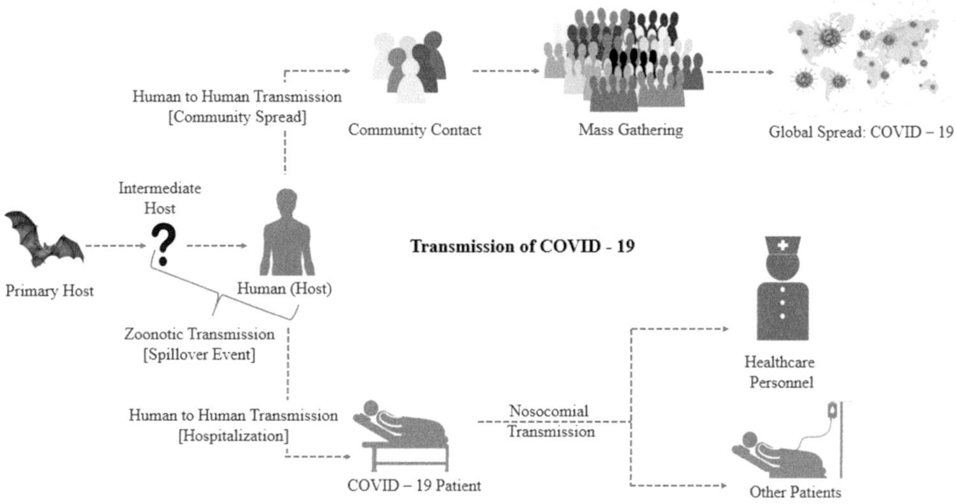

Figure 1.5 Sequence of Transmission of COVID-19.

contact (generally within one meter) with the infected person. The infected person may transmit the virus through a cough or sneeze or sometimes just by talking (without protective masks) and, as a result, the mucosa (nose and mouth) and conjunctiva (eyes) of the healthy person may be exposed to potentially infective respiratory droplets (Ong et al., 2020). The virus can also get transmitted through fomites (Ong et al., 2020). Fomites are objects that are contaminated with infectious agents (in this case, SARS-CoV-2) and serve in their transmission (Merriam-Webster, n.d.). Therefore, direct contact with the infected individual and indirect contact with fomites are the major ways by which SARS-CoV-2 is transmitted. Airborne transmission is when the droplet nuclei (containing the pathogen) remain in the air for a long period of time and are transmitted to individuals over distances greater than one meter. Airborne transmission of COVID-19 is possible under specific circumstances in which procedures that lead to aerosol production are carried out. Endotracheal intubation, non-invasive positive pressure ventilation, and disconnecting a patient from a ventilator are some of the situations (among many) that can lead to airborne transmission (WHO, 2020) (Figure 1.5).

SYMPTOMS ASSOCIATED WITH COVID-19

The words signs and symptoms are commonly used interchangeably but understanding their differences are very important for clinicians. According to the National Cancer Institute at the National Institutes of Health, a "symptom" is a physical or mental problem that a person experiences that may indicate a disease or a condition. Symptoms cannot be seen and do not show up on medical tests (NCI Dictionary of Cancer Terms, n.d.). A medical sign is a physical response linked to a medical fact or characteristic that is detected by a physician, nurse, or medical device during the examination of a patient (Felman, 2018).

Whenever we are dealing with any kind of disease, having a clear understanding of the signs and symptoms is very important for the practice of medicine. The COVID-19 disease is

TABLE 1.3 SYMPTOMS OF COVID–19

Clinical Presentation of COVID-19 (World Health Organization, 2020; Hollimon, 2020)	
Signs and Symptoms	**Percentage**
Fever/pyrexia (An increase in the body temperature of an individual)	83–99%
Cough (Expelling air from the lungs with a sudden sharp sound)	59–82%
Fatigue (Extreme tiredness resulting from mental or physical exertion or illness)	44–70%
Anorexia (Lack or loss of appetite for food)	40–84%
Dyspnea (Shortness of breath)	31–40%
Myalgia (Muscle aches and pain)	11–35%
Mucus/phlegm	27%

Source: www.who.int and www.cdc.gov, 2020.

caused when a person is infected with SARS-CoV-2. Following infection into a host cell, the virus requires a certain amount of time to acclimatize with the host cell's internal environment. This time required by the virus to acclimatize inside the host cells is called the incubation period. The incubation period can technically be defined as the time period between the infection of an individual by a pathogen and the manifestation of the illness or disease it causes in the form of signs and symptoms. The documented incubation period for SARS-CoV-2 is generally about five to six days but may extend up to 14 days. This time period may sometimes be called a "pre-symptomatic period". Fever, dry cough, and tiredness are the most common symptoms associated with COVID-19. The less common symptoms may include loss of smell or taste, nasal congestion, diarrhea, sore throat, conjunctivitis, body ache, and skin rashes. Persistent heaviness and pains in the chest, shortness of breath, loss of appetite, confusion, irritability, impaired consciousness, depression-associated disorders, sleep disorders, stroke, brain inflammation, delirium, and nerve damage have also been reported as the less common symptoms associated with COVID-19 (WHO, 2020; CDC, 2020). It is to be understood that all the symptoms listed in this section may or may not be present in every patient in equal intensity and that presenting signs and symptoms of COVID-19 may vary (Table 1.3).

GRADATION OF THE SYMPTOMS ASSOCIATED WITH COVID-19

As we have a basic idea of the general symptoms that are reported from patients suffering from COVID-19, it is now important to understand the classification of COVID-19 symptoms. There are two aspects based on which COVID-19 symptoms are graded or classified. The first and primary approach is based on the level of disease severity and the second approach is to determine the extent of pulmonary involvement using imaging techniques. Let us now understand each of these approaches systematically and realize how these two systems complement each other in the process of clinical management.

CLASSIFICATION BASED ON DISEASE SEVERITY

According to the guidelines provided by the World Health Organization, based on disease severity, symptoms can be grouped into five categories: mild disease, moderate disease (having mild pneumonia), severe disease (having severe pneumonia), critical disease (with acute respiratory distress syndrome), and critical disease (with sepsis and septic shock) (WHO Headquarters, 2021).

1. **Mild disease.** A person has symptoms like fever, loss of taste and smell, cough and cold, fatigue, loss of appetite, shortness of breath, and muscle and joint pain (and many other symptoms mentioned in the previous sections) that meet the definition of COVID-19. Also, it is to be confirmed that there is no evidence of viral pneumonia or hypoxia. The case can then be classified as mild disease (WHO Headquarters, 2021).
2. **Moderate disease (mild pneumonia).** An adolescent or adult having clinical signs of mild pneumonia (pyrexia, dyspnea, tachypnea) with general symptoms of COVID-19 mentioned in the previous sections along with an oxygen saturation percentage (SpO_2) greater than or equal to 90% under normal room conditions. A child showing clinical signs of mild pneumonia (cough, dyspnea, tachypnea) and there is no evidence of severe pneumonia (to be confirmed using an appropriate chest radiograph or CT scan). The cases can be classified as moderate disease (WHO Headquarters, 2021).
3. **Severe disease (severe pneumonia).** An adolescent or adult having clinical signs of pneumonia with the general symptoms of COVID-19 mentioned in the previous sections along with a respiratory rate greater than 30 breaths/minute or severe respiratory distress or an oxygen saturation percentage (SpO_2) less than 90% under normal room condition. If a child is showing clinical signs of advanced stages of pneumonia (cough, dyspnea, tachypnea) (to be confirmed using an appropriate chest radiograph or CT scan) along with central cyanosis or the SpO_2 level is less than 90% of normal room condition, or severe respiratory distress, an inability to breastfeed or drink, unconsciousness, or convulsions. Then cases can be classified as severe disease (WHO Headquarters, 2021).
4. **Critical disease (acute respiratory distress syndrome [ARDS]).** The patient is categorized under this category if the following criteria are fulfilled.
    - Progressive worsening of respiratory symptoms.
    - Chest imaging may reveal bilateral opacities not fully explained by volume overload, lobar or lung collapse, or nodules.
    - Respiratory failure not fully explained by cardiac failure or fluid overload. Objective assessment is advised for excluding hydrostatic cause of oedema if no risk factor is present.
    - In adults, the parameters are:

Mild ARDS	200 mmHg $< PaO_2/FiO_2 \leq$ 300 mmHg (with PEEP or CPAP $\geq$ 5 cmH_2O)
Moderate ARDS	100 mmHg $< PaO_2/FiO_2 \leq$ 200 mmHg (with PEEP $\geq$ 5 cmH2O)
Severe ARDS	$PaO_2/FiO_2 \leq$ 100 mmHg (with PEEP $\geq$ 5 cmH_2O)

PEEP: positive end expiratory pressure.

CPAP: continuous positive airway pressure.

5. **Critical disease (sepsis and septic shock).**
   a. **Sepsis**. Sepsis is the body's extreme response to an infection and is a life-threatening medical condition (Sepsis is a medical emergency. ACT FAST, 2021; WHO Headquarters, 2021).
      i. If adults present with the following signs and symptoms, then they are considered as conditions of septic shock:
         - Acute life-threatening organ dysfunction caused by a dysregulated host response to suspected or proven infection.
         - Signs of organ dysfunction that include altered mental status, difficult or fast breathing, low oxygen saturation, reduced urine output, fast heart rate, weak pulse, cold extremities or low blood pressure, skin mottling, confirmed coagulopathy, thrombocytopenia, acidosis, high lactate, or hyperbilirubinemia.
      ii. If children present with the following signs and symptoms, then they are considered as conditions of septic shock:
         - Suspected or proven infection associated with age-based systemic inflammatory response syndrome (SIRS) (including abnormal white blood cell count and body temperature).
   b. **Septic shock**. Septic shock is a subset of sepsis in which profound circulatory, cellular, and metabolic abnormalities are associated with a greater risk of mortality than with sepsis alone.
      i. If adults present with the following signs and symptoms, then they are considered as conditions of septic shock.
         - Persistent hypotension despite volume resuscitation.
         - Vasopressors are required for maintaining mean arterial pressure (MAP) greater than equals to 65 mmHg and serum lactate level greater than 2 mmol/L (WHO Headquarters, 2021).
      ii. If children present with the following signs and symptoms, then they are considered as conditions of septic shock:
         - Hypotensive state along with conditions like altered mental status, bradycardia (<90 or >160 beats per minute in infants) or tachycardia (<70 or >150 beats per minute in infants), fast breathing, hyperthermia or hypothermia, petechial or purpuric rash, high lactate concentration, or low urine output (WHO Headquarters, 2021).

CLASSIFICATION BASED ON CO-RADS

The word CO-RADS means COVID-19 Reporting and Data System. It is used in the standardized assessment of pulmonary involvement. It helps in simplifying the pulmonary involvement of COVID-19 in chest computed tomography (CT) with a five-point scale of suspicion. CO-RADS can be implemented in moderate to critical cases. CO-RADS helps clinicians to categorize a given non-enhanced chest CT scan into specific groups or categories. These seven categories are named CO-RADS 0 to 6 (Table 1.4).

REASONS BEHIND THE SEVERITY OF COVID-19

COVID-19 in totality is a new disease. The scientific community has been studying human coronaviruses for a long time but the outcome of exposure to the novel coronavirus SARS-CoV-2 and the

TABLE 1.4 CATEGORIES OF CO-RADS AND THE CORRESPONDING LEVELS OF SUSPICION FOR PULMONARY INVOLVEMENT IN COVID-19

Category of CO-RADS	Pulmonary Involvement of COVID-19: Levels of Suspicion	Interpretation
CO-RADS 0	Not interpretable	Insufficient for assignment of scores.
CO-RADS 1	Very low	Non-infectious or normal.
CO-RADS 2	Low	Typical for non-COVID-19 infections.
CO-RADS 3	Equivocal	Features compatible with COVID-19, as well as other diseases.
CO-RADS 4	High	Suspicious for COVID-19.
CO-RADS 5	Very high	Typical COVID-19.
CO-RADS 6	Proven	RT-PCR tests positive for SARS-CoV-2.

disease it causes is a bit different compared with SARS-CoV, MERS-CoV, and so on. There are a number of different viruses (rhinoviruses, coronaviruses, etc.) that appear every year and cause the symptoms of flu in humans. For years, the same family of viruses has been appearing but with increased virulence in the subsequent year. The virulence of the same virus changes over time because of the mutations they acquire. The human immune system has the ability to generate immunologic memory. If a pathogen (virus) infects an individual, the immune system develops a protective response as well as a memory response directed against the same pathogen. Previous exposure to a certain pathogen (virus) produces immunologic memory which is present in the form of antibodies that are designed to recognize and neutralize the specific pathogen. When the virulent form of the same pathogen infects the previously exposed individual, the components of immunologic memory take over and eliminate the threat before symptoms manifest. Thus, previous exposure to a pathogen provides human beings with a certain degree of protection. SARS-CoV-2, on the other hand, has not been around in the environment previously and human beings are not habituated with the virus. So when an individual comes in contact with SARS-CoV-2, the immune system recognizes it as a completely new threat and mounts a completely new set of immune responses. The development of an immune response against a pathogen that is completely new takes a long time to engage. This longer lag time is the reason behind the severity of the SARS-CoV-2 infection. Since the human body has to create a completely new set of immune memory responses, the virus gets enough time and better opportunities to manifest itself and thus give rise to the observable symptoms. So, if the virus is relatively new to the human population, then the outcome of that infection will be severe as compared with the infections caused by viruses that appear annually. New viruses (SARS-CoV-2) have serious symptomatology because the immune system is modifying itself to protect the system against the virus as well as developing immunological memory against it (Lipton, 2020).

REFERENCES

Almeida J (2008-06-26). "June Almeida (née Hart)". *BMJ*. **336** (7659): 1511. doi:10.1136/bmj.a434. ISSN 0959-8138. PMC 2440895.

Almeida JD, Tyrrell DA (April 1967). "The morphology of three previously uncharacterized human respiratory viruses that grow in organ culture". *Journal of General Virology*. **1** (2): 175–8. doi:10.1099/0022-1317-1-2-175. PMID 4293939.

Almeida JD, Berry DM, Cunningham CH, Hamre D, Hofstad MS, Mallucci L, McIntosh K, Tyrrell DA (November 1968). "Virology: Coronaviruses". *Nature.* **220** (5168): 650. Bibcode:1968Natur.220.650. doi:10.1038/220650b0.

Bruce. H Lipton. PhD (2020, March 30). *Bruce Lipton on COVID-19, Coronavirus Pandemic & Evolution [Video]* https://www.youtube.com/watch?v=oyijHfL-W7w&t=2728s Accessed on 27th June 2020.

Burke RM, Midgley CM, Dratch A, Fenstersheib M, Haupt T, Holshue M, et al. (January–February 2020). "Active monitoring of persons exposed to patients with confirmed COVID-19: United States". *MMWR Morb Mortal Wkly Rep.* 2020 doi:10.15585/mmwr.mm6909e1external icon.

CDC. (2020, March 28). *COVID Data Tracker.* Centers for Disease Control and Prevention. Retrieved June 12, 2021, from https://covid.cdc.gov/covid-data-tracker/#global-variant-report-map

Centers for Disease Control and Prevention. (2020). *Coronavirus Disease 2019 (COVID – 19) – Symptoms of Coronavirus* Retrieved June 22, 2020, from: https://www.cdc.gov/coronavirus/2019-ncov/symptoms-testing/symptoms.html

Chan J, Yuan S, Kok K et al. (2020). "A familial cluster of pneumonia associated with the 2019 novel coronavirus indicating person-to-person transmission: a study of a family cluster". *Lancet.* 2020. doi: 10.1016/S0140-6736(20)30154-9.

Chen L, Liu W, Zhang Q, Xu K, Ye G, Wu W, et al. "RNA based mNGS approach identifies a novel human coronavirus from two individual pneumonia cases in 2019 Wuhan outbreak". *Emerg Microb Infect.* 2020;9:313–319. doi: 10.1080/22221751.2020.1725399.

Decaro N (2011). "Gammacoronavirus". In Tidona C, Darai G (eds.). *Gammacoronavirus‡: Coronaviridae. The Springer Index of Viruses.* Springer. pp. 403–413. doi:10.1007/978-0-387-95919-1_58. ISBN 978-0-387-95919-1. PMC 7176155.

Dimmock, N.J., Easton, A.J., & Leppard, K.N. (2007). *Introduction to Modern Virology* (6th ed.). Blackwell Publishing.

Dutta, J., Goswami, S., & Mitra, A. (Eds.). (2021). *Multidimensional Approaches to Impacts of Changing Environment on Human Health* (1st ed.). CRC Press. https://doi.org/10.1201/9781003095422

Estola T (1970). "Coronaviruses, a New Group of Animal RNA Viruses". *Avian Diseases.* **14** (2): 330–336. doi:10.2307/1588476. ISSN 0005-2086. JSTOR 1588476.

Fabricant, J. (1998). "The Early History of Infectious Bronchitis". *Avian Diseases.* **42** (4): 648–650.

Fabricant J (1998). "The Early History of Infectious Bronchitis". *Avian Diseases.* **42** (4): 648–650. doi:10.2307/1592697. ISSN 0005-2086. JSTOR 1592697.

Felman, A. (2018, February 22). Why do signs and symptoms matter? *Medical News Today.* Retrieved June 18, 2021, from https://www.medicalnewstoday.com/articles/161858#medical-signs

Hamre D, Procknow JJ (January 1966). "A new virus isolated from the human respiratory tract". *Proceedings of the Society for Experimental Biology and Medicine.* Society for Experimental Biology and Medicine. **121** (1): 190–3. doi:10.3181/00379727-121-30734. PMID 4285768.

Hollimon, N. (2020, March 18). Symptoms of Coronavirus. *WebMD.* Retrieved June 17, 2021, from https://www.webmd.com/lung/covid-19-symptoms#1

Huang C, Wang Y, Li X, et al. (2020). Clinical features of patients infected with 2019 novel coronavirus in Wuhan, China. *Lancet.* 395(10223): 497–506. https://doi.org/10.1016/s0140-6736(20)30183-5

Kahn JS, McIntosh K (November 2005). "History and recent advances in coronavirus discovery". *The Pediatric Infectious Disease Journal.* **24** (11 Suppl) Suppl: S223–7, discussion S226. doi:10.1097/01.inf.0000188166.17324.60. PMID 16378050.

Kendall EJ, Bynoe ML, Tyrrell DA (July 1962). "Virus isolations from common colds occurring in a residential school". *British Medical Journal.* **2** (5297): 82–6. doi:10.1136/bmj.2.5297.82. PMC 1925312. PMID 14455113.

Knapp, Alex. "The Secret History of the First Coronavirus". *Forbes.* Retrieved May 6, 2020.

Li Q, Guan X, Wu P, et al. Early transmission dynamics in Wuhan, China, of novel coronavirus-infected pneumonia. *N Engl J Med* 2020; doi:10.1056/NEJMoa2001316.

Liu J, Liao X, Qian S et al. Community transmission of severe acute respiratory syndrome coronavirus 2, Shenzhen, China, 2020. *Emerg Infect Dis* **2020** doi:10.3201/eid2606.200239.

Lu R, Zhao X, Li J, Niu P, Yang B, Wu H, et al. Genomic characterisation and epidemiology of 2019 novel coronavirus: implications for virus origins and receptor binding. *Lancet.* 2020;395:565–574. doi: 10.1016/S0140-6736(20)30251-8.

Mahase E (April 2020). "The BMJ in 1965". *BMJ*. **369**: m1547. doi:10.1136/bmj.m1547. PMID 32299810.

McIntosh K (1974). "Coronaviruses: A Comparative Review". In Arber W, Haas R, Henle W, Hofschneider PH, Jerne NK, Koldovský P, Koprowski H, Maaløe O, Rott R (eds.). *Current Topics in Microbiology and Immunology / Ergebnisse der Mikrobiologie und Immunitätsforschung. Current Topics in Microbiology and Immunology / Ergebnisse der Mikrobiologie und Immunitätsforschung*. Berlin, Heidelberg: Springer. p. 87. doi:10.1007/978-3-642-65775-7_3. ISBN 978-3-642-65775-7.

McIntosh K, Becker WB, Chanock RM (December 1967). "Growth in suckling-mouse brain of "IBV-like" viruses from patients with upper respiratory tract disease". *Proceedings of the National Academy of Sciences of the United States of America*. **58** (6): 2268–73. Bibcode:1967PNAS...58.2268M. doi:10.1073/pnas.58.6.2268. PMC 223830. PMID 4298953.

Merriam-Webster. (n.d.). Fomite. In *Merriam-Webster.com dictionary*. Retrieved June 13, 2020.

Merriam-Webster. (n.d.). Incubation period. In *Merriam-Webster.com dictionary*. Retrieved June 24, 2020, from https://www.merriam-webster.com/dictionary/incubation%20period

NCI Dictionary of Cancer Terms. (n.d.). National Cancer Institute. Retrieved June 18, 2021, from https://www.cancer.gov/publications/dictionaries/cancer-terms/def/symptom

Ong SW, Tan YK, Chia PY, Lee TH, Ng OT, Wong MS, et al. Air, surface environmental, and personal protective equipment contamination by severe acute respiratory syndrome coronavirus 2 (SARS-CoV-2) from a symptomatic patient. *JAMA*. 2020 Mar 4 [Epub ahead of print].

Paraskevis D, Kostaki EG, Magiorkinis G, Panayiotakopoulos G, Sourvinos G, Tsiodras S. (2020). Full-genome evolutionary analysis of the novel corona virus (2019-nCoV) rejects the hypothesis of emergence as a result of a recent recombination event. *Infect Genet Evol*. 79:104212. doi: 10.1016/j.meegid.2020.104212.

Rehman, S. U., Shafique, L., Ihsan, A., & Liu, Q. (2020). Evolutionary Trajectory for the Emergence of Novel Coronavirus SARS-CoV-2. *Pathogens*, 9(3), 240. doi:10.3390/pathogens9030240.

Richmond C (2005-06-18). "David Tyrrell". *BMJ: British Medical Journal*. **330** (7505): 1451. doi:10.1136/bmj.330.7505.1451. PMC 558394

Sepsis is a medical emergency. ACT FAST. (2021, May 10). Centers for Disease Control and Prevention. Retrieved June 18, 2021, from https://www.cdc.gov/sepsis/what-is-sepsis.html

Su S, Wong G, Shi W, Liu J, Lai AC, Zhou J, et al. (June 2016). "Epidemiology, Genetic Recombination, and Pathogenesis of Coronaviruses". *Trends in Microbiology*. **24** (6): 490–502. doi:10.1016/j.tim.2016.03.003. PMC 7125511. PMID 27012512.

Tyrrell DA, Byone ML (June 1965). "Cultivation of a Novel Type of Common-Cold Virus in Organ Cultures". *British Medical Journal*. **1** (5448): 1467–70. doi:10.1136/bmj.1.5448.1467. PMC 2166670. PMID 14288084.

WHO Headquarters (2021, January 25). *COVID-19 Clinical management: living guidance*. World Health Organization. Retrieved October 20, 2021, from https://www.who.int/publications/i/item/WHO-2019-nCoV-clinical-2021-1

World Health Organization (2020). Naming the Coronavirus Disease (COVID-19) and the virus that causes it; 2020. Retrieved June 24, 2020, from https://www.who.int/emergencies/diseases/novel-coronavirus-2019/technical-guidance/naming-the-coronavirus-disease-(covid-2019)-and-the-virus-thatcauses-it

World Health Organization. (2020a, January 30). Pneumonia of unknown cause – China. Retrieved May 27, 2021, from https://www.who.int/csr/don/05-january-2020-pneumonia-of-unkown-cause-china/en/

World Health Organization. Infection prevention and control of epidemic- and pandemic-prone acute respiratory infections in health care. Geneva: World Health Organization; 2014 https://apps.who.int/iris/bitstream/handle/10665/112656/9789241507134_eng.pdf?sequence=1

World Health Organization. (2020, January 30) *Modes of Transmission of Virus Causing COVID -19 implications for IPC Precautions Recommendations*; 2020. Retrieved June 22, 2020, from https://www.who.int/news-room/commentaries/detail/modes-of-transmission-of-virus-causing-covid-19-implications-for-ipc-precaution-recommendations

World Health Organization (2020d). Report of the WHO-China Joint Mission on Coronavirus Disease 2019 (COVID-19) 16–24 February 2020 [Internet]. Geneva: World Health Organization; 2020 Available from: https://www.who.int/docs/default- source/coronaviruse/who-china-joint-mission-on-covid-19-final-report.pdf.

World Health Organization. Symptoms of COVID – 19; 2020. Retrieved June 22, 2020, from https://www.who.int/emergencies/diseases/novel-coronavirus-2019/question-and-answers-hub/q-a-detail/q-a-coronaviruses#:~:text=symptoms

Zhang Y, Chen C, Zhu S et al. [Isolation of 2019-nCoV from a stool specimen of a laboratory-confirmed case of the coronavirus disease 2019 (COVID-19)]. *China CDC Weekly*. 2020;2(8):123–4. (In Chinese).

Zhu N, Zhang D, Wang W, Li X, Yang B, Song J, et al. (February 2020). "A Novel Coronavirus from Patients with Pneumonia in China, 2019". *The New England Journal of Medicine*. 382(8): 727–733. doi:10.1056/NEJMoa2001017

Chapter 2

SARS-CoV-2 Morphology, Genomic Organisation and Lifecycle

Srijan Goswami* and Ushmita Gupta Bakshi

CONTENTS

INTRODUCTION

The basic understanding of the origin and development of a coronavirus infection calls for a clear understanding of pathogen biology. The characteristic features that form the foundation are fundamental structural and functional characteristics of the pathogen, including the lifecycle, are discussed in this chapter. Research related to the novel coronavirus strain SARS-CoV-2 or nCoV-2019 is emerging and rapidly evolving with new findings every day. This section discusses the established scientific communication until June 2020 after the discovery of the novel strain in January 2020. It is to be understood that similar findings might rapidly change and open an altogether new vista in front of us with a deeper understanding and groundbreaking research on the virulent strain.

DOI: 10.1201/9781003178514-3

1. Structure and function of the pathogen
2. The lifecycle of the pathogen – mechanism of entry, replication of genome, assembly of viral particles, formation of viral progeny

These concepts provide an understanding of how the organisms function and how the structures and functions are modified during the course of the disease. Understanding the lifecycle and underlying biochemical processes of the pathogen helps in designing specific sophisticated diagnostic tests to facilitate healthcare professionals in examining patients efficiently. And most importantly, it helps in understanding the underlying biochemical pathways that can be used to develop targeted therapies.

THE BASIC STRUCTURE OF SARS-CoV-2

As discussed in Chapter 1, the coronaviruses are classified into four genera: alphacoronavirus, betacoronavirus, gammacoronavirus and deltacoronavirus. SARS-CoV-2, the enveloped virus responsible for COVID-19, belongs to genera betacoronavirus and shares structural similarities with SARS-CoV and MERS-CoV (the other two members of the same genera) (Lu et al., 2020). The genome of coronaviruses consists of positive-sense single-stranded RNA (+ssRNA) and are around 29,881 bp in length (GenBank no. MN908947) with 9860 amino acids (Chen et al., 2020; Wang, 2020). The genome consists of gene sequences encoding structural proteins and non-structural proteins. The electron microscopic analysis of SARS-CoV-2 revealed that it has a spherical body with a diameter of approximately 60 nm to 140 nm and a crown-like spike structure of approximately 9 nm to 12 nm in length (Zhu et al., 2020). These crown-like spike structures are common to all the representative members of the coronavirus family. There are also various kinds of structural proteins that are present on the outer surface of coronaviruses (Astuti & Ysrafil, 2020). SARS-CoV-2 possess four major structural proteins on the outer surface similar to other coronaviruses, namely the spike protein (S), envelope protein (E), membrane protein (M) and nucleocapsid protein (N) (Figure 2.1). Let us now understand each of these four proteins in detail.

Spike (S) Protein

The spike (S) protein of SARS-CoV-2, the most outward envelope protein, is a glycosylated transmembrane structure, made up of 1162 to 1452 amino acid residues. The spike protein facilitates the attachment of SARS-CoV-2 with the receptors on the host cell membranes, leading to the fusion of the two structures. The spike protein of SARS-CoV-2 is not only responsible for the tropism of the virus but also aids in the induction of the host immune response (Masters, 2006; Hulswit et al., 2016 Li, 2016; Tortorici & Veesler, 2019). Tropism is the ability of a pathogenic microorganism to infect a particular host (host tropism) (McFadden et al., 2009). This makes the spike protein a structure of medical concern. Based on topology, the spike protein can be divided into three basic regions (domains). These are the cytoplasmic domain, the helical (transmembrane) domain and the extracellular domain. The cytoplasmic domain, also known as the endodomain or the intracellular tail, presents at the virion interior (residues 1235–1273, UniProtKB – P0DTC2, n.d.). The helical (transmembrane) domain consists of only a small N-terminal segment (residues 1214–1234, UniProtKB – P0DTC2, n.d.). The extracellular domain, also known as the Ectodomain, presents at the virion exterior (residues 13–1213, UniProtKB – P0DTC2, n.d.)

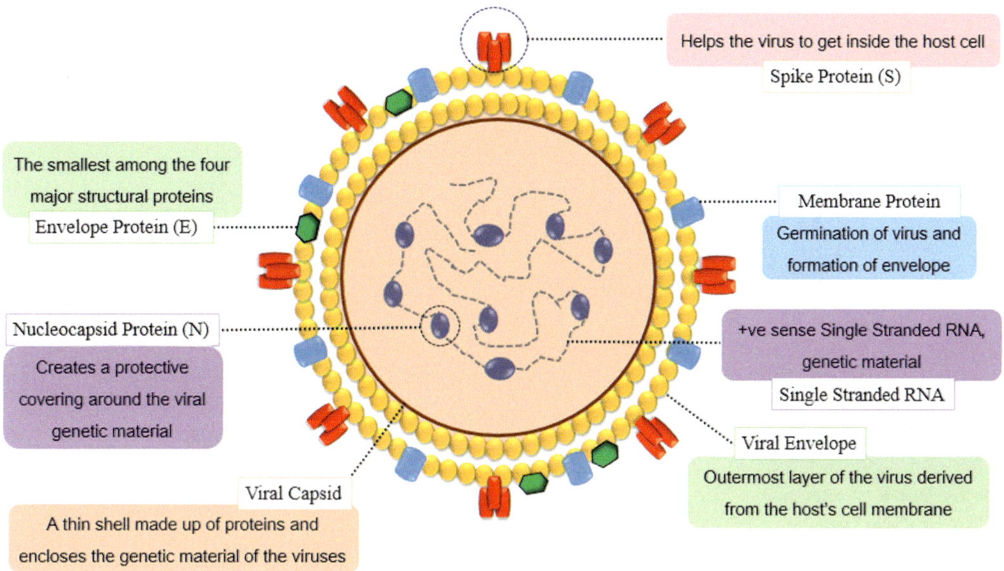

Figure 2.1 The basic structure of SARS-CoV-2.

(Masters, 2006; Li, 2016). Apart from that, the fundamental structure of the spike protein can be divided into two major subunits, S1 and S2. Subunit 1 (S1) also known as the receptor-binding domain, helps coronaviruses bind to host cell receptors (UniProtKB – P59594, n.d.; Hulswit et al., 2016; Tortorici & Veesler, 2019). The receptor-binding domain (RBD) of SARS-CoV-2 recognises a specific receptor known as the angiotensin converting enzyme receptor-2 (ACE-2). These ACE-2 receptors are located in the lungs, heart, kidneys and intestines inside the human body. The affinity of the RBD of SARS-CoV-2 for ACE-2 has been found to be 20 times higher as compared with a normal SARS virus. This increased affinity makes SARS-CoV-2 a global concern. The second functional portion, known as subunit 2 (S2) (as shown in Figure 2.2), mediates the fusion reaction between the virus and the host cell membrane. Subunit 2 can be considered as a class I viral fusion protein having a fusion peptide (FP), heptad repeat 1 (HR1), a central helix (CH), a connector domain (CD), heptad repeat 2 (HR2), a transmembrane domain (TM) and a cytoplasmic tail (CT) (UniProtKB – P59594, n.d.; Hulswit et al., 2016; Tortorici & Veesler, 2019) (Figure 2.3).

HR1 and HR2 collectively form a six helical bundle important for membrane fusion and increased infectivity, thus making the structure a potential drug target. The S1 subunit is composed of two separate domains known as the N-terminal domain (S1-NTD) and the C-terminal domain (S1-CTD). Depending on the virus, one or both of these domains may bind to receptors and function as an RBD. The RBD of the SARS-CoV-2 spike protein is responsible for the recognition of ACE-2 on the host cell membrane. The RBD is made up of two distinct portions, first the highly conserved core subdomain, and second, the external subdomain. The core of RBD contains an important region called the receptor-binding motif (RBM) containing the major binding sites for ACE-2 (Lan et al., 2020). The S1-NTDs are responsible for binding sugar receptor molecules except for the betacoronavirus, the S1-NTD of which binds a protein receptor called CEACAM1 (carcinoembryonic antigen-related cell adhesion molecule 1/CD66a). The roles of the S1-CTDs are

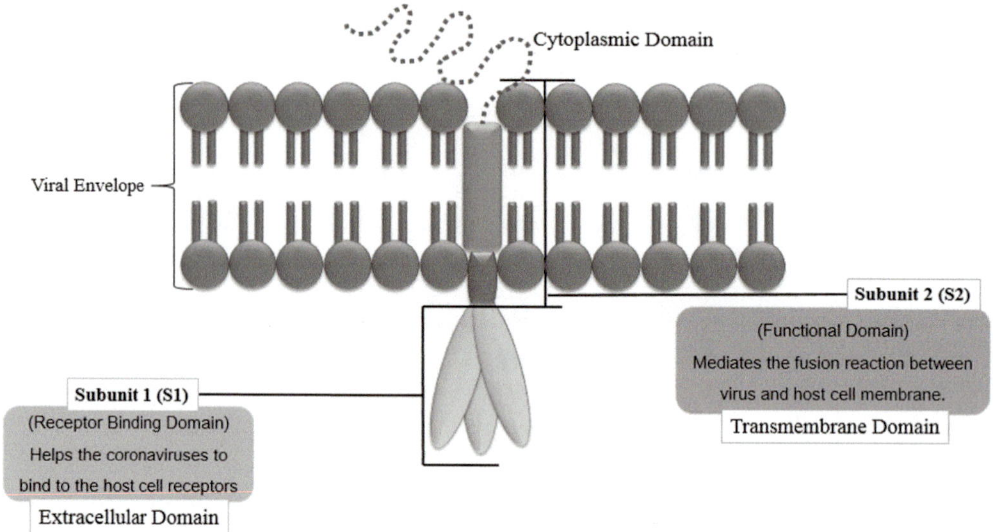

Figure 2.2 The basic structure of the SARS-CoV-2 spike protein.

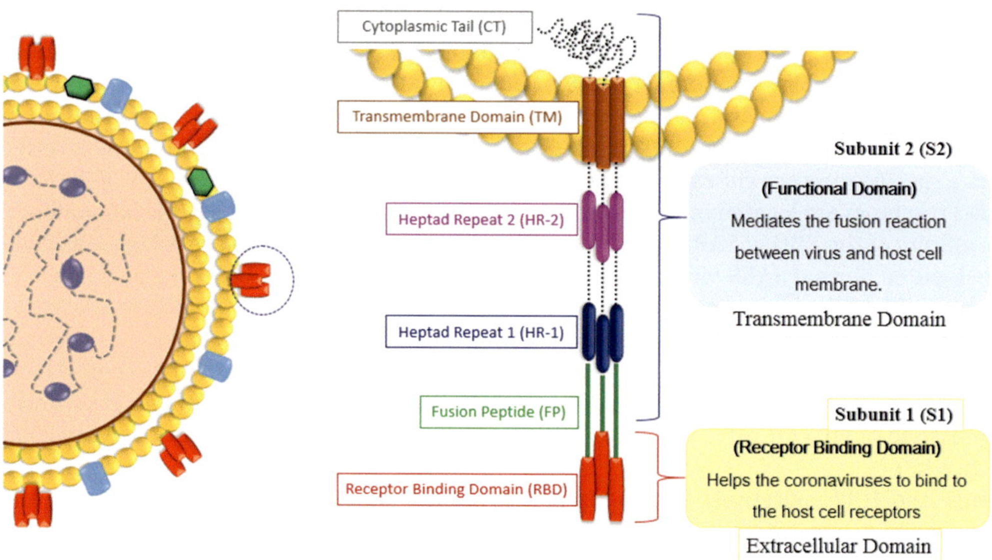

Figure 2.3 Functional units of the spike protein.

to bind to protein receptors ACE-2, Aminopeptidase N (APN) and dipeptidyl peptidase 4 (DPP4) (Li, 2016; Ou et al., 2020). Structurally, the S1 subunit of the betacoronavirus spike protein is divided into four distinct β-rich domains, A, B, C and D. Domains A and B are suggested to serve as RBD. The core structure of domain A shows a galectin-like β-sandwich fold. Domain B contains a core subdomain of antiparallel β-sheets decorated with an extended loop on the viral membrane-distal side. The domains A and B are linked by a linker region. Domain A is located within the functionally S1-NTD, whereas the domains B, C and D are located within the S1-CTD. The domains C and D form β-sheet-rich structures adjacent to the S2 subunit (Hulswit et al., 2016). Structural studies of SARS-CoV RBD revealed that the RBD contains a core and a motif termed RBM that is critical for forming contact with the receptor. The researchers reported that the S2 subunit undergoes three basic conformational changes, namely a pre-fusion native state, a pre-hairpin intermediate state, and a post-fusion hairpin state. The sequential conformational changes promote the alignment and subsequent fusion of viral and host cell membranes (UniProtKB – P59594, n.d.). Because of the critical role they play in binding to target cells and mediating the entry, both subunit 1 and subunit 2 of the spike protein are fundamental factors in relation to the designing of vaccines and also for creating synthetic drugs for the treatment of COVID-19 (UniProtKB – P59594, n.d.).

Membrane (M) Protein

Membrane proteins or M-proteins are the most abundant structural proteins present on the surface of coronaviruses and play a central role in morphogenesis and the assembly of the virus (see Figure 2.1). The shape of the viral envelope is determined by this protein and also acts as a central organiser for the assembly of coronaviruses by interacting with other structural proteins (Chan et al., 2020). The possible structural arrangement is shown in Figure 2.4 (UniProtKB – P59596, n.d.; UniProtKB – P0DTC2, n.d.).

1. Virion surface domain (2 to 19 amino acids; marked as 1 in Figure 2.4)
2. Helical (transmembrane) domain (20 to 40 amino acids; marked as 2 in Figure 2.4)
3. Intravirion domain (41 to 50 amino acids; marked as 3 in Figure 2.4)

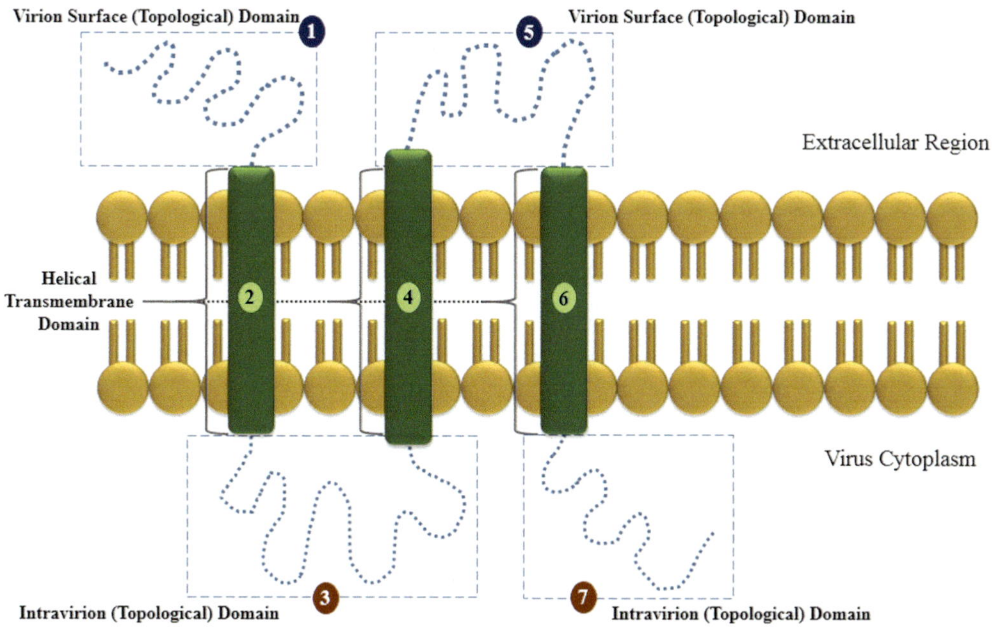

Figure 2.4 The basic structure of the SARS-CoV-2 membrane protein.

4. Helical (transmembrane) domain (51 to 71 amino acids; marked as 4 in Figure 2.4)
5. Virion surface domain (72 to 79 amino acids; marked as 5 in Figure 2.4)
6. Helical (transmembrane) domain (80 to 100 amino acids; marked as 6 in Figure 2.4)
7. Intravirion domain (101 to 222 amino acids; marked as 7 in Figure 2.4)

Envelope (E) Protein

Envelope proteins or E-proteins are the smallest of all major structural proteins present on SARS-CoV-2. The major functions of the envelope protein are as follows:

- First, it helps in the assembly and release of viruses from host cells.
- Second, during the process of viral replication, it is largely located at the regions of intracellular trafficking, for example, near the endoplasmic reticulum and Golgi apparatus.
- It functions as a viroporin and self-assembles in host membranes forming pentameric protein-lipid pores that allow ion transport and plays a role in the induction of apoptosis (UniProtKB – P59637, n.d.).
- It is known to activate the host NLR family pyrin domain containing 3 (NLRP3) inflammasome, leading to interleukin-1 beta (IL-1β) overproduction.

So, both membrane and envelope proteins play an integral role in transforming the host cell apparatus into viral workshops where the virus and host cells work together for making new viral particles (UniProtKB – P59637, n.d.). It is divided into three basic domains, the virion surface (topological) domain, the helical (transmembrane) domain and the intravirion (transmembrane) domain (UniProtKB – P59637, n.d.) (Figure 2.5).

Viral Envelope

The viral envelope is present just under the surface proteins and is the outermost layer of the virus derived from the host's cell membrane. Since the host's cell membrane is made up of phospholipids and proteins, the fundamental composition of the viral envelope is the same as the host

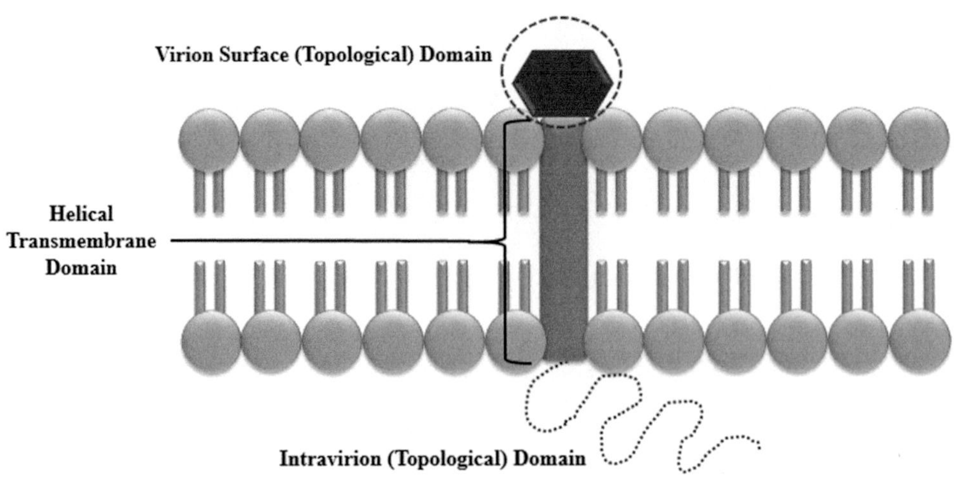

Figure 2.5 The basic structure of the SARS-CoV-2 envelope protein.

cell membrane. The only distinguishing feature is that, in viruses, these membrane structures are incorporated with viral glycoproteins instead of host cell glycoproteins. The phospholipid-protein complex of the viral envelope gets denatured when treated with soap, which in turn destroys the virus. This is the reason that the World Health Organization recommended thorough handwashing with soap as an important preventive measure.

The Viral Capsid and the Nucleocapsid (N) Protein

The capsid, located just below the viral envelope, is a thin shell made up of proteins and encloses the genetic material of the virus. Nucleocapsid proteins are located below the capsid, associated with the viral genetic material, and thus create a protective covering around it. The nucleocapsid plays three critical roles in the virus lifecycle (UniProtKB – P59595, n.d.). First, it protects viral particles by inhibiting the host's defence mechanisms, second, it assists viral RNA in replicating itself, and third, it aids in the generation of new viral particles (UniProtKB – P59595, n.d.).

GENOMIC ORGANISATION OF SARS-CoV-2

The members of the coronavirus family possess a large genome containing approximately 30,000 nucleotides (29,891 nucleotides to be exact according to Chan et al., 2020). The genome is capable of synthesising around 9860 amino acids and 38% is the total G+C content (Chan et al., 2020). According to the Baltimore classification of viruses, coronaviruses belong to 'Class-4', which means these viruses have +ssRNA as their genetic material (Dimmock et al., 2016). The genetic material of coronaviruses is a single-stranded, linear chain, with a positive-sense structure having a 5' cap and 3' poly-A tail. One of the important features to consider is that in comparison with other coronaviruses, SARS-CoV-2 lacks the hemagglutinin esterase (HE) gene (Chan et al., 2020). The 5' end of the genetic material has an array of numerous structural components and functional genes, some of which we will be considering are 5'-leader sequence, open reading frame 1a (ORF-1a), open reading frame 1b (ORF-1b), ribosomal frameshift site (present at the junction of ORF-1a and ORF-1b), spike protein (S)-gene, envelope protein (E)-gene, membrane protein (M)-gene, nucleocapsid protein (N)-gene and 3' untranslated region (3' UTR) (Figure 2.6). ORF-1a and ORF-1b along with the ribosomal frameshift site fall under the group of genes that encodes replicase polyproteins (also known as non-structural proteins or NSPs) and S, E, M and N belong to the group of genes coding for structural proteins (Swiss Institute of Bioinformatics, 2020). These polyproteins are further processed and broken down into 16 distinct non-structural protein forms (classified as nsp1 to nsp16) by the action of viral proteins. Apart from all these, the genome also consists of genes for accessory proteins namely ORF 3, ORF 6, ORF 7a, ORF 7b, ORF 8 and ORF 9b (as shown in Figures 2.6 and 2.7) (Chan et al., 2020).

THE LIFECYCLE OF SARS-CoV-2

Mechanism of Cell Entry

Coronaviruses belong to the group of spherical enveloped viruses having single-stranded positive-sense RNA as their genetic material. The viral envelope is composed of lipoproteins and expresses three important structures, namely S-protein, E-protein and M-protein (Dimmock et al., 2016). Like any other viruses, the members of the coronavirus family also require a host

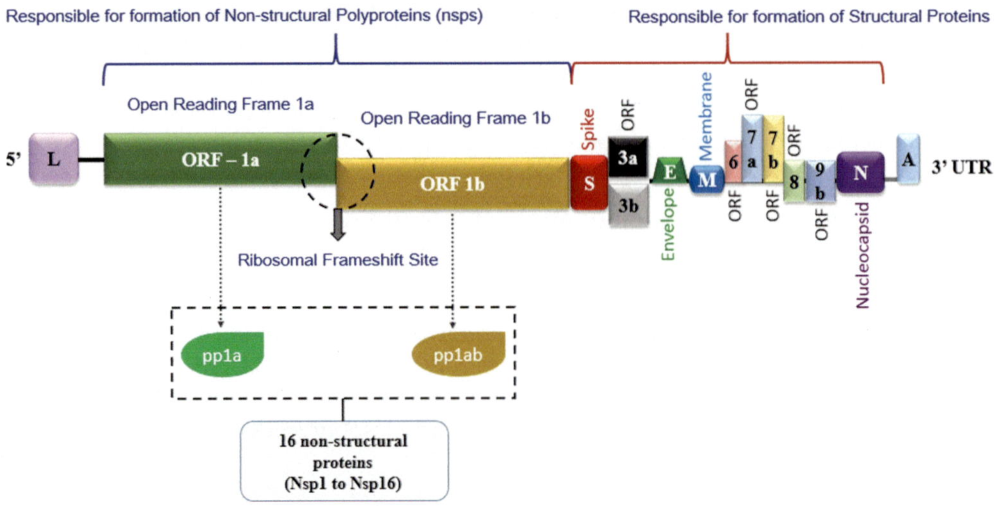

Figure 2.6 The basic structure of the SARS-CoV-2 genome.

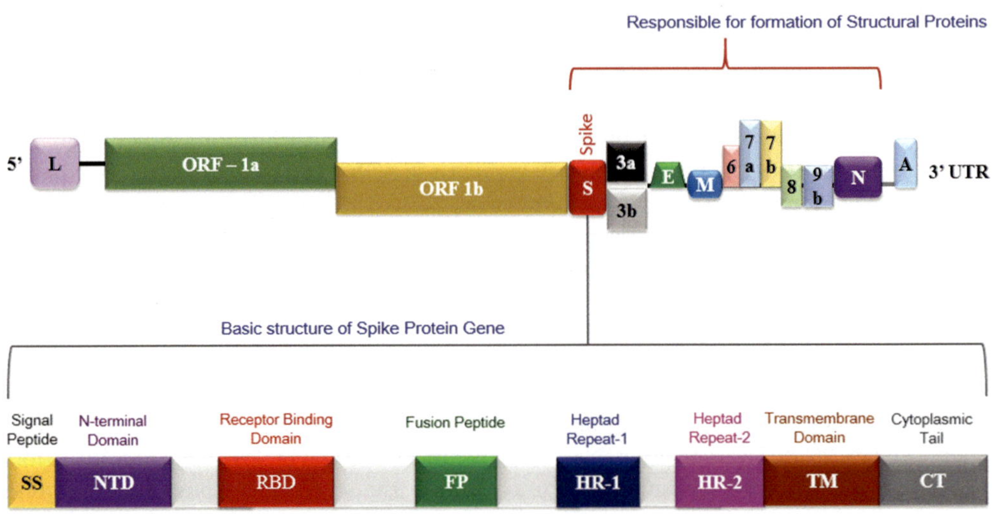

Figure 2.7 The basic structure of the SARS-CoV-2 spike protein sequence.

cell for their multiplication. In order for the virus to be able to utilise the host cell's replication machinery, it must first be able to establish interaction and subsequently infect the host cell. So let us understand the mechanism by which SARS-CoV-2 enters host cells.

It is known that SARS-CoV-2 spreads mainly by respiratory droplets through coughing or sneezing which aerosolises the virus, allowing it to enter into the nasal and oral cavity and this is the reason behind symptoms like nasal congestion, headache, sore throat and so on (WHO, 2020a). Studies have shown that the multiplication of viral particles occurs within the epithelial cells of the upper respiratory tract. Just like SARS, SARS-CoV-2 can enter deep inside the lungs

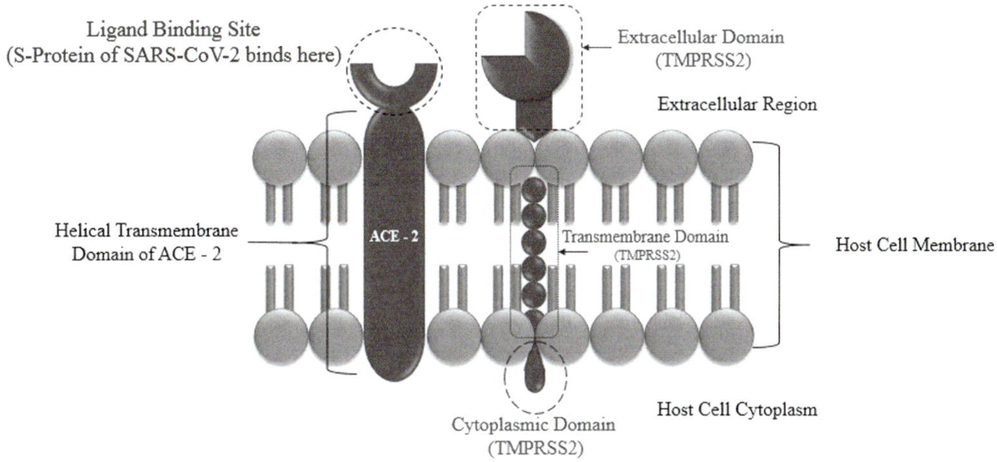

Figure 2.8 The basic structure of ACE-2 and TMPRSS2 on the cell membrane.

and damage the alveolar epithelial cells by replicating inside them. ACE-2 is present on the membrane of the epithelial cells of alveoli (of the host cell) in the lungs. SARS-CoV-2 uses its S-proteins to bind to these ACE-2 receptors present on the membrane of host cells. This mechanism of binding of SARS-CoV-2 with ACE-2 receptors is similar to the mechanism of binding in the SARS virus. Figure 2.8 represents the basic structure of the ACE-2 receptor and transmembrane serine protease 2 (TMPRSS2) present in the host cell membrane. Once the S-protein recognises the ACE-2 receptor, another important enzyme on the host cell, TMPRSS 2, present near the ACE-2 receptors, activates the S-protein by cleaving it at a specific site (see Figure 2.9 A and B).

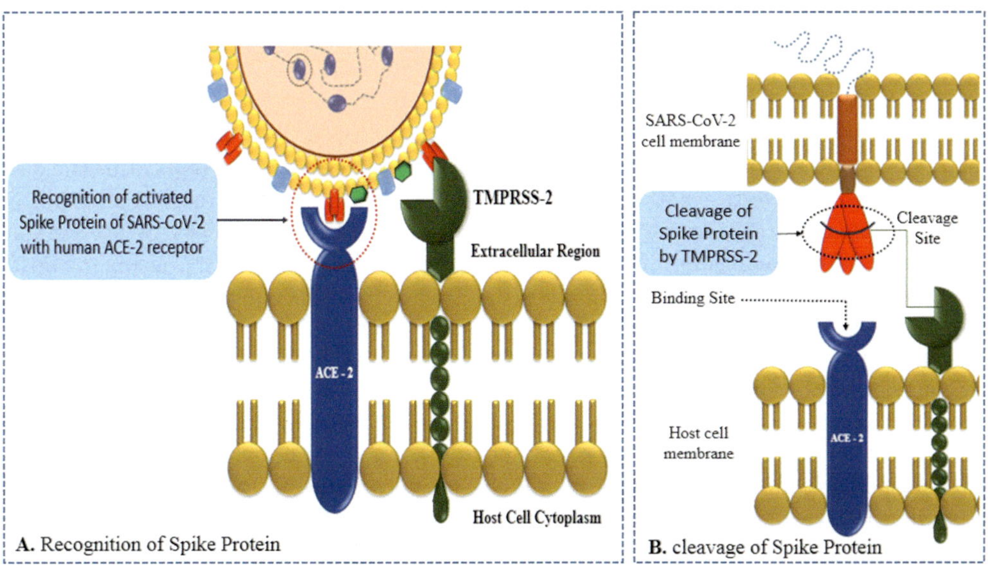

Figure 2.9 (A) Recognition of ACE -2 by the S-protein. (B) Cleavage and activation of the S-protein by TMPRSS2.

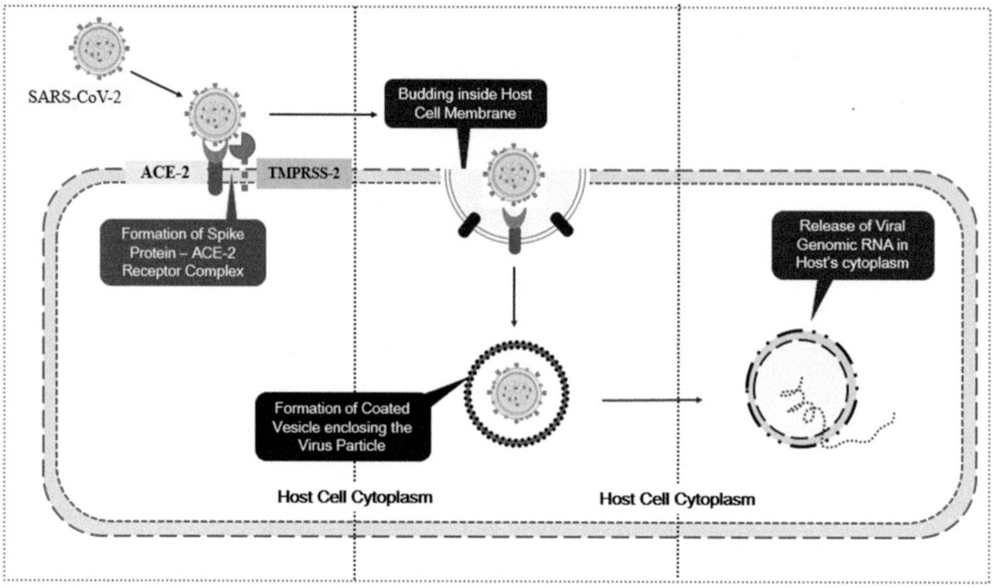

Figure 2.10 ACE-2 mediated endocytosis of SARS-Cov-2 and the release of viral genomic RNA.

Following the cleavage, the S-protein binds to the ACE-2 receptor, thus forming a spike protein–ACE-2 receptor complex (see Figure 2.10). This cleavage of the S-protein by TMPRSS 2 and the subsequent formation of the spike protein–ACE-2 receptor complex promotes the fusion of the viral envelope with the host cell membrane and results in subsequent endocytosis of the virus particle (see Figure 2.11) (Fung & Liu, 2019).

Endocytosis is the process by which materials (in this case the virus itself) enter the cell after being surrounded by an area of the cell membrane (of the host) which then buds off inside the cell and forms a vesicle. After the viral particle is endocytosed, the genomic RNA is released into the host's cytoplasm. The virus then uses the host's ribosomes and enzymes for replicating the viral genomic RNA and also for translating viral genomic RNA into proteins. As a result, virus-specific mRNA and proteins are synthesised inside the cytoplasm of host cells. Further viral proteins are then assembled with blueprints of information contained within the viral RNA using the host's cellular machinery. The endoplasmic reticulum and Golgi apparatus together not only assemble the newly synthesised RNA and proteins but also package them inside an envelope (composed of a phospholipid bilayer and glycoproteins). Finally. the newly assembled viral particles leave the Golgi apparatus by forming a vesicle made up of a phospholipid membrane of the Golgi apparatus itself and is released from the host cell by the process of cellular exocytosis Thus, it is clear that wherever the ACE-2 enzyme is present, the coronavirus can gain entry into these cells, so that it is responsible for the tissue tropism of the coronavirus (specific organs which the SARS-CoV-2 will be able to affect). This ACE-2 enzyme is expressed on tissues like alveolar cells in the lungs (responsible for pulmonary complications), small intestinal epithelial cells (responsible for GI symptoms), cardiac tissues, kidneys, liver and blood vessels. SARS-CoV-2 has ten to 20 times more affinity to a human cell's ACE-2 as compared with the SARS virus (Liu et al., 2020) (Lim et al., 2016).

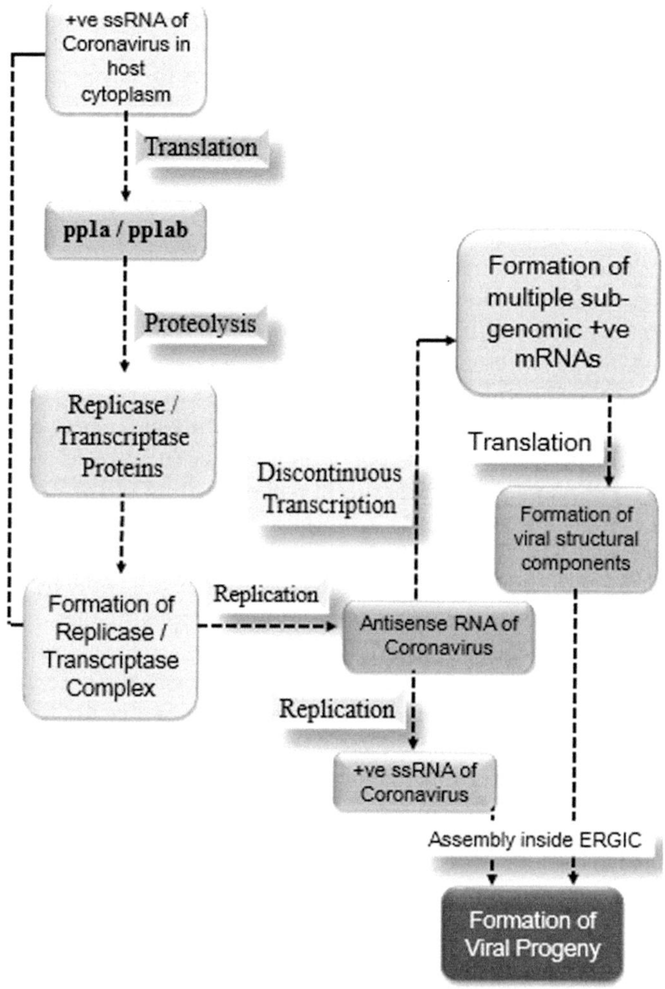

Figure 2.11 Ribosomal frameshifting and synthesis of SARS-CoV-2 polyproteins.

The Replication Cycle of SARS-CoV-2

Studies have shown that the replication cycle of coronaviruses undergoes two important biochemical mechanisms. First, ribosome frameshifting during genome translation. This can be observed during the initial production of polyproteins, which are actually used to generate most of the protein machinery of the replisome or transcriptosome. Second, synthesis of both genomic and multiple subgenomic RNA species.

So, the hallmark of the coronavirus transcription process is the production of many subgenomic mRNAs. Subgenomic mRNAs are differently sized mRNAs that are created from the original RNA genome (Dimmock et al., 2016). The ACE-2 protein present on the host cell membrane is influential in the SARS-CoV-2 infection process. The SARS-CoV-2 spike protein possesses the ability to recognise and bind to ACE-2 receptors on host cell membranes. This binding of the SARS-CoV-2 spike protein generates a conformational change of the human ACE-2 receptor which facilitates receptor-mediated endocytosis. This receptor-mediated endocytosis pulls the virus inside the host cell. Once inside the host cell, the uncoating of the viral particle begins. During the process of uncoating the protein covering, the virus particle dissolves and the genomic RNA of the virus is released into the host cell cytoplasm.

The viral genomic RNA then utilises the host cell machinery, primarily the ribosomes, for translating the viral genomic RNA strand in order to generate several open reading frames (ORFs) essential for the virus lifecycle. As the genomic RNA of the coronavirus undergoes the process of translation utilising the host ribosomes, two important polyproteins (among many) are synthesised. These are very large proteins that come from viral genomic RNA. The two polyproteins are named polyprotein-1a (pp1a) and polyprotein-1ab (pp1ab). These two major polyproteins are synthesised through the process of 'frameshifting' during translation (Figure 2.6). In Figure 2.6, the region designated ORF1a represents open reading frame 1a and ORF1b represents open reading frame 1b. The irregular junction between ORF1a and ORF1b represents the frameshift site (marked with a dotted circle). ORF1a, ORF1b and the frameshift site in between are responsible for the production of the polyproteins. The polyproteins generated are referred to as replicase polyproteins because they play an important role in replication and further transcription. As the translation progresses through ORF1a, pp1a is synthesised.

But if the translation process while proceeding through OFR1a frameshifts to a region of ORF1b, the resultant protein thus formed is pp1ab. Polyprotein 1ab is the hybrid of ORF1a and ORF1b. These polyproteins are further proteolyzed into numerous smaller proteins and play a critical role in viral replication and transcription. Proteins involved in replication are called replicase complex while the proteins involved in transcription are called transcriptase complex. All these proteins combine with viral genomic RNA (sense strand) and facilitate replication. When the +ssRNA of the coronavirus replicates, an antisense RNA is produced. The conversion of the sense RNA into antisense RNA is very much important for the lifecycle of the virus. The antisense RNA is important because:

- It can be replicated back to sense RNA, which is essentially the same thing that entered with the original virus during uncoating.
- This antisense RNA can be transcribed through a method called discontinuous transcription. Discontinuous transcription of antisense RNA generates a diverse range of mRNAs that can then be translated into different proteins.

Reconversion to Positive-Sense Single-Stranded RNA

It is known that the coronavirus genome is +ssRNA. After the virus enters the host cell RNA dependent RNA polymerase are produced by transcription of the original viral genomic RNA. This viral polymerase is attached to the 3' end of the original viral genomic RNA (+ssRNA) and transcribes an antisense RNA. The RNA dependent RNA polymerase again binds to the 3' end of antisense RNA and synthesises multiple copies of +ssRNA (original form). This original form of viral genomic RNA is further repackaged into the viral offspring (virions). Virions are then released by the process of exocytosis and infect other cells (Figure 2.12).

Discontinuous Transcription of Antisense RNA

Coronaviruses utilise RNA dependent RNA synthesis to generate mRNAs to be transcribed by host cell machinery. The RNA dependent RNA polymerase is synthesised from sense RNA

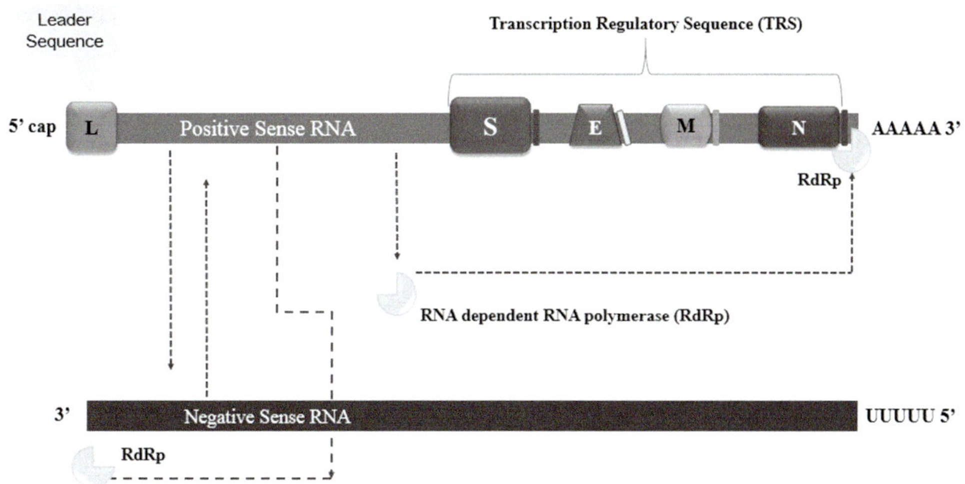

Figure 2.12 Reconversion to positive-sense single-stranded RNA.

(original genomic RNA). This viral polymerase is attached to the 3' end of the original viral genomic RNA (+ssRNA) and initiates the transcription process. During this transcription process, the RNA dependent RNA polymerase synthesises a series of positive-sense subgenomic mRNAs that vary in their length. This occurs by discontinuous transcription.

The RNA dependent RNA polymerase copies the +ssRNA starting from the 3' end up until it reaches the first transcription regulatory sequence (TRS), for example, the gene for nucleocapsid designated as N in Figure 2.13. From that TRS (corresponding to N gene), the viral polymerase

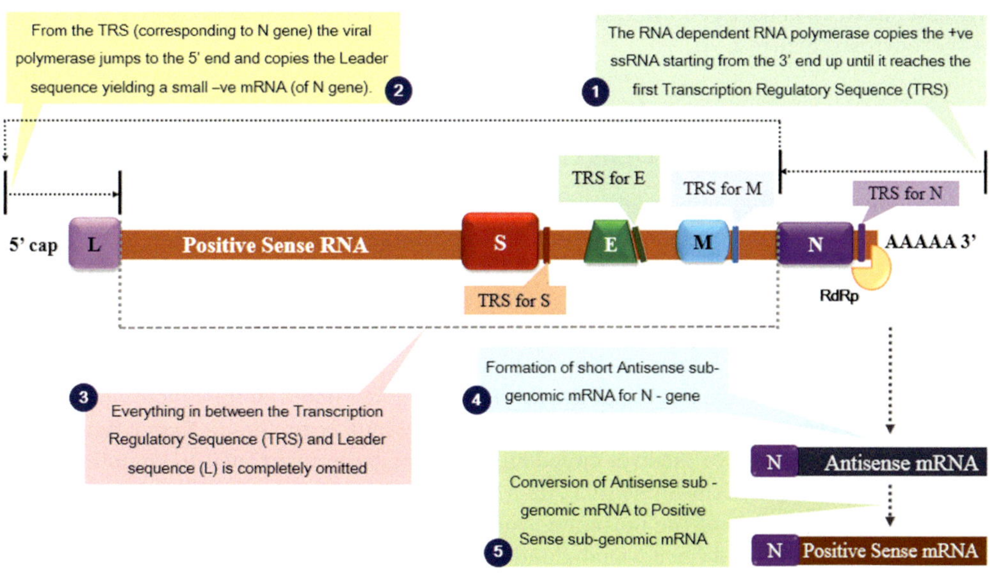

Figure 2.13 Discontinuous transcription of antisense RNA of SARS-CoV-2.

jumps to the 5' end and copies the leader sequence, yielding a small negative mRNA (of N gene). Again, the viral polymerase starts copying from the 3' end of +ssRNA, and this time it ignores the first TRS (i.e., the N gene) and instead recognises the second TRS, for example, the gene for membrane protein designated as M. From that TRS (corresponding to the M gene), the viral polymerase jumps to the 5' end and again copies the leader sequence, yielding another small negative mRNA (of M gene). That means everything in between the TRS and leader sequence (L) is completely omitted. This discontinuous transcription process continues until all the different types of negative subgenomic mRNAs are synthesised that are important for the viral lifecycle. All these newly synthesised negative mRNAs of varying size come from the same strand of original RNA, therefore, they are called subgenomic. The negative subgenomic mRNAs are then converted back to respective positive subgenomic mRNAs, and these are an actual form of subgenomic mRNA that encodes viral structural proteins. These viral structural proteins are combined with original genomic sense genomic RNA to make progeny.

Assembly and Release of Viral Particles

The assembly of newly synthesised viral particles begins with the systematic aggregation of +ssRNA and viral structural components. During this phase of the virus lifecycle, the nucleocapsid bound to +ve ssRNA interacts with other structural proteins (example: S, E and M proteins) to form the intact virus particle (Lim et al., 2016). The assembly of newly synthesised coronavirus particles is accomplished through the budding of nucleocapsid through membranes early in the secretory pathway from the endoplasmic reticulum to the Golgi intermediate compartment (ERGIC). The contribution of the host cell during this process is still under investigation. Studies have shown that M-protein controls and regulates the process of viral assembly by mediating the interaction with nucleocapsid to allow the budding of newly synthesised virus particles (Neuman et al., 2011). The M-protein also interacts with E-protein and S-protein to complete the assembly of mature virus particles (Shang et al., 2020). Following assembly and budding, the newly assembled viral particles are transported in vesicles and eventually released by the process of exocytosis (Figure 2.14).

RENIN–ANGIOTENSIN–ALDOSTERONE SYSTEM AND SARS-CoV-2

The interconnection of the renin–angiotensin system with the kidneys, liver, lungs, blood vessels and adrenals are essential for understanding the importance of ACE-2 in relation to COVID-19. The renin–angiotensin system is a closed-loop feedback mechanism that helps maintain normal renal blood flow. The kidneys are designed to filter nitrogenous waste products of protein metabolism in our bodies. To function normally, kidneys need a steady flow of blood, receiving about 25% of total cardiac output. A drop in blood pressure either systematically from heart failure or locally from the narrowing of the arteries supplying blood to the kidneys stimulates the kidneys to secrete a chemical called renin into the bloodstream. Renin then reacts with a protein hormone produced in the liver called angiotensinogen converting it to angiotensin I. A second enzyme produced in the lungs, ACE, then links angiotensin I, converting it to angiotensin II, the active configuration of the hormone. Angiotensin II acts on both the peripheral arteries throughout the body and the adrenal glands. The arteries constrict and the adrenal glands produce another hormone called aldosterone, which causes the kidneys to resorb more salt and

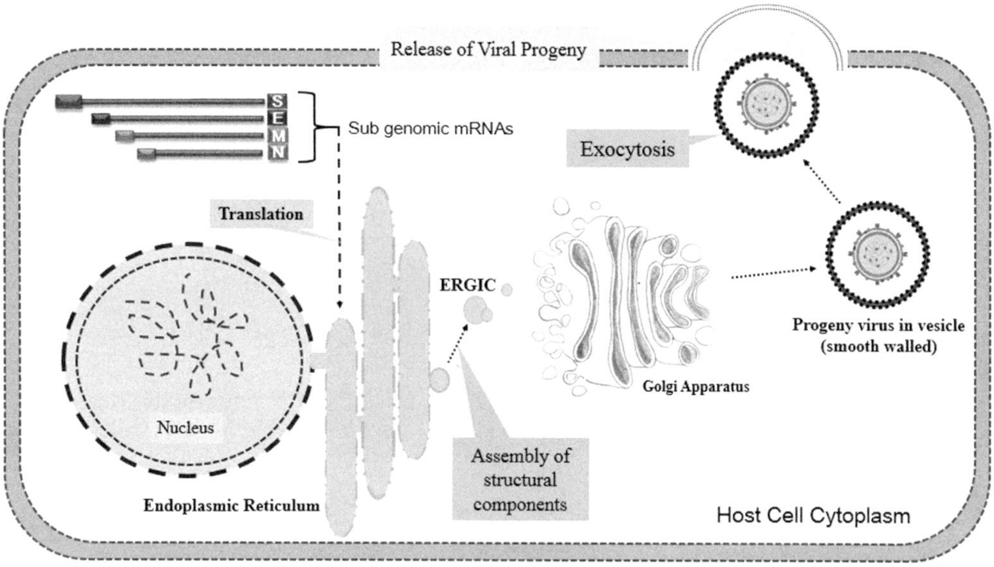

Figure 2.14 Assembly and release of SARS-CoV-2 progenies.

water from the urine. The combination of vascular constriction and saltwater retention raises the systemic blood pressure and restores blood flow to the compromised kidneys. This is the basic idea about the renin–angiotensin system (Wiese et al., 2020)(Lanza et al., 2020).

ACE-2 and the Renin–Angiotensin System: The Connection

This section describes how the renin–angiotensin system is related to the human ACE-2 membrane protein that SARS-CoV-2 uses to locate and infect particular cells in the human body for reproduction. In previous sections, we discussed the basic model of an intact human ACE-2 membrane protein. The active form of protein is formed by an additional enzyme called sheddase. Sheddase cleaves the external component of the ACE-2 protein and releases it into the bloodstream. The cleaved ACE-2 then interacts with angiotensin II, converting it into angiotensin 1–7. Angiotensin 1–7 is a powerful antioxidant and vasodilator that dilates the peripheral blood vessel of the body and eliminates the action of angiotensin II on the adrenals. Angiotensin 1–7 lowers the blood pressure and counterbalance the renin–angiotensin system. There is medication that also counteracts the renin–angiotensin system, for example, angiotensin converting enzyme inhibitors (ACEI) and angiotensin II receptor blockers (ARB) (Wiese et al., 2020; Lanza et al., 2020).

- **ACEIs** are industrially synthesised drug molecules that block ACE from transforming angiotensin I to angiotensin II. This drug molecule causes relaxation of blood vessels and thus helps in lowering blood pressure. ACEIs are generally prescribed to patients suffering from hypertension, chronic kidney diseases, cardiac failure and diabetes with associated renal failure. Some common examples are benazepril, captopril and ramipril.

TABLE 2.1 NAMES OF HORMONES, ENZYMES AND MEDICATIONS IN RELATION TO ACE-2 AND THE RENIN–ANGIOTENSIN SYSTEM

Hormones Involved
• Angiotensin I • Angiotensin II • Angiotensin 1–7
Enzymes that Modify the Hormones
• Renin from the kidneys • Angiotensin converting enzyme (ACE) from the lungs • Angiotensin converting enzyme-2 (ACE-2) from the lungs, kidneys and blood vessels
Medications Involved
• Angiotensin converting enzyme inhibitors (ACEIs) • Angiotensin receptor blockers (ARBs)

- **ARBs** work along the system a little further down the line by blocking angiotensin II from binding to receptors on blood vessels and adrenal glands. Like ACEIs, this drug molecule causes relaxation of blood vessels and thus helps in lowering blood pressure. ARBs are generally prescribed to patients suffering from hypertension, coronary artery disease, cardiac failure and diabetes. Some common examples are telmisartan, olmesartan and eprosartan (Table 2.1).

Let us consider the SARS-CoV-2 receptor. The goal of the virus is to reproduce and infect as many hosts as possible to ensure its existence. Once the virus establishes a reproductive cycle in the cytoplasm of host cells, the ribosomes of the host cell synthesise the proteins, which creates new copies of virus particles that bud out. These newly synthesised viral particles can either infect other cells in the host's body or they can pass from one individual into the environment to infect another host. Studies have shown that ACE-2 surface proteins are located predominantly in the lungs, kidneys, blood vessels and GI tract, as such, when the new virus buds from the host cell, it can either be coughed out through the lungs, urinated out through the kidneys, defecated from the GI tract or absorbed from the bloodstream of the infected host. With all these potential routes of transmission, the chances of being infected by this particular virus are high and thus personal hygiene and handwashing are imperative. Let us now understand the presumed risk factors of COVID-19 infection and how these may be related to the ACE-2 surface protein. The initial viral load, integrity and strength of the immune system and number and configuration of ACE-2 surface proteins are three dominant factors that may determine the clinical response to SARS-CoV-2 infection. SARS-CoV-2 gains entry to the cytoplasm and commands host ribosomes and other proteins making machinery in the cytoplasm to make new copies of viruses with a limited initial viral load; a new particle enters the host cell, reproduces, and new viral particles can then be detected by our immune system. As a result, the immune system then produces antibodies against the virus which keeps the virus in check. These patients are asymptomatic carriers of SARS-CoV-2. However, with a large initial viral load and a weakened immune system, there is an abundance of viral genetic material available in the cytoplasm for reproduction and to produce an overwhelming number of new viral particles that can then infect other cells in the body starting a chain reaction and COVID-19 infection. Like any chain reaction, there needs to be an initial critical mass of genetic material to sustain the process which may explain a 10–14 days incubation period observed in many COVID-19 cases. Epidemiological analysis of COVID-19 patients over the year has revealed some of the risk factors associated with a severe clinical response to SARS-CoV-2, including advanced age, baseline health, physical fitness and diet. Theoretically, excluding initial viral load and immune system integrity factor, initial data suggests all of these may be explained by the ACE-2 surface protein and its relation to the renin–angiotensin system. It is known that the two dominant active hormone configurations in the renin–angiotensin system are angiotensin II and angiotensin 1–7. Angiotensin II raises blood pressure in response to limited blood flow to the kidneys and appears to have inflammatory and atherogenic properties (causes plaques to form in vessels of our body). Angiotensin 1–7, on the other hand, lowers blood pressure and appears to have an anti-inflammatory and antioxidant effect, reducing atherosclerotic disease in blood vessels. It is evident that these two key hormones have direct competition, and the dominant one is probably determined by an individual's baseline health status. In young healthy and physically fit individuals, angiotensin 1–7 is high, however, in sedentary elderly individuals with heart failure, hypertension, diabetes and malnutrition, angiotensin II increases. In a situation where Angiotensin 1–7 is the dominant hormone, the enzyme sheddase may become highly active, cleaving the external component of ACE-2 metalloprotein and thereby converting angiotensin II to angiotensin 1–7. Finally, let us assume the spike protein on the SARS-CoV-2 viral particle specifically recognises the intact transmembrane ACE–2 protein on our cell membrane. In healthy individuals, with an abundance of angiotensin 1–7, most of the ACE–2 protein would have been cleaved, reducing the potential number of viral gateways to our cells and limiting the chance of cytoplasm reaching the critical genetic mass. However, in chronically ill patients where angiotensin II dominates, most of the ACE-2 surface proteins would remain intact, allowing many viral particles entry points, increasing the likelihood of COVID-19 infection. The binding of spike proteins further reduces the availability of the ACE–2 enzyme increasing the vascular inflammation, resulting in the local thrombosis of arteries in the body which could explain the finding of stroke and ischemia in the finger and toes of some patients (digital ischemia). If that turns out to be true, exogenous sheddase enzyme may be a powerful medication in the treatment of both hypertension and SARS-CoV-2 infection (Mascolo et al., 2020).

ACEIs, ARBs and Susceptibility to COVID-19

There were significant concerns among the scientific community that ACEIs and ARBs may increase an individual's susceptibility to SARS-CoV-2 as well as increasing the possibility of severe COVID-19 illness (Wiese et al., 2020; Lanza et al., 2020). As reported by Wan et al., the concern of the scientific community regarding the relation of ACEIs and ARBs with COVID-19 is based on analysis of biological plausibility (Wiese et al., 2020; Lanza et al., 2020). The word biological plausibility refers to the result of research or a trial which are believable in terms of current scientific biological knowledge. An article published by the World Health Organization, titled 'COVID-19 and the Use of Angiotensin Converting Enzyme Inhibitors and Receptor Blockers: A Scientific Brief', dated 7 May 2020 (WHO, 2020b), concluded the following:

- The researchers did not find any studies that were designed to directly evaluate whether the susceptibility to COVID-19 is related to ACEIs or ARBs (WHO, 2020a).
- There were no studies that addressed the potential benefits and harm of initiating ACEIs or ARBs as a treatment for patients with COVID-19 (WHO, 2020a).
- There is low certainty evidence that patients on long-term therapy with ACEIs or ARBs are not at higher risk of poor outcomes from COVID-19 (WHO, 2020a).

REFERENCES

Astuti, I., & Ysrafil (2020). Severe acute respiratory syndrome coronavirus 2 (SARS-CoV-2): An overview of viral structure and host response. *Diabetes & Metabolic Syndrome, 14*(4), 407–412. Advance online publication. https://doi.org/10.1016/j.dsx.2020.04.020.

Chan J, Yuan S, Kok K et al. (2020). A familial cluster of pneumonia associated with the 2019 novel coronavirus indicating person-to-person transmission: A study of a family cluster. *Lancet*. https://doi.org/10.1016/S0140-6736(20)30154-9.

Chen, L., Liu, W., Zhang, Q., Xu, K., Ye, G., Wu, W., Sun, Z., Liu, F., Wu, K., Zhong, B., Mei, Y., Zhang, W., Chen, Y., Li, Y., Shi, M., Lan, K., & Liu, Y. (2020). RNA based mNGS approach identifies a novel human coronavirus from two individual pneumonia cases in 2019 Wuhan outbreak. *Emerging Microbes & Infections, 9*(1), 313–319. https://doi.org/10.1080/22221751.2020.1725399

Dimmock, N. J., Easton, A. J., & Leppard, K. N. (2016). *Introduction to Modern Virology* (7th Ed.). Wiley-Blackwell.

Fung, T. S., & Liu, D. X. (2019). Human coronavirus: Host-pathogen interaction. *Annual Review of Microbiology, 73*, 529–557. https://doi.org/10.1146/annurev-micro-020518-115759

Hulswit, R. J., de Haan, C. A., & Bosch, B. J. (2016). Coronavirus spike protein and tropism changes. *Advances in Virus Research, 96*, 29–57. https://doi.org/10.1016/bs.aivir.2016.08.004

Lan, J., Ge, J., Yu, J. et al. (2020). Structure of the SARS-CoV-2 spike receptor-binding domain bound to the ACE2 receptor. *Nature, 581*, 215–220. https://doi.org/10.1038/s41586-020-2180-5

Lanza, K., Perez, L. G., Costa, L. B., Cordeiro, T. M., Palmeira, V. A., Ribeiro, V. T., & Simões E Silva, A. C. (2020). Covid-19: The renin-angiotensin system imbalance hypothesis. *Clinical Science* (1979), *134*(11), 1259–1264. https://doi.org/10.1042/CS20200492

Li, F. (2016). Structure, function, and evolution of coronavirus spike proteins. *Annual Review of Virology, 3*(1), 237–261. https://doi.org/10.1146/annurev-virology-110615-042301

Lim, Y. X., Ng, Y. L., Tam, J. P., & Liu, D. X. (2016). Human coronaviruses: A review of virus-host interactions. *Diseases, 4*(3), 26. https://doi.org/10.3390/diseases4030026.

Liu, J, Liao, X, Qian, S et al. (2020). Community transmission of severe acute respiratory syndrome coronavirus 2, Shenzhen, China, 2020. *Emerging Infectious Diseases, 26*(6), 1320. doi.org/10.3201/eid2606.200239.

Lu, R., Zhao, X., Li, J., Niu, P., Yang, B., Wu, H., Wang, W., Song, H., Huang, B., Zhu, N., Bi, Y., Ma, X., Zhan, F., Wang, L., Hu, T., Zhou, H., Hu, Z., Zhou, W., Zhao, L., . . . Tan, W. (2020). Genomic characterisation and epidemiology of 2019 novel coronavirus: Implications for virus origins and receptor binding. *Lancet, 395*(10224), 565–574. https://doi.org/10.1016/s0140-6736 (20)30251-8

Mascolo, A., Scavone, C., Rafaniello, C., Ferrajolo, C., Racagni, G., Berrino, L., Paolisso, G., Rossi, F., & Capuano, A. (2020). Renin-angiotensin system and coronavirus disease 2019: A narrative review. *Frontiers in Cardiovascular Medicine, 7*, 143. https://doi.org/10.3389/fcvm.2020.00143

Masters P. S. (2006). The molecular biology of coronaviruses. *Advances in Virus Research, 66*, 193–292. https://doi.org/10.1016/S0065-3527(06)66005-3

McFadden, G., Mohamed, M., Rahman, M. et al. (2009). Cytokine determinants of viral tropism. *Nature Reviews Immunology 9*, 645–655. https://doi.org/10.1038/nri2623

Neuman, B. W., Kiss, G., Kunding, A. H., Bhella, D., Baksh, M. F., Connelly, S., Droese, B., Klaus, J. P., Makino, S., Sawicki, S. G., Siddell, S. G., Stamou, D. G., Wilson, I. A., Kuhn, P., & Buchmeier, M. J. (2011). A structural analysis of M protein in coronavirus assembly and morphology. *Journal of Structural Biology, 174*(1), 11–22. https://doi.org/10.1016/j.jsb.2010.11.021.

Ou, X., Liu, Y., Lei, X. et al. (2020). Characterization of spike glycoprotein of SARS-CoV-2 on virus entry and its immune cross-reactivity with SARS-CoV. *Nature Communications 11*, 1620. https://doi.org/10.1038/s41467-020-15562-9.

Shang, J., Wan, Y., Luo, C., Ye, G., Geng, Q., Auerbach, A., & Li, F. (2020). Cell entry mechanisms of SARS-CoV-2. *Proceedings of the National Academy of Sciences, 117*(21), 11727–11734. https://doi.org/10.1073/pnas.2003138117

Swiss Institute of Bioinformatics. Retrieved from https://viralzone.expasy.org/764?outline=all_by_species Accessed on 10th June 2020.

Tortorici, M. A., & Veesler, D. (2019). Structural insights into coronavirus entry. *Advances in Virus Research, 105*, 93–116. https://doi.org/10.1016/bs.aivir.2019.08.002

UniProtKB – P59637. (n.d.). E: Envelope small membrane protein: Severe acute respiratory syndrome coronavirus (SARS-CoV): E gene & protein. *UniProt*. Retrieved November 18, 2021, from https://www.uniprot.org/uniprot/P59637

UniProtKB – P59596. (n.d.). M: Membrane protein: Severe acute respiratory syndrome coronavirus (SARS-CoV): M gene & protein. *UniProt*. Retrieved November 18, 2021, from https://www.uniprot.org/uniprot/P59596

UniProtKB – P59595. (n.d.). N: Nucleoprotein: Severe acute respiratory syndrome coronavirus (SARS-CoV): N gene & protein. *UniProt*. Retrieved November 18, 2021, from https://www.uniprot.org/uniprot/P59595

UniProtKB – P0DTC2. (n.d.). S: Spike glycoprotein precursor: Severe acute respiratory syndrome coronavirus 2 (2019-nCoV): S gene & protein. *UniProt*. Retrieved November 18, 2021, from https://www.uniprot.org/uniprot/P0DTC2

UniProtKB – P59594. (n.d.). S: Spike glycoprotein precursor: Severe acute respiratory syndrome coronavirus (SARS-CoV): S gene & protein. *UniProt*. Retrieved November 18, 2021, from https://www.uniprot.org/uniprot/P59594

Wang, M. (2020, November 25). SARS-CoV-2: Structure, biology, and structure-based therapeutics development. *Frontiers in Cellular and Infection Microbiology*. Retrieved June 17, 2021, from https://www.frontiersin.org/articles/10.3389/fcimb.2020.587269/full

WHO. (2020a). *WHO Clinical Care Severe Acute Respiratory Illness (SARI) Training*. World Health Organization. Retrieved June 22, 2020, from https://openwho.org/courses/severe-acute-respiratory-infection

WHO. (2020b). *COVID-19 and the Use of Angiotensin-Converting Enzyme Inhibitors and Receptor Blockers*. World Health Organization. Retrieved March 6, 2022, from https://www.who.int/news-room/commentaries/detail/covid-19-and-the-use-of-angiotensin-converting-enzyme-inhibitors-and-receptor-blockers

Wiese, O. J., Allwood, B. W., & Zemlin, A. E. (2020). COVID-19 and the renin-angiotensin system (RAS): A spark that sets the forest alight? *Medical Hypotheses, 144*, 110231. https://doi.org/10.1016/j.mehy.2020.110231

Zhu, N., Zhang, D., Wang, W., Li, X., Yang, B., Song, J., Zhao, X., Huang, B., Shi, W., Lu, R., Niu, P., Zhan, F., Ma, X., Wang, D., Xu, W., Wu, G., Gao, G. F., & Tan, W. (2020). A novel coronavirus from patients with pneumonia in China, 2019. *New England Journal of Medicine, 382*(8), 727–733. https://doi.org/10.1056/nejmoa2001017

Chapter 3

Molecular Pathophysiology and the Clinical Presentation of COVID-19

The Comparison between Reductionistic and Holistic Approaches

Srijan Goswami* and Ushmita Gupta Bakshi

CONTENTS

INTRODUCTION

The subject of pathophysiology is made up of two medical disciplines: physiology and pathology. It is a branch of science that deals with the physiology of abnormal states or the functional changes that accompany a particular syndrome or disease. The scientific discipline of pathophysiology enables us to understand why and how diseases develop and various clinical manifestations that appear. Science is a tool that we use to understand how nature works. There are two ways to achieve this understanding – the reductionistic approach and the holistic approach. In conventional or modern medicine, we conservatively follow the reductionistic approach. Many of us do not even understand the science behind the holistic approach or how it relates to existing medical practices. Unfortunately, in conventional settings, just because we have been conditioned to believe that "reductionism is the only gold standard for scientific studies" we tend to make vague assumptions that medical practices that fall under the category of complementary and alternative medicine systems (CAMS) are all unscientific, baseless, and are not worthy to be considered or talked about. This is an example of the conceptual bias and monopoly that exists in our medical education and healthcare system. The Father of Medicine, Great Hippocrates taught us that "Never make money in the sick room", but even after taking an oath in his name, we intentionally teach and mandate those medical practices and protocols from which huge profits can be generated. This conceptual bias and half-hearted understanding of human existence

DOI: 10.1201/9781003178514-4

is and will keep holding us back from getting closer to actual patient-centric solutions (Null, 2011; Hegde, 2014). It is high time that we practice science as science and not as a religion. The approach we take to study science determines the outcome. Through this chapter, the author intends to explain the pathophysiology of COVID-19 or severe acute respiratory illnesses (SARI) or influenza-like illnesses (ILIs) from both reductionistic and holistic perspectives. The understanding of COVID-19 pathophysiology from both perspectives will not only enable the reader to have a complete picture of the concepts but will help them make sense of both medical systems, their individual merits and demerits, and the ways through which they can be integrated to design patient-centric COVID-19 prevention, treatment, and management protocols.

UNDERSTANDING THE HUMAN BODY: REDUCTIONISTIC AND HOLISTIC APPROACHES

Reductionism views the universe (for example, nature or the human body) as a machine made out of various parts that are discretely functional and each of these component parts can be isolated and studied separately. This ideology believes the addition or removal of various parts does not produce a significant effect on the overall functioning of the system. In case the system breaks down, efforts are made only to detect and fix the part that appears to have malfunctioned and does whatever it takes to fix the issue and does not consider the overall effect the approach makes on the system (Goswami & Gupta Bakshi, 2020; Hegde, 2014; Lipton, 2016).

Holism views the universe (for example, nature or the human body) as a system made out of interrelated and inseparable parts that function in a synchronized manner. Each component is inseparably interconnected with each other and thus cannot be studied in isolation. The addition or removal of components generate a dynamic effect on the overall functioning of the system. In case the system breaks down, detecting and fixing the part that appeared to have malfunctioned will not solve the issue. The emphasis is made to identify the actual cause that resulted in the malfunctioning and thus restoring overall balance (Goswami & Gupta Bakshi, 2020; Hegde, 2014; Lipton, 2016) (Figure 3.1).

FUNCTIONAL ANATOMY OF RESPIRATORY SYSTEM: A BRIEF OVERVIEW

Respiration means the action of breathing. It is a biological process involving the production of energy, typically with the intake of oxygen and the release of carbon dioxide from the oxidation of complex organic substances. Respiration is classified into two types (see Figure 3.2). External respiration involves the exchange of oxygen and carbon dioxide between the lungs and blood, while internal respiration involves the exchange of gases between the blood and tissues. Also, respiration occurs in two phases (see Figure 3.2). Inspiration (breathing in), an active process during which air enters the lungs from the atmosphere. Expiration (breathing out), a passive process during which air leaves the lungs (Hall, 2015; Ralston et al., 2018).

The respiratory system is the network of organs, such as the airways, lungs, blood vessels, and the muscles associated with the lungs, which helps in breathing in and breathing out. These parts work together to move oxygen throughout the body and expel gases like carbon dioxide (Hall, 2015; Ralston et al., 2018). Figure 3.3 represents the fundamental aspects of the human respiratory system.

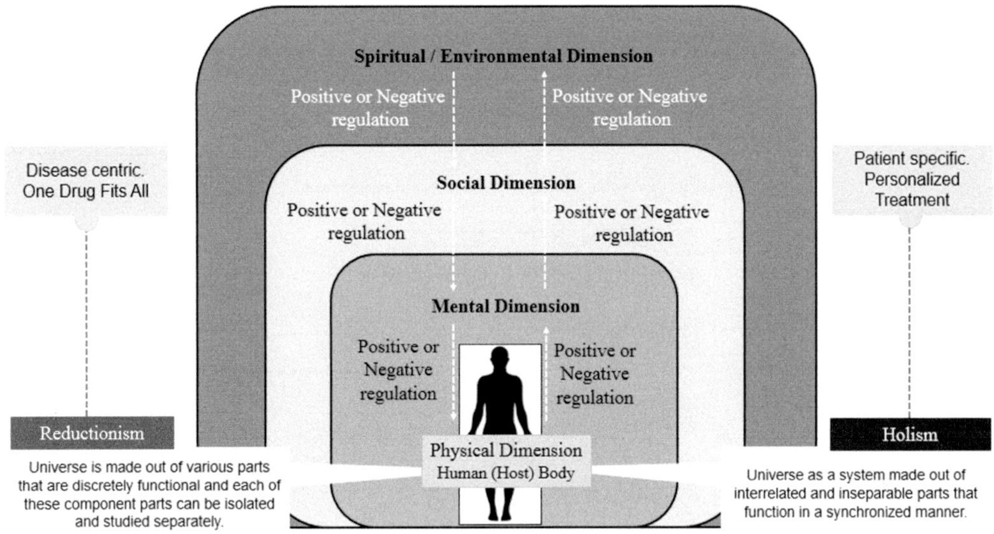

Figure 3.1 Representation of human existence from reductionistic and holistic perspectives.

The lungs occupy the upper two-thirds of the thorax, bounded medially by the vertebral column, the heart, and the mediastinum, and inferiorly by the diaphragm. Based on the arrangement, the respiratory system is divided into two regions, the upper respiratory tract consisting of nose, nasal cavities, and the pharynx, and the lower respiratory tract consisting of the larynx, trachea, and the lungs (bronchi, bronchioles, and alveoli). Also, based on functions, the mentioned structures

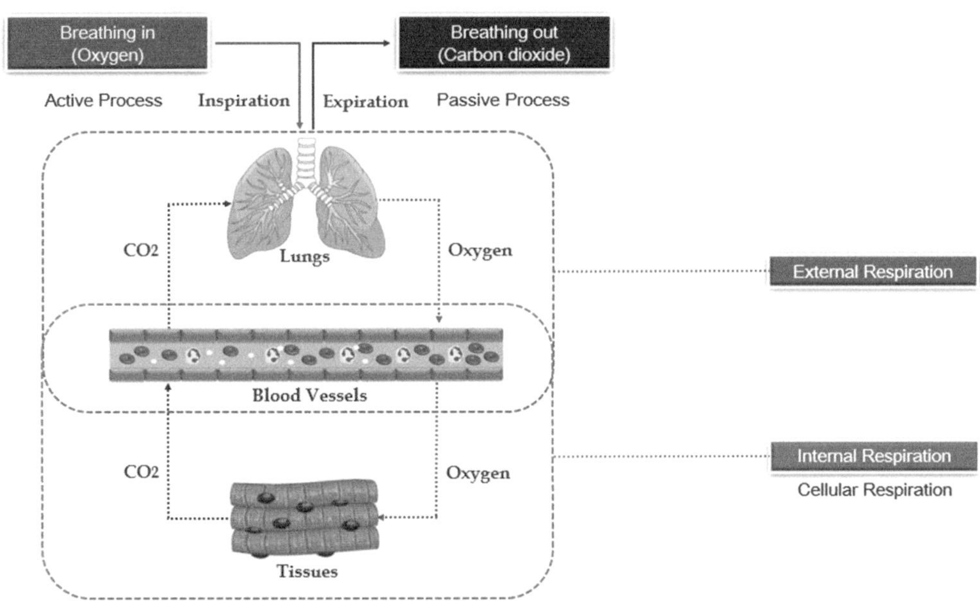

Figure 3.2 Types and phases of respiration.

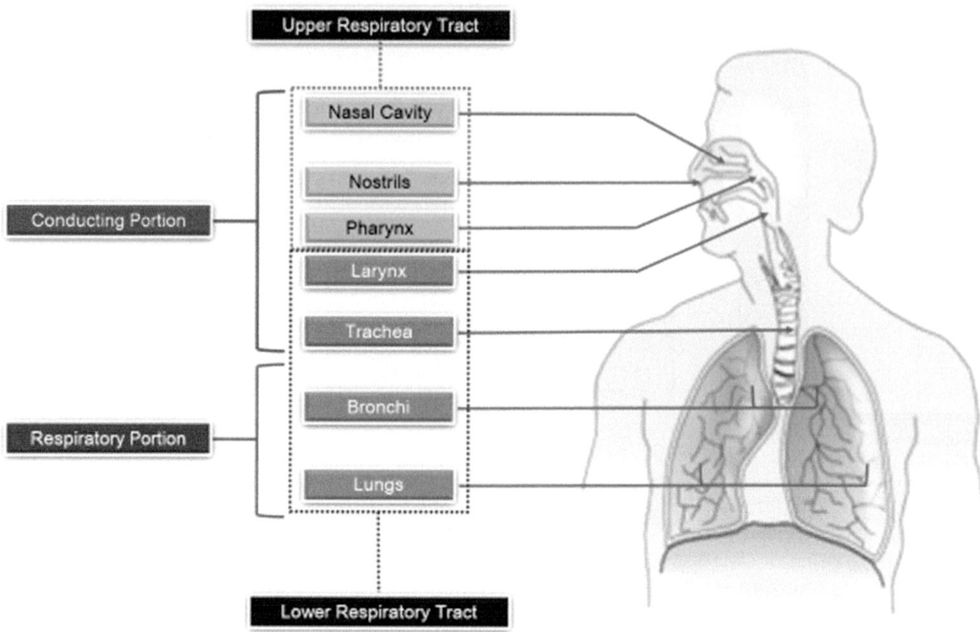

Figure 3.3 Fundamental aspects of the human respiratory system.

are divided into two portions, the first is the conducting portion (involved in the transportation of air) consisting of the nose, nasal cavity, pharynx, larynx, trachea, and airways, and the second is the respiratory portion (involved in actual gas exchange), which includes respiratory bronchioles, alveolar ducts, and alveoli (air sacs). Each lung is covered by a bilayered serous membrane called the pleura or pleural sac (see Figure 3.4). The pleura has two layers, namely inner visceral and outer parietal layers. The visceral pleura and parietal pleura are separated by a space called the intrapleural space or pleural cavity that contains a thin film of serous fluid called intrapleural fluid, which is secreted by the visceral layer of the pleura. The intrapleural fluid performs several functions like providing lubrication to prevent friction between pleural layers and the creation of negative pressure called intrapleural pressure within intrapleural space. In some pathological conditions, the pleural cavity expands with the accumulation of air (pneumothorax), water (hydrothorax), blood (hemothorax), or pus (pyothorax) (Hall, 2015; Ralston et al., 2018).

The trachea separates into two primary (main) bronchi called right and left bronchi. Inside the lungs, each primary bronchus separates into secondary bronchi which are further subdivided into tertiary bronchi. These tertiary bronchi form bronchioles. Bronchioles having a diameter of 1 mm or less are known as terminal bronchioles. The trachea and bronchi are together called the tracheobronchial tree. The structural and functional unit of lungs, known as the respiratory unit, consists of respiratory bronchioles, alveolar ducts, alveolar sacs, antrum, and alveoli, and is responsible for the actual exchange of gases between lungs and blood. Each *alveolus* is lined by epithelial cells called alveolar cells or pneumocytes. Pneumocytes are of two types (Hall, 2015; Ralston et al., 2018):

- **Type I alveolar cells.** Type I alveolar cells are the squamous epithelial cells forming about 95% of the total number of cells. These cells form the site of gaseous exchange between the alveolus and blood (Hall, 2015; Ralston et al., 2018).

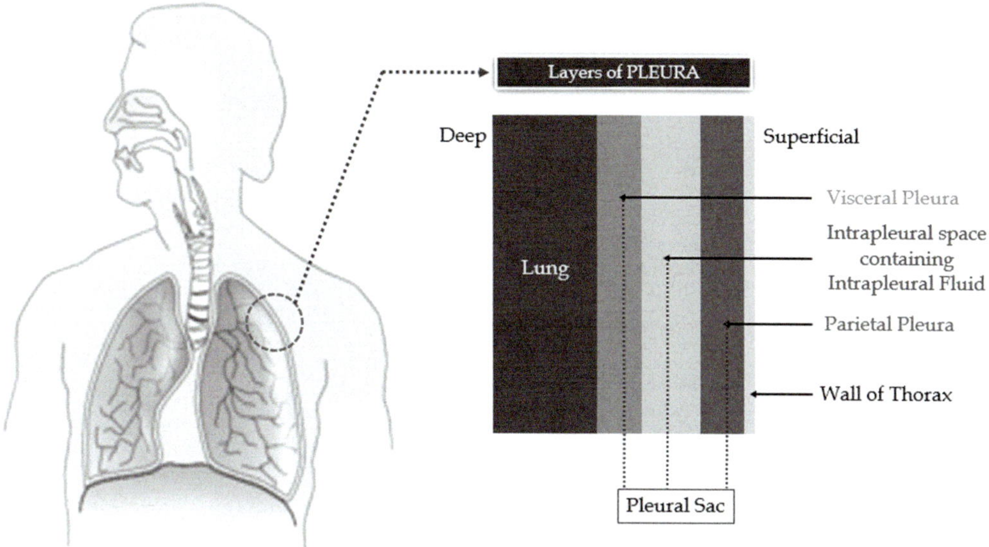

Figure 3.4 Layers of the pleura or pleural sac.

- **Type II alveolar cells.** Type II alveolar cells are cuboidal in nature and form about 5% of alveolar cells. These cells are also called granular pneumocytes. Alveolar fluid and surfactant are secreted by these cells (Hall, 2015; Ralston et al., 2018) (Figure 3.5).

The exchange of gases occurs through the respiratory membrane, the fundamental region of the respiratory unit that keeps air in the alveoli and the circulating blood in the capillaries separated.

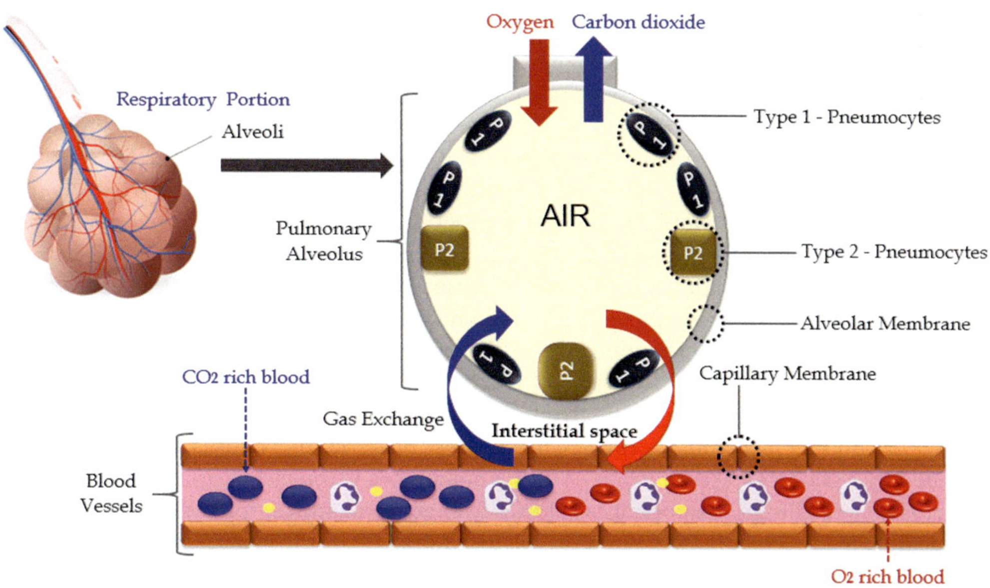

Figure 3.5 Fundamental representation of the respiratory unit.

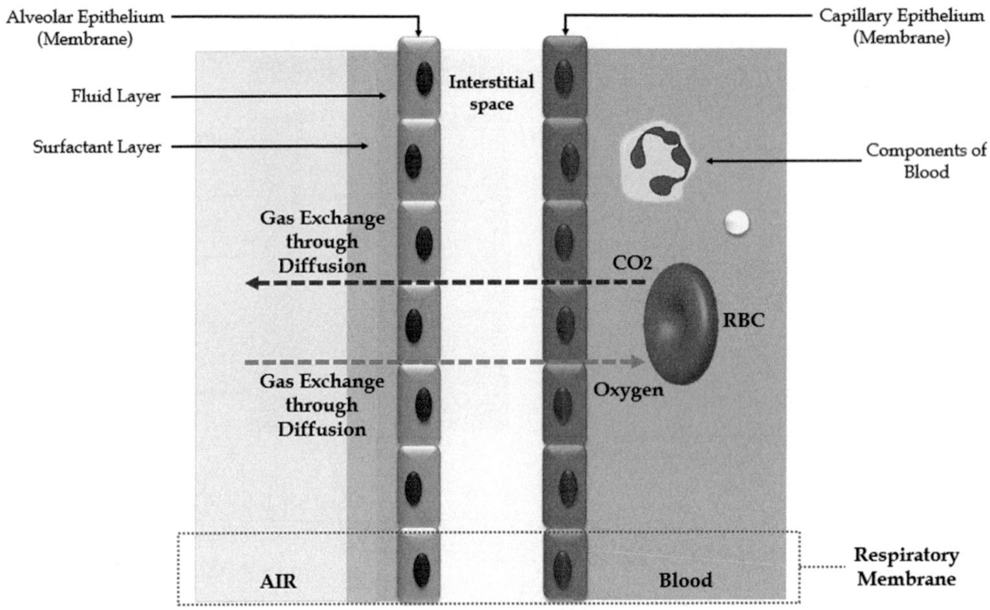

Figure 3.6 Basic arrangement of the respiratory membrane.

The respiratory membrane is composed of the alveolar membrane and capillary membrane separated by thin interstitial space. The respiratory membrane has a surface area of 70 square meters and a thickness of 0.5 microns. Figure 3.6 represents the basic arrangement of the respiratory membrane.

Besides respiration, the respiratory system performs several critical non-respiratory functions.

- **Olfaction**. The sense of smell. The mucus membrane of the nostrils contains olfactory receptors that aid in the sensation and characterization of smell.
- **Vocalization**. The ability to speak or generate the voice. The larynx (voice box) and its associated structures form the speech apparatus that helps in the generation and modulation of the voice.
- **Filtration**. Nasal hairs and the mucus membrane filter dust and pathogen particles entering the respiratory tract from the air. The foreign particles are expelled by the ciliary movements of hair trapped by the secretory action of mucus and if these mechanisms fail, the particles are phagocytosed by alveolar macrophages.
- **Immunological action**. Components of the respiratory tract along with cells of the immune system help in the defense of the body. Defensins, cathelicidins, and other potent antimicrobial proteins secreted by epithelial cells of the lungs form a part of the innate immune mechanism. The defense against bacteria and viruses is mainly provided by leucocytes like neutrophils and lymphocytes through the process of phagocytosis. In the lungs, macrophages act as scavengers and antigen-presenting cells. The invading pathogen or foreign particles are phagocytosed by the macrophages and antigen processing and presentation are initiated. Macrophages secrete interleukins, tumor necrosis factors (TNF), and chemokines that help activate the general immune system of the body and attract immune cells toward the site of any inflammation. Mast cells

secrete heparin, histamine, serotonin, and hydrolytic enzymes that lead to hypersensitivity reactions like allergy and anaphylaxis. Natural killer cells, the first line of defense in specific immunity, particularly against viruses, produces interferons and tumor necrosis factors that destroy the viruses and viral infected or damaged cells. Inside the lungs, dendritic cells along with the macrophages act as antigen-presenting cells (Kumar et al., 2014).

- **Coughing.** Protective reflex caused by irritation of the respiratory tract and some other areas such as the external auditory canal. A cough begins with a deep inspiration followed by forced expiration with closed glottis. It causes the expulsion of irritant substances out of the respiratory tract.
- **Sneezing.** Protective mechanism caused by irritation of nasal mucous membrane because of dust particles, debris, mechanical obstruction of the airway, and excess fluid accumulation in the nasal passages. Sneezing starts with deep inspiration, followed by a forceful expiratory effort with opened glottis resulting in the expulsion of irritant agents out of the respiratory tract.
- **Swallowing apnea.** Deglutition (swallowing) apnea is a protective mechanism during which respiration is temporarily arrested, which prevents food particles from entering the respiratory tract.
- **Water balance.** The respiratory tract plays a role in the water loss mechanism. During expiration, water evaporates through the expired air and an amount of body water is lost by this process.
- **Thermoregulation.** During expiration, along with water, heat is also lost from the body. Thus, the respiratory tract plays a role in the heat loss mechanism.
- **Acid-base balance.** The lungs play a role in the maintenance of the acid-base balance of the body by regulating the carbon dioxide content in the blood.
- **Enzyme secretion.** The angiotensin converting enzyme (ACE) secreted by endothelial cells of pulmonary capillaries plays an important role in the regulation of extracellular fluid volume and blood pressure by converting angiotensin I to angiotensin II.
- **Blood pressure regulation.** Lung tissues regulate blood pressure by synthesizing various kinds of chemicals like hormonal substances, prostaglandins, acetylcholine, and serotonin, which have several physiological actions

MOLECULAR PATHOPHYSIOLOGY AND CLINICAL MANIFESTATIONS OF COVID-19: THE REDUCTIONISTIC PERSPECTIVE OF CONVENTIONAL MEDICINE

SARS-CoV-2, after entering the lower respiratory tract, damages the alveoli, the structure responsible for gas exchange between the lungs and circulating blood. There are two types of alveolar cells – type I pneumocytes and type II pneumocytes. The genetic material of SARS-CoV-2 is replicated, translated, and reassembled into small viral particles inside type II pneumocytes (see Chapter 2). The release of newly synthesized virus progenies results in permanent destruction of the alveolar cells. Progressive and exponential damage to alveolar cells leads to a spectrum of severe complications such as pneumonia, acute respiratory distress syndrome (ARDS), consolidation, sepsis, septic shock, multi-system organ failure, and even death (World Health Organization, 2020; Lim et al., 2016; Jian et al., 2020; Yuki et al., 2020; Mason, 2020; Fehr & Perlman, 2015; Abbas et al., 2004).

Specific inflammatory mediators capable of triggering and stimulating macrophages are released by the damaged type II pneumocytes. Cytokines such as interleukin–1 (IL-1), interleukin–6 (IL-6), and tumor necrosis factor-α (TNF-α) secreted by macrophages cause the dilation of endothelial cells and increases capillary permeability. This leads to the leaking and accumulation of plasma into interstitial space and alveoli leading to its compression. The accumulation of excess fluid inside alveoli results in alveolar edema, a condition that leads to the drowning out of the surfactants, which results in increased surface tension. An increase in surface tension increases the collapsing pressure, thus resulting in alveolar collapse. The accumulation of an excessive amount of fluid around the alveoli damages the respiratory membrane, this results in decreased gas exchange and hypoxemia, which can be indicated as an increased effort in breathing (acute respiratory distress syndrome) (World Health Organization, 2020; Lim et al., 2016; Jian et al., 2020; Yuki et al., 2020; Mason, 2020; Fehr & Perlman, 2015; Abbas et al., 2004). These inflammatory mediators trigger and regulate the recruitment of neutrophils at the site of infection inside alveoli. The destruction of pathogens induced by inflammatory mediators releases proteases and reactive oxygen species (ROS) that damages the virus (pathogen) and type I and type II pneumocytes. This results in a significant decrease in gas exchange and an increase in alveolar surface tension. The overcrowding caused by the accumulation of fluids, proteins, and cellular debris inside the alveoli leads to consolidation. Consolidation means the pathological alteration of lung tissue from an aerated condition to one of a solid consistency. This consolidation alters the rate of gas exchange, leading to hypoxemia, which results in a cough with mucus (World Health Organization, 2020; Lim et al., 2016; Jian et al., 2020; Yuki et al., 2020; Mason, 2020; Fehr & Perlman, 2015; Abbas et al., 2004). The hypothalamus (a part of the central nervous system involved in thermoregulation) under the influence of interleukin-1 (IL-1) and interleukin-6 (IL-6) releases specific prostaglandins that increase the body temperature (fever or pyrexia). Also, specific chemoreceptors are activated by the decrease in the partial pressure of oxygen which triggers a reflex of the sympathetic nervous system (stimulated) and increases the patient's respiratory rate (tachypnea) and heart rate (tachycardia) (World Health Organization, 2020; Lim et al., 2016; Jian et al., 2020; Yuki et al., 2020; Mason, 2020Fehr & Perlman, 2015; Abbas et al., 2004). The degeneration of lungs caused by the leaking of cellular inflammatory components into the bloodstream leads to systemic inflammatory response syndrome (SIRS) and sepsis. Leaking and accumulation of fluid in tissue spaces decrease the overall blood volume which results in vasodilation, which in turn leads to a decrease in total peripheral resistance. A decrease in total peripheral resistance leads to a decrease in blood volume, resulting in lowering blood pressure (hypotension). This state of hypotension decreases the flow of blood to multiple organs causes septic shock which ultimately leads to multi-system organ failure (MSOF) (World Health Organization, 2020; Lim et al., 2016; Jian et al., 2020; Yuki et al., 2020; Mason, 2020; Fehr & Perlman, 2015; Abbas et al., 2004).

HOLISTIC UNDERSTANDING OF PATHOPHYSIOLOGY: COVID-19/INFLUENZA-LIKE ILLNESSES/SEVERE ACUTE RESPIRATORY ILLNESSES

SARS-CoV-2 is the coronavirus known to cause a type of severe acute respiratory illness called COVID-19. There are basically two ways by which a pathogen gains entry inside the respiratory tract, one is through the nasopharyngeal route and the other is through the oropharyngeal route. When any respiratory pathogen, be it a bacteria, a fungus, or a virus (in this case, SARS-CoV-2) enters the upper respiratory tract, it first makes contact with the epithelial cells of the nasal mucosa. Anatomically, the nasopharynx is one of the routes that creates a connection between the outside environment and the host's respiratory system. The intelligence of the body knows that there is a good chance that pathogenic microorganisms may try to gain entry to the respiratory tract through this route. So, strong innate and adaptive immune components are present throughout this system. When a respiratory pathogen enters the nasopharynx, the cellular intelligence recognizes the threat and initiates protective responses like watery discharge from the nostrils, the sneezing reflex, increased secretion of mucus from the nose, and the swelling of nasal polyps giving rise to a collection of responses that cause discomfort in the upper respiratory tract.

ILIs are non-specific respiratory illnesses (synonym: acute respiratory illness [ARI]) having clinical presentation like that of classical influenza. The major signs and symptoms include fever, cough, sore throat, runny or stuffy nose, muscle or body aches, fatigue (tiredness), loss of taste, loss of appetite, diarrhea or vomiting, and fast breathing with shortness of breath (in moderate to severe cases). If observed carefully, we will find that the signs and symptoms of COVID-19 and ILI are the same, thus COVID-19 may be categorized as a type of ILI. For designing and planning a proper curative treatment regimen, it is very important to have a clear understanding of the reasons behind the signs and symptoms. The way we approach understanding science determines the way we interpret clinical outcomes. Unfortunately, conventional medical science has always considered signs and symptoms as the reason for a disease and tries to suppress the symptoms by using industrially synthesized chemical drugs, surgical interventions, or any means possible. But the whole scenario becomes different if the signs and symptoms of a disease (be it a common cold or COVID-19) are observed from the perspective of holistic CAMS.

We know that ILIs and COVID-19 are diseases that affect a person's respiratory system. This means the causative organism of the ILI (in this case, SARS-CoV-2) gains access to the host's respiratory system through the upper respiratory tract and subsequently reaches

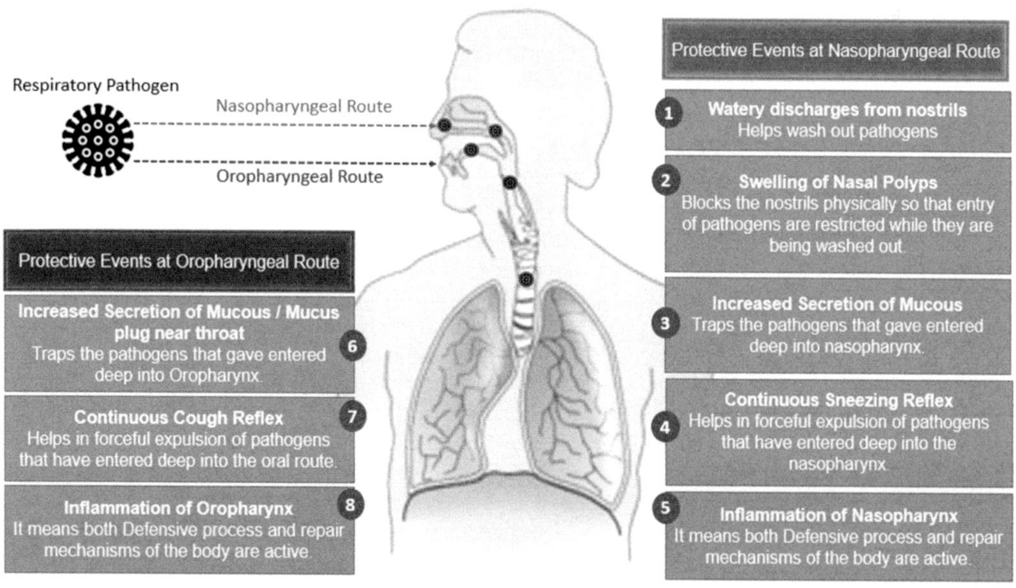

Figure 3.7 Protective events at the oropharyngeal and nasopharyngeal routes.

TABLE 3.1 COMPARISON OF THE MENTIONED SIGNS AND SYMPTOMS FROM THE PERSPECTIVE OF REDUCTIONISTIC CONVENTIONAL MEDICINE AND CAMS

Signs and Symptoms	Conventional Approach to ILI	Holistic Approach to ILI
Runny or stuffy nose (associated sneezing)	A runny and stuffy nose is considered a disease and thus over the counter (OTC) or prescription medications are provided to stop the nasal discharge and open up the blocked nostrils.	The foreign agent causing respiratory tract infections may enter the respiratory system through the nasopharyngeal route. Thus, Mother Nature created a defense mechanism to block and expel the pathogen trying to enter the system. The swelling of nasal polyps (as a result of local inflammation) blocks the passage and excessive discharge from the nose washes out the foreign substance, thus alarming the individual about an incoming threat as well as performing a defense mechanism. To ensure the proper clearing of the foreign substance, the defense mechanism of the body triggers the sneezing reflex in order to forcefully expel the threat. By stopping the catarrh, opening the nasal passage, and suppressing the sneeze reflex forcefully, we may feel that we have addressed the issue, but it should be noted, in the absence of these barriers, foreign pathogens will be able to easily enter the respiratory tract as well as the digestive tract without any barrier.
Cough and sore throat	Cough causes discomfort and prolonged coughing causes a sore throat, and thus OTC or prescription medications are provided to stop the cough reflex and palliate the soreness or pain in the throat.	The oropharynx is another way to gain access to the respiratory system. So, when the pathogen tries to enter the system through the mouth, the cough reflex is triggered in order to expel the threat forcefully. The continuous coughing produces strain on the soft inner lining of the throat, causing the soreness. A mucus plug also forms in the throat, thus trapping the threat and eliminating it through the cough reflex. By stopping the cough reflex, we may feel that we have addressed the issue, but it should be noted, in the absence of a cough, foreign pathogens will be able to enter the respiratory tract as well as the digestive tract without any barrier.
Fever and body aches	Fever or rise in body temperature beyond the normal range is considered as an illness and thus temperature lowering medications are prescribed to bring down the fever by force. Body aches associated with fever are also dealt with industrially synthesized painkillers.	Fever is not a disease, but the defense mechanism of the human body. When the foreign pathogen enters the human body, it requires a certain amount of time to acclimatize. The intelligence of the human body raises the temperature to an extent, which makes it inhabitable for the foreign pathogen and aids in its disintegration, thus protecting the body from the threat. The rise in body temperature and pain are attributes of inflammation, and inflammation is the defense mechanism of the body. It should be clinically regulated but not suppressed at any cost. So, lowering the fever by force with medications means stopping our defense mechanism and allowing the foreign pathogen to act freely inside the system.

(*Continued*)

TABLE 3.1 (CONTINUED) COMPARISON OF THE MENTIONED SIGNS AND SYMPTOMS FROM THE PERSPECTIVE OF REDUCTIONISTIC CONVENTIONAL MEDICINE AND CAMS

Signs and Symptoms	Conventional Approach to ILI	Holistic Approach to ILI
Loss of appetite and loss of taste	With conventional medication, we may or may not treat this issue, as loss of appetite and taste is not a big concern.	Digestion of food is an energy-consuming process. During active infection, the majority of the body's energy is utilized by the immune system to fight off the infection and promote healing mechanisms. Consumption of heavy foods forces the body to divert the majority of the energy toward the digestion process and thus halting the ongoing defense and healing process, as defending the human system from the active infection and healing it from the damage caused is a high priority compared with the process of digestion. To address this issue, the intelligence of the human body stops the hunger reflex and turns off the activity of the taste buds in order to ensure that the individual does not take in the type of food that requires digestion, which leads to unnecessary energy loss. The intelligence of the body does not stop the thirst reflex, indicating that nutritional substances should be taken only in liquid form so that optimum nutrition can be obtained and utilized without the misuse of energy in the digestion of food.

the lower respiratory tract. The upper respiratory tract includes the nostrils, nasal cavity, mouth, and pharynx while the lower respiratory tract includes the larynx, trachea, bronchi, and lungs. The infectious agent causing ILI (in this case, SARS-CoV-2) can enter the respiratory tract either through the nostrils and nasal cavity (the nasopharyngeal route) or through the mouth (the oro-pharyngeal route). Mother Nature is intelligent enough to understand the gravity of this situation and bestowed us with a strong innate immune system to act as the first line of defense. The innate immune response is not only responsible for defending our body from possible threats but also designed to raise an SOS alarm to the consciousness of the individual in the form of signs and symptoms so that health-promoting measures can be taken (see Figure 3.7). We have to understand the signs and symptoms such as fever, cough and sore throat, runny or stuffy nose, muscle or body aches, fatigue (tiredness), loss of taste, loss of appetite, diarrhea, or vomiting are not our enemies but a defense mechanism and SOS alarm raised by an individual's innate immune system. Table 3.1 provides a comparison of the mentioned signs and symptoms from the perspective of reductionistic conventional medicine and CAMS.

REFERENCES

Abbas, A. K., Aster, J. C., & Kumar, V. (2004). *Robbins and Cotran Pathologic Basis of Disease* (7th ed.). Philadelphia, PA: Elsevier Saunders.

Fehr, A. R., & Perlman, S. (2015). Coronaviruses: An overview of their replication and pathogenesis. *Methods in Molecular Biology, 1282*, 1–23. https://doi.org/10.1007/978-1-4939-2438-7_1.

Goswami, S., & Gupta Bakshi, U. (2020). Understanding classical naturopathy: The Hippocratic way of healing. In A. Sharma et al. (Ed.), *Herbal Product Development Formulation and Applications* (1st ed., pp. 293–320). Palm Bay, FL: Apple Academic Press. https://doi.org/10.1201/9781003003182

Hall, J. (2015). *Guyton and Hall Textbook of Medical Physiology* (13th ed.). India: Elsevier Saunders.

Hegde, B. M. (2014). *What Doctors Don't Get to Study in Medical School.* India: Paras Medical Publisher.

Kumar, V., Abbas, A., & Aster, J. (2014). *Robbins & Cotran Pathologic Basis of Disease* (9th ed.). United States: Elsevier.

Lim, Y. X., Ng, Y. L., Tam, J. P., & Liu, D. X. (2016). Human coronaviruses: A review of virus-host interactions. *Diseases, 4*(3), 26. https://doi.org/10.3390/diseases4030026.

Lipton, B. H. (2016) *The Biology of Belief, Unleashing the Power of Consciousness, Matter & Miracles* (18th Reprint). India: Hay House Publishers.

Mason, R. J. (2020). Pathogenesis of COVID-19 from a cell biology perspective. *European Respiratory Journal, 55*(4), 2000607. https://doi.org/10.1183/13993003.00607-2020

Null, G. (2011) *Death by Medicine* (Revised Paperback ed.). Edindurg, VA: Praktikos Books.

Ralston, S., Penman, I., Strachan, M., & Hobson, R. (2018). *Davidson's Principles and Practice of Medicine* (23rd ed.). United States: Elsevier.

Shang, J., Wan, Y., Luo, C., Ye, G., Geng, Q., Auerbach, A., & Li, F. (May 2020). Cell entry mechanisms of SARS-CoV-2. *Proceedings of the National Academy of Sciences, 117*(21), 11727–11734. https://doi.org/10.1073/pnas.2003138117.

World Health Organization. (2020). *WHO Clinical Care Severe Acute Respiratory Illness (SARI) Training.* World Health Organization, Retrieved from https://openwho.org/courses/severe-acute-respiratory-infection on 22 June 2020.

Yuki, K., Fujiogi, M., & Koutsogiannaki, S. (2020). COVID-19 pathophysiology: A review. *Clinical Immunology, 215*, 108427. https://doi.org/10.1016/j.clim.2020.108427.

Chapter 4

SARS-CoV-2 and Its Variants

Definitions and Classifications

Srijan Goswami, Ushmita Gupta Bakshi*, and Shreya Bhattacharya

CONTENTS

INTRODUCTION

The first variant of the original SARS-CoV-2 (D641G, reported around January–February 2020), originated in China, spread throughout the world, and has been undergoing constant mutations, leading to an increase in its variants (World Health Organization, 2021a). The word "variant" is derived from the *Latin* word "*variantem*", which means "tending to change" (Variant | Online Etymology Dictionary, n.d.). Constant change through mutations is one of the characteristic features of viruses (Coronavirus Disease 2019 (COVID-19), 2020a). Thus, the genomic sequence of a virus variant always differs from that of the original virus as a result of one or more mutations (Racaniello, 2021). The same phenomenon is applicable to SARS-CoV-2, the virus responsible for COVID-19. Throughout the pandemic, multiple variants of the original SARS-CoV-2 have been reported and documented worldwide. Globally, scientists and researchers from various domains are working day and night to compare differences in genomic sequences, identify variants, and establish relations among each other (Coronavirus Disease 2019 (COVID-19), 2020a). So, having a

DOI: 10.1201/9781003178514-5

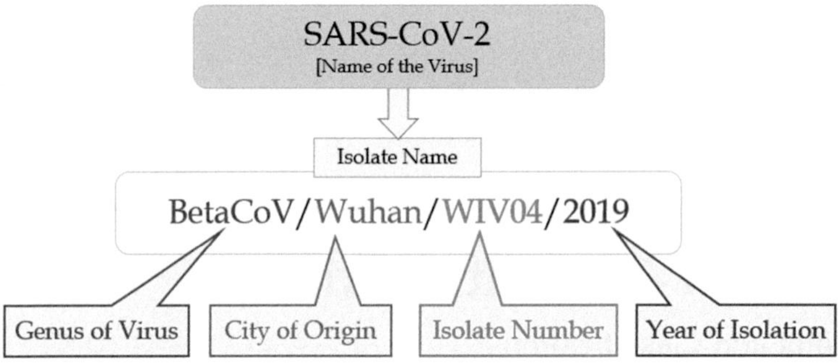

Figure 4.1 Virus isolate nomenclature (Racaniello, 2021).

sound understanding of the definitions, classifications, and molecular details about SARS-CoV-2 variants is very important for predicting their global impact and planning countermeasures accordingly (World Health Organization, 2021a).

The present chapter focuses on the definition and classification of SARS-CoV-2 variants, and SARS-CoV-2 Sequencing for Public Health Emergency Response, Epidemiology, and Surveillance (SPHERES). The chapter also provides a basic description of three specific variants, namely B.1.1.7, B.1.351, and P.1. But before moving on, it is essential that we learn about basic terminologies related to virology. According to an article published in "Virology Blog", virology terms like virus isolates, variants, and strains are being used inappropriately during the pandemic by people who do not have an in-depth understanding of virology, and thus are creating confusion (Racaniello, 2021).

- **Virus isolate**. When a sample containing a suspected virus is isolated from a host, and then grown in a specific viral culture medium. When the virus present in the host sample proliferates in the culture medium, those viruses can be called virus isolates. The isolates are named to indicate the origin (Figure 4.1).
- **Virus variant**. These are the viruses whose genome sequences differ from the original (reference) virus. The change in the genome sequence varies from one type to another (Racaniello, 2021).
- **Virus strain**. These are variants having unique and stable phenotypic features (Racaniello, 2021).
- **Serotype**. These are viruses of the same species but have different antigenic properties (Racaniello, 2021).
- **Genotype**. Represents the genetic makeup of the virus (Racaniello, 2021).

In order to understand SARS-CoV-2 variants properly, it is important to have a brief idea about the replication and life cycle of the original SARS-CoV-2 virus. Once we do that, then we will talk about the variants, their classification, and the genetic changes or mutations that contrast from the original SARS-CoV-2 virus and how those mutations may increase transmissibility, viral production, viral replication, lethality, severity, or mortality associated with these variants.

REPLICATION AND LIFECYCLE OF THE ORIGINAL SARS-CoV-2: A QUICK OVERVIEW

In Chapter 2, the author described the morphology, genomic organization, and life cycle of the original SARS-CoV-2 in detail. In this section, the authors provide a quick and brief overview of the replication and life cycle of the original SARS-CoV-2, which is necessary to understand the context of the present chapter. SARS-CoV-2 possesses an important structure called the spike (S) protein on its outer covering made of a phospholipid bilayer. Inside the virus, there is positive-sense single-stranded RNA as genetic material. These two components are vital in relation to the formation of variants.

For transferring the viral genetic material, SARS-CoV-2 has to infect the host cells. The spike protein on SARS-CoV-2 recognizes and binds to a specific structure expressed on host cells known as angiotensin converting enzyme-2 (ACE-2) receptors. The formation of the spike protein–ACE-2 receptor complex activates another protein called transmembrane serine protease-2 (TMPRSS-2) that cleaves a portion of the spike protein. This cleave results in successful infection by the process of receptor-mediated endocytosis, which brings the viral genetic material into the cell in a vesicle (Zhou et al., 2021).

Once inside the cell, the vesicle breaks and the viral genetic material (positive-sense single-stranded RNA) is released into the cytoplasm where it interacts with host cell components. The positive-sense single-stranded RNA of SARS-CoV-2 possesses multiple genes for the production of viral RNA polymerase, replicases, various proteases, and viral structural proteins (like S, M, N, and E). In this section, we are concerned only with the SARS-CoV-2 spike protein and its associated genetic sequences because the SARS-CoV-2 variants reported have major mutations in the sequences of this particular gene. The alteration in the sequence of the spike protein gene results in the formation of spike proteins having increased infectivity, transmissibility, and ability to evade host immune defenses. After successful infection, and replication of the mutated genes, virions will be produced containing the mutated spike proteins, which will be released and spread.

Thus, mutation in the gene encoding the spike protein and the spike protein variant itself are the two critical components of SARS-CoV-2 that the scientific community are worried about.

DEFINITION AND CLASSIFICATION

In March 2020, a SARS-CoV-2 Interagency Group (SIG) (Coronavirus Disease 2019 (COVID-19), 2020a) or COVID-19 Scientific Interest Group (SIG) (COVID-19 Scientific Interest Group | NIH Office of Intramural Research, n.d.) was established by the United States Department of Health and Human Services (HHS) in order to strengthen the coordination among various global regulatory authorities. The organizations that are part of SIG include the Centers for Disease Control and Prevention (CDC), the National Institutes of Health (NIH), the Food and Drug Administration (FDA), the Biomedical Advanced Research and Development Authority (BARDA), and the Department of Defense (DoD). The objectives of SIG include rapid characterization of emerging variants and monitoring their potential impact on critical SARS-CoV-2 countermeasures, including vaccines, therapeutics, and diagnostics (Coronavirus Disease 2019 (COVID-19), 2020a; COVID-19 Scientific Interest Group | NIH Office of Intramural Research, n.d.) (Figure 4.2).

The United States SIG, assigned a classification system for variants, according to this, SARS-CoV-2 variants are grouped into three categories, variants of interest (VOI), variants of concern (VOC), and variants of high consequences (VOHC).

Category 1: Variants of Interest

According to the CDC, variants having mutations in their receptor-binding domain leading to changes in receptor-binding properties, reduced antibody generation and efficiency, and a

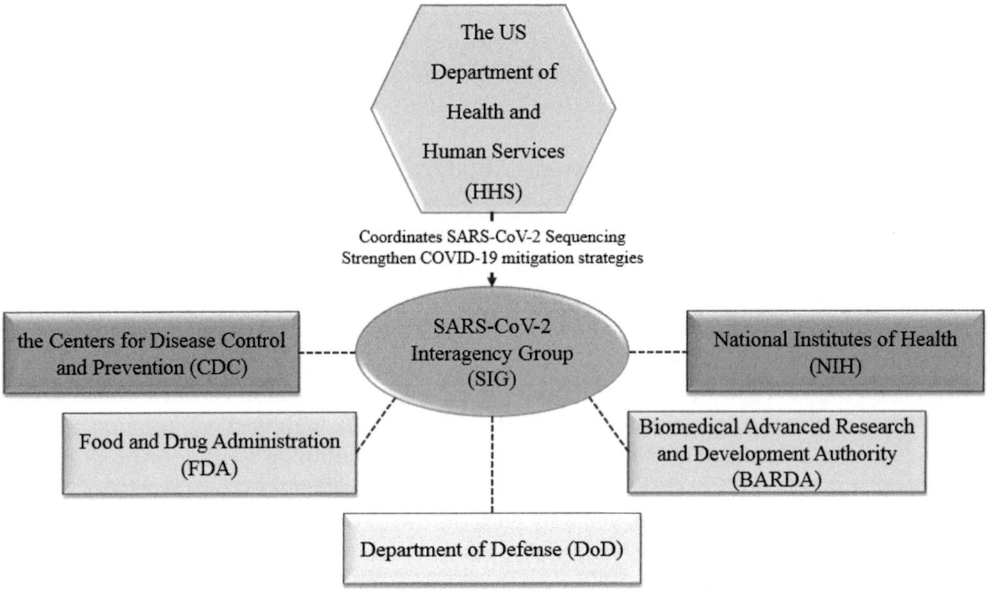

Figure 4.2 The United States Department of Health and Human Services (HHS) SARS-CoV-2 Interagency Group (SIG).

reduced response to treatment and disease management are grouped under this category. Sophisticated sequence surveillance, laboratory procedures, and epidemiological assessment are implemented for their investigation and characterization (Coronavirus Disease 2019 (COVID-19), 2020a). One sequence change designated as D614G is reported to be common in many of the variants detected worldwide. The name of some of the common VOI are:

- **B.1.525**. First detected in the UK and Nigeria in December 2020. This variant has several mutations in the spike protein sequences like D614G, 69del, 70del, 144del, E484K, Q677H, and F888L (Coronavirus Disease 2019 (COVID-19), 2020a).
- **B.1.526**. First detected in the United States in November 2020. This variant has several mutations in the spike proteins among which are T95I and D253G (Coronavirus Disease 2019 (COVID-19), 2020a).
- **B.1.526.1**. First detected in the United States in October 2020. D80G, 144del, F157S, L452R, D614G, and D950H are some of the major sequence changes reported for this type (Coronavirus Disease 2019 (COVID-19), 2020a).
- **B.1.617**. First detected in India in February 2021. Three notable changes reported in this variant are L452R, E484Q, and D614G (Coronavirus Disease 2019 (COVID-19), 2020a).
- **B.1.617.1**. First detected in India in December 2020. T95I, G142D, E154K, L452R, E484Q, D614G, P681R, and Q1071H are some of the notable changes detected in this particular variant (Coronavirus Disease 2019 (COVID-19), 2020a).
- **B.1.617.2**. First detected in India in December 2020. T19R, G142D, 156del, 157del, R158G, L452R, T478K, D614G, P681R, and D950N are some of the notable changes detected (Coronavirus Disease 2019 (COVID-19), 2020a).

- **B.1.617.3**. First detected in India in October 2020. T19R, G142D, L452R, D614G, D950N, and P681R are some of the notable changes in the spike protein sequence. The changes have similarities with B.1.617.2 (Coronavirus Disease 2019 (COVID-19), 2020a).
- **P.2**. First detected in Brazil in April 2020. E484K, V1176F, and D614G are the most prominent changes recorded in this variant (Coronavirus Disease 2019 (COVID-19), 2020a).

Category 2: Variants of Concern

Increased viral transmissibility, increased disease severity, reduced antibody generation and efficiency, and reduced response to treatment and disease management are grouped under this category. Researchers have reported evidence for reduced vaccine-induced protection from severe disease along with reduced production of effective neutralizing antibodies in response to natural infection (Coronavirus Disease 2019 (COVID-19), 2020a). The name of some of the common VOCs are:

- **B.1.1.7**. First detected in the UK: 69del, 70del, 144del, N501Y, A570D, D614G, P681H, T716I, and S982A are the major sequence changes reported in this variant (Coronavirus Disease 2019 (COVID-19), 2020a).
- **B.1.351**. First detected in South Africa. D80A, D215G, 241del, 242del, 243del, K417N, E484K, N501Y, D614G, and A701V are major sequences reported in this variant (Coronavirus Disease 2019 (COVID-19), 2020a).
- **B.1.427**. First detected in the United States in March 2021. L452R and D614G are major sequence changes reported in this variant (Coronavirus Disease 2019 (COVID-19), 2020a).
- **B.1.429**. First detected in the United States in March 2021, possess sequence changes like S13I, W152C, L452R, and D614G (Coronavirus Disease 2019 (COVID-19), 2020a).
- **P.1**. First detected in Japan and Brazil. L18F, T20N, P26S, D138Y, R190S, K417T, E484K, N501Y, D614G, H655Y, and T1027I are the notable sequence changes reported in this variant (Coronavirus Disease 2019 (COVID-19), 2020a).

Category 3: Variants of High Consequences

According to the CDC, the members of this category are thought to have characteristics like increased severe disease presentation and increased impact. As of 12 June 2021, there are no variants classified under this category (Coronavirus Disease 2019 (COVID-19), 2020a) (Figure 4.3).

THE WORLD HEALTH ORGANIZATION'S NOMENCLATURE OF SARS-CoV-2 VARIANTS

WHO, in collaboration with partners, expert networks, national authorities, institutions, and researchers has been monitoring and assessing the evolution of SARS-CoV-2 since January 2020 (Tracking SARS-CoV-2 Variants, 2021). To assist with public discussions of variants, WHO proposed using labels consisting of the Greek alphabet, that is, alpha, beta, gamma, as a practical way to discuss variants by non-scientific audiences (Coronavirus Disease 2019 (COVID-19), 2020a). The nomenclature is given in Table 4.1.

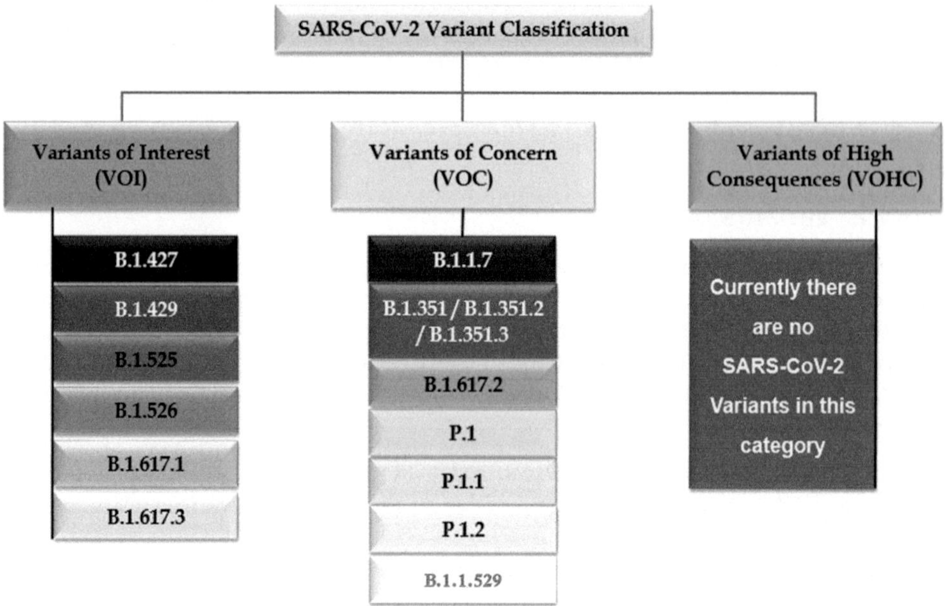

Figure 4.3 SARS-CoV-2 variant classification.

TABLE 4.1 GENERAL NOMENCLATURE OF SARS-COV-2 VARIANTS AS GIVEN BY THE WHO

SARS-CoV-2 Variants	Common Geek Nomenclature
B.1.525	Eta
B.1.526	Iota
B.1.617.1	Kappa
P.2	Zeta
B.1.1.7	Alpha
B.1.351	Beta
B.1.427	Epsilon
B.1.617.2	Delta
P.1	Gamma
B.1.1.529	Omicron

SARS-CoV-2 SEQUENCING FOR PUBLIC HEALTH EMERGENCY RESPONSE, EPIDEMIOLOGY, AND SURVEILLANCE

The Advanced Molecular Detection (AMD) Program of the CDC established SPHERES, a collaboration of experts from various clinical and public health laboratories, academic institutions, and authorized public sector organizations. The primary goal of this initiative is to coordinate and expand the implementation of pathogen genomics and associated technological advancements in order to

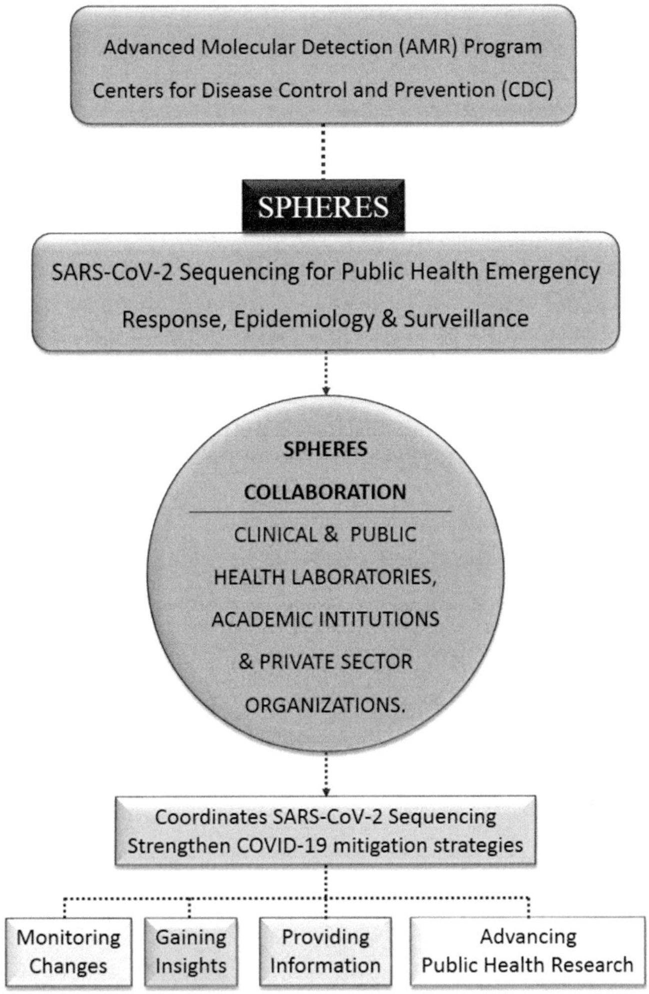

Figure 4.4 SARS-CoV-2 Sequencing for Public Health Emergency Response, Epidemiology, and Surveillance (SPHERES).

strengthen infectious disease surveillance and outbreak response (Cases, Data, and Surveillance, 2020). The SPHERES initiative promotes regulated collaboration among 60 federal, state, county, and local public health laboratories, several large regional and national clinical diagnostic corporations, and academic and non-profit leaders in pathogen genomics, bioinformatics, and public health from across the United States. The aims and objectives of SPHERES are presented in Figure 4.4.

UNDERSTANDING THE SPECIFIC VARIANTS

In previous sections, we learned that all the variants of SARS-CoV-2 have single or multiple mutations in the spike protein gene sequence. A change in the morphology of the spike protein of SARS-CoV-2 could potentially lead to the increased ability to evade the immune system, increased capability of infection, replication, and reproduction inside host cells, and increased transmissibility. In this section, we will be discussing three major variants: B.1.1.7, B.1.351, and P.1. These three variants are classified as VOCs.

B.1.1.7

The variant B.1.1.7 (UK variant), classified as a VOC, was first detected in the UK (September 2020), and has become the most prominent SARS-CoV-2 variant; 69del, 70del, 144del, N501Y, A570D, D614G, P681H, T716I, S982A, and D1118H are some of the major sequence changes (single nucleotide polymorphism [SNPs]) in the spike protein gene of SARS-CoV-2 reported in this particular variant. E484K, S494P, and K1191N are not uniformly present in all members (Lineage B.1.1.7, 2021; Coronavirus Disease 2019 (COVID-19), 2020a; Rambaut, 2021) (Table 4.2).

One of the major SNPs is N501Y, that is, substitution between two amino acids (asparagine [N] and tyrosine [Y]) at the 501st position of the spike protein. This substitution leads to an important

TABLE 4.2 SEQUENCES CHANGES OF B.1.1.7, THE ALPHA VARIANT

S. No	Spike Protein Sequence Change	Interpretation of the Sequence Change
Common sequence changes B.1.1.73		
1.	69del	Deletion at the 69th amino acid position
2.	70del	Deletion at the 70th amino acid position
3.	144del	Deletion at the 144th amino acid position
4.	N501Y	Substitution between two amino acids (asparagine [N] and tyrosine [Y]) at the 501st position.
5.	A570D	Substitution between two amino acids (alanine [A] and aspartic acid [D]) at the 570th position.
6.	D614G	Substitution between two amino acids (aspartic acid [D] and glycine [G]) at the 614th position.
7.	P681H	Substitution between two amino acids (proline [P] and histidine [H]) at the 681st position.
8.	T716I	Substitution between two amino acids (threonine [T] and isoleucine [I]) at the 716th position.
9.	S982A	Substitution between two amino acids (serine [S] and alanine [A]) at the 982nd position.
10.	D1118H	Substitution between two amino acids (aspartic acid [D] and histidine [H]) at the 1118th position.
Less common sequence changes (not present in all)		
12.	E484K	Substitution between two amino acids (glutamic acid [E] and lysine [K]) at the 484th position.
13.	S494P	Substitution between two amino acids (serine [S] and proline [P]) at the 494th position.
14.	K1191N	Substitution between two amino acids (lysine [K] and asparagine [N]) at the 1191st position.

structural change in the spike protein. The spike protein structure has three basic components: the S1 region, the S2 region, and the receptor-binding domain (RBD). N501Y changes the structure of the RBD. Let us now understand why this change is a global concern. The RBD is the main portion that interacts with the ACE-2 receptor. This mutation in SARS-CoV-2, particularly in the UK variant, increased the entry, binding, and endocytosis of the virus into the cell. So, the mutated RBD increased the affinity between the spike protein and the ACE-2 receptor protein, which resulted in increased infectivity. The increase in viral infectivity increases the chances of replication and viral load inside the host cells and this may lead to a potential problem. With an increase in viral load, the body triggers innate immune responses through sneezing, coughing, and mucus secretion, and that could increase the transmissibility. Thus, N501Y increases the changes of infectivity and transmissibility. The N501Y mutation is present in the South Africa variant (B.1.351) and the Brazil variant (P.1) (Lineage B.1.1.7, 2021; Coronavirus Disease 2019 (COVID-19), 2020a; Rambaut, 2021). The next major SNPs are 69del (deletion at 69th amino acid position) and 70del (deletion at 70th amino acid position), having the ability to change the structure of S1 and S2 regions of the spike protein. Let us now understand the factors that make these changes a concern. The immune system of the host produces neutralizing antibodies directed toward the spike protein of the original SARS-CoV-2 as a result of natural infection by the virus or by immunization through COVID-19 vaccines. The host's neutralizing antibodies (generated through natural infection or by artificial immunization [vaccines]) perform their functions and provide immunity by specifically recognizing and binding to the S1 and S2 regions of the spike protein. The concern with these deletions is that the portion of neutralizing antibodies that bind with spike proteins has weak affinity and binding capability and this may lead to an increased ability to evade the neutralizing antibodies and the host's immune system by the concerned variant (Lineage B.1.1.7, 2021; Coronavirus Disease 2019 (COVID-19), 2020a; Rambaut, 2021). The next notable mutation is P618H, that is, substitution between two amino acids (proline [P] and histidine [H]) at the 618th position of the spike protein. This mutation also results in the structural modification of the S1 and S2 regions of the spike protein. The RBD interacts with the ACE-2 receptor and the S1 and S2 region of the spike protein interacts with TMPRSS-2 and facilitates receptor-mediated endocytosis (taking the virus inside the host cell). The P618H mutation may increase the activity of the cleavage site as it may increase viral entry into the cell, as a result of increased interaction with TMPRSS-2 and the spike protein region (Lineage B.1.1.7, 2021; Coronavirus Disease 2019 (COVID-19), 2020a; Rambaut, 2021).

B.1.351

The variant B.1.351 (South Africa variant) was first detected in South Africa (September 2020). D80A, D215G, 241del, 242del, 243del, K417N, E484K, N501Y, D614G, and A701V are some of the major sequence changes (SNPs) in the spike protein gene of SARS-CoV-2 reported in this particular variant. This variant shares similarity with the UK variant in having N501Y and D614G sequence changes (Lineage B.1.351, 2021) (Table 4.3).

One of the prominent sequence changes in both the South African and Brazilian variants is E484K. E484K is a substitution between two amino acids (glutamic acid [E] and lysine [K]) at the 484th position of the spike protein. The RBD has a particular portion that specifically comes in contact with ACE-2. This mutation leads to a sequence change in the receptor-binding motif of the RBD of the spike protein. This sequence change increases the affinity and interaction between the RBM of RBD and ACE-2. This increases the viral entry into the host cell, the viral load, and the transmissibility (Lineage B.1.351, 2021).

TABLE 4.3 SEQUENCES CHANGES OF B.1.351, THE BETA VARIANT

S. No	Spike Protein Sequence Change	Interpretation of the Sequence Change
Common sequence changes B.1.351		
1.	D80A	Substitution between two amino acids (aspartic acid [D] and alanine [A]) at the 80th position.
2.	D215G	Substitution between two amino acids (aspartic acid [D] and glycine [G]) at the 215th position.
3.	241del	Deletion at the 241st amino acid position
4.	242del	Deletion at the 242nd amino acid position
5.	243del	Deletion at the 243rd amino acid position
6.	K417N	Substitution between two amino acids (lysine [K] and asparagine [N]) at the 417th position.
7.	D614G	Substitution between two amino acids (aspartic acid [D] and glycine [G]) at the 614th position.
8.	E484K	Substitution between two amino acids (glutamic acid [E] and lysine [K]) at the 484th position.
9.	N501Y	Substitution between two amino acids (asparagine [N] and tyrosine [Y]) at the 501st position.
10.	A701V	Substitution between two amino acids (alanine [A] and valine [V]) at the 701st position.

P.1

The variant P.1 was first detected in Brazil and Japan. L18F, T20N, P26S, D138Y, R190S, K417T, E484K, N501Y, D614G, H655Y, and T1027I are some of the major sequence changes (SNPs) in the spike protein gene of SARS-CoV-2 reported in this particular variant. The combination of K417T, E484K, and N501Y substitutions is present in this particular variant (Table 4.4).

SARS-CoV-2 VARIANTS AND VACCINE EFFICACY

Now the question that is a concern for the scientific community worldwide is, will the (original) COVID-19 vaccines be able to provide protection against these variants? For this, we have to understand the basic mechanism of action of the major vaccines. Vaccines (designed for COVID-19) have mRNA enclosed in a lipid nanoparticle which helps the mRNA enter the cell, and once it has been taken into the cell, the lipid nanoparticle disintegrates and releases the mRNA. The mRNA of interest then binds to the ribosome of the host cell and translates the viral mRNA into viral proteins (specifically the S-peptide). The portions of the newly produced S-protein (derived from the mRNA of vaccines) are expressed on the host cell. This mechanism activates the major histocompatibility complex-II (MHC-II) pathway.

These MHC-II molecules are only found on antigen-presenting cells abbreviated as APCs (for example, macrophages, b-cells, and dendritic cells). Once the MHC-II complex presents the piece of the S-peptide to naive T-helper cells (T_H-cells), the T-cell receptor (TCR) on naïve T_H-cells interacts with the MHC-II complex. Once the interaction occurs, it starts releasing cytokines. These cytokines cause the naive T_H-Cell to start proliferating, thus making more T_H-cells that are primed and able to recognize the S-peptide if they ever come into contact again in the future

TABLE 4.4 SEQUENCES CHANGES OF P.1, THE GAMMA VARIANT

S. No:	Spike Protein Sequence Change	Interpretation of the Sequence Change
Common sequence changes P.1		
1.	L18F	Substitution between two amino acids (leucine [L] and phenylalanine [F]) at the 18th position.
2.	T20N	Substitution between two amino acids (threonine [T] and asparagine [N]) at the 20th position.
3.	P26S	Substitution between two amino acids (proline [P] and serine [S]) at the 26th position.
4.	D138Y	Substitution between two amino acids (aspartic acid [D] and tyrosine [Y]) at the 138th position.
5.	R190S	Substitution between two amino acids (arginine [R] and serine [S]) at the 190th position.
6.	K417T	Substitution between two amino acids (lysine [K] and threonine [T]) at the 570th position.
7.	E484K	Substitution between two amino acids (glutamic acid [E] and lysine [K]) at the 484th position.
8.	N501Y	Substitution between two amino acids (asparagine [N] and tyrosine [Y]) at the 501st position.
9.	D614G	Substitution between two amino acids (aspartic acid [D] and glycine [G]) at the 614th position.
10.	H655Y	Substitution between two amino acids (Histidine [H] and tyrosine [Y]) at the 655th position.
11.	T1027I	Substitution between two amino acids (threonine [T] and isoleucine [I]) at the 102nd position.

(memory T-cells). These T-cells release more cytokines, which activate another set of cells, called B-cells. These B-cells from the cytokines are converted to antibody-secreting plasma cells. These antibodies are particularly primed toward the S-peptide of SARS-CoV-2. The human system has memory T-cells and antibody-secreting plasma cells. The B-cells are stimulated and take two pathways where plasma cells become effector B-cells and memory B-cells. The memory B-cells produce a specific type of antibody on their cell's membrane. These antibodies are primed for the S-peptide of SARS-CoV-2. The question is, is this immune response strong enough to battle off the actual variants? If the viral (the S-peptide of virus) peptide is mutated (with small change), the preformed antibodies (vaccine) are still able to recognize the variants because of the existing conserved sequences. There might be a small reduction in efficacy, but for the most part, it is expected that there will be a considerable degree of effectiveness with neutralizing antibodies. However, rigorous clinical studies and thorough research are required to validate the hypotheses (Nixon & Ndhlovu, 2021; Bian et al., 2021; SARS-CoV-2 Variants vs. Vaccines, 2021).

REFERENCES

Bian, L., Gao, F., Zhang, J., He, Q., Mao, Q., Xu, M., & Liang, Z. (2021). Effects of SARS-CoV-2 variants on vaccine efficacy and response strategies. *Expert Review of Vaccines*, *20*(4), 365–373. https://doi.org/10.1080/14760584.2021.1903879

Cases, Data, and Surveillance. (2020, February 11). Centers for Disease Control and Prevention. Retrieved June 12, 2021, from https://www.cdc.gov/coronavirus/2019-ncov/variants/spheres.html

Coronavirus Disease 2019 (COVID-19). (2020a, February 11). Centers for Disease Control and Prevention. Retrieved June 5, 2021, from https://www.cdc.gov/coronavirus/2019-ncov/variants/variant-info.html

COVID-19 Scientific Interest Group | NIH Office of Intramural Research. (n.d.). National Institutes of Health, Office of Intramural Research. Retrieved June 5, 2021, from https://oir.nih.gov/sigs/covid-19-scientific-interest-group

Lineage B.1.1.7. (2021). *PANGO Lineages*. Retrieved June 13, 2021, from https://cov-lineages.org/global_report_B.1.1.7.html

Lineage B.1.351. (2021, June 14). *PANGO Lineage*. Retrieved June 14, 2021, from https://cov-lineages.org/global_report_B.1.351.html

Nixon, D. F., & Ndhlovu, L. C. (2021) Vaccine breakthrough infections with SARS-CoV-2 variants.. *New England Journal of Medicine*, 385, e7. https://doi.org/10.1056/nejmc2107808

Racaniello, V. (2021, February 25). Understanding virus isolates, variants, and strains. *Virology Blog*. Retrieved June 5, 2021, from https://www.virology.ws/2021/02/25/understanding-virus-isolates-variants-strains-and-more/

Rambaut, A. (2021, February 4). Preliminary genomic characterisation of an emergent SARS-CoV-2 lineage in the UK defined by a novel set of spike mutations. *Virological*. Retrieved June 13, 2021, from https://virological.org/t/preliminary-genomic-characterisation-of-an-emergent-sars-cov-2-lineage-in-the-uk-defined-by-a-novel-set-of-spike-mutations/563

SARS-CoV-2 Variants vs. Vaccines. (2021, March 3). *ASM.Org*. Retrieved July 3, 2021, from https://asm.org/Articles/2021/February/SARS-CoV-2-Variants-vs-Vaccines

Tracking SARS-CoV-2 Variants. (2021, May 31). World Health Organization. Retrieved June 15, 2021, from https://www.who.int/en/activities/tracking-SARS-CoV-2-variants/

Variant | Online Etymology Dictionary. (n.d.). *Online Etymology Dictionary*. Retrieved June 5, 2021, from https://www.etymonline.com/search?q=variant&ref=searchbar_searchhint

World Health Organization. (2021a, January 22). *SARS-CoV-2 Variants*. Retrieved June 5, 2021, from https://www.who.int/csr/don/31-december-2020-sars-cov2-variants/en/

Zhou, B., Thao, T. T. N., Hoffmann, D., Taddeo, A., Ebert, N., Labroussaa, F., Pohlmann, A., King, J., Steiner, S., Kelly, J. N., Portmann, J., Halwe, N. J., Ulrich, L., Trüeb, B. S., Fan, X., Hoffmann, B., Wang, L., Thomann, L., Lin, X., . . . Beer, M. (2021). SARS-CoV-2 spike D614G change enhances replication and transmission. *Nature*, *592*(7852), 122–127. https://doi.org/10.1038/s41586-021-03361-1

Part II

Conventional Treatment Strategies for COVID-19 and Associated Public Health Concerns

Chapter 5

Epidemiology of COVID-19

Rehab A. Rayan*, Christos Tsagkaris, Imran Zafar, and Aikaterini Tata

CONTENTS

INTRODUCTION

Coronaviruses are significant animal and human pathogens. In late 2019, a new coronavirus was discovered as the causative agent of a series of unusual pneumonia infections in Wuhan, China (Li et al., 2020). This was a zoonotic coronavirus that showed person-to-person spread (Xie & Chen, 2020). It quickly transmitted into outbreaks and sporadic infections and caused an epidemic all over China, followed by a growing number of infected patients in many countries worldwide. In early 2020, the World Health Organization (WHO) declared the new disease caused by coronaviruses as COVID-19 (WHO, 2020b; Zhu et al., 2020). The virus leads to severe acute respiratory syndrome coronavirus 2 (SARS-CoV-2) as named by the International Committee on Taxonomy of Viruses (ICTV)-4; earlier, it was known as 2019-nCoV. SARS-CoV-2 belongs to the family of coronaviruses that infect the human species. The viruses of this family were six in total with the new virus ranking as the seventh. Four (229 E, OC 43, NL 63, and HKU 1) are quite common and usually cause flu-like symptoms in people with weakened immune systems. The other two strains of the virus are associated with severe acute respiratory syndrome (SARS- CoV-1) and Middle East respiratory syndrome (MERS-CoV), inflicting serious and often

DOI: 10.1201/9781003178514-7

fatal diseases. SARS-CoV was identified as the causative agent of the disease that caused acute respiratory distress incidents in 2002–2003 in China while the MERS-CoV was the responsible pathogen for another spate of similar diseases in the Middle East in 2012. After gene mapping, the new coronavirus was found to be 82% identical with the first and 50% with the second (Zhu et al., 2020). The COVID-19 infection is transmittable, and this virus adds a severe burden on population health. For the lack of unique antiviral therapeutics globally, many serious conditions cause deaths daily. This chapter discusses the virology, clinical features, epidemiology, diagnosis, pathogenesis, and promising vaccines and treatments for the COVID-19 infection.

Virology

The coronavirus COVID-19 is a betacoronavirus in the same subgenus as a severe SARS virus, but it has seen full sequencing and phylogenetic analysis. The receptor-binding region of the cell has been found to use the same receptor to enter the cell and the angiotensin converting enzyme-2 (ACE-2) (Zhou et al., 2020) (Figure 5.1).

The International Taxonomy of Viruses Coronavirus Research Group has shown that this virus is a severe coronavirus-2 acute syndrome (SARS-CoV-2) (Gorbalenya et al., 2020). A packaged, non-segmented RNA virus of 29,891 to 29,903 nucleotides is the genomic form of SARS-CoV-2. It belongs to the β-CoV subfamily of the orthocoronaviridae family. There are 14 Open Reading Frames (ORFs) in the SARS-CoV-2 genome that encode 27 proteins. The pP1ab and pp1a proteins including nsp1 to nsp10 and nsp12 to nsp16 were encrypted at the end of five by orf1ab and orph1a genes. The third end of the genome is composed of four structural proteins (S, E, M, N) and eight more (3a, 3b, p6, 7a, 7b, 8b, 9b, and orf14) (Wu et al., 2020). SARS-CoV-2 is a crucial stage and determinant of tropism in tissue and host cell and virus infection. SARS-CoV has a CoV-2 identity of 79.6%, and MERS-CoV has a CoV-2 identity of 51.8%. SARS-CoV-2 is anchored in the viral

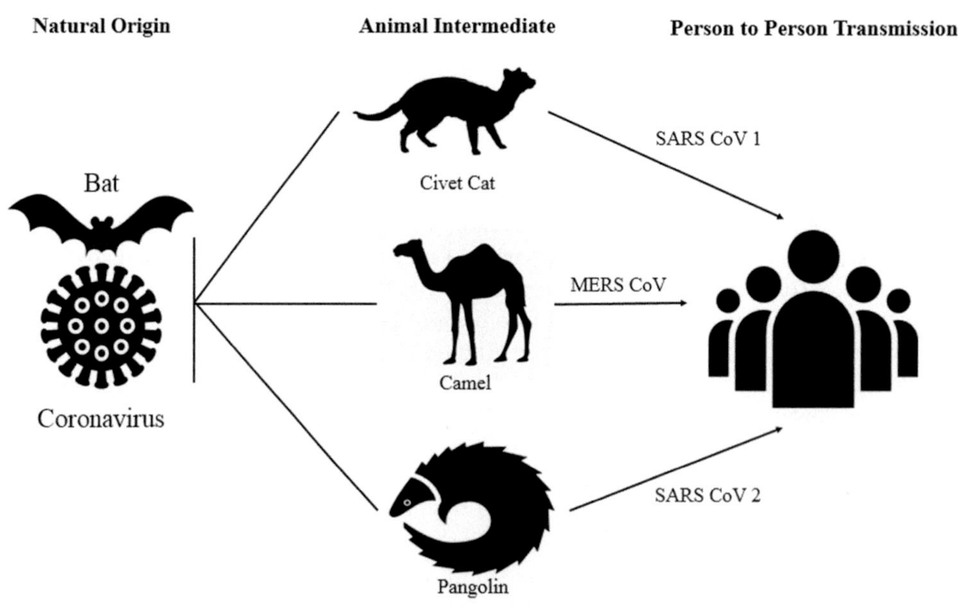

Figure 5.1 The natural habitat of arising coronaviruses SARS-CoV-1, MERS-CoV, and SARS-CoV-2.

membrane, using nail protein (S) like SARS-CoV (Wrapp et al., 2020). SARS-CoV-2 protein S is a new feature that differentiates between SARS-CoV-2 and SARS-CoV and has a site polybase cleavage at the S1 and S2 boundary (fusion of viruses and cell membranes) handled during biogenesis (Walls et al., 2020). The subunit S1 contains the receptor-binding domain (RBD), while the molecule movement S2 involves the membrane fusion driving regions. RBD is the RBD trend. The entry of SARS-CoV-2 into cells is based on the impact of ACE-2 and Transmembrane Serine Protease 2 (Human) (TMPRSS2), and these are promising candidates for anti-SARS-CoV-2 therapy. Both SARS-CoV-2 and SARS-CoV use ACE-2 as a receptor to mediate cellular entry of TMPRSS2, but differentiation in the host entry phase can explain certain differences in transmission and pathogenesis of the two viruses. SARS-CoV-2 is quite pathogenic because it is 10–20 times higher than the SARS-CoV protein S for ACE-2 binding (Hoffmann et al., 2020). A greater distribution in the kidneys, gastrointestinal tract, or brain may be related to the expression of local ACE-2 (Bourgonje et al., 2020). Increased expression and ACE-2 gene polymorphism can also contribute to increased SARS-CoV-2 susceptibility and an improvement in the risk of unfavorable findings from COVID-19 (Devaux et al., 2020). Protease adhesion to protein S is vital for the mixing of viral cells and the release into the cytoplasm of genome RNA, and the structural release of viral and SARS-CoV virus and RNA translation, replication, and packaging (Kupferschmidt & Cohen, 2020).

EPIDEMIOLOGY: FREQUENCY OF SYMPTOMS

Most patients experience mild-to-moderate symptoms and may not seek medical attention. Because of this, it is projected that actual COVID-19 cases are up to ten times more than the recorded cases. Patients with COVID-19 may experience one or more of the following symptoms in order of decreasing frequency: cough (51%), fever (41%), myalgia (38%), anosmia and/or loss of taste (15–16%), shortness of breath, fatigue, headache, confusion, and gastrointestinal symptoms. Studies have shown that up to 20% of confirmed cases can be completely asymptomatic, with this percentage increasing in younger age groups. Complications of the disease include severe pneumonia, acute respiratory distress syndrome (ARDS), acute cardiac failure, acute renal failure, sepsis, and multi-organ failure (multiple organ dysfunction syndrome, MODS) (Pongpirul et al., 2020) as shown in Figure 5.2.

TRANSMISSION OF THE DISEASE

The mode of transmission of the virus has not yet been fully elucidated with current data showing that human-to-human transmission occurs primarily through nasal or oral droplets. Many studies also suggest airborne transmission of the virus, which need to be documented more thoroughly (Wiersinga et al., 2020). Wiersinga et al. (2020) reported the confluence of the first cases to the WHO on December 31, 2019, while on January 12, 2020, the cause of the disease became known and was attributed to the new coronavirus SARS-CoV-2. The disease has spread rapidly to over 8,200 confirmed cases causing 171 deaths in China until January 30, with another 112 cases being diagnosed outside China in 21 other countries, including the United States. Facing the growing spread of the new coronavirus (2019- nCoV), the WHO declared the COVID-19 epidemic a global health emergency (Public Health Emergency of International Concern, PHEIC) on January 30, 2020, and then issued interim guidance to China and other countries on detecting, managing, and containing the virus (WHO, 2020a; Worldometer, 2021). Despite the efforts of all countries to

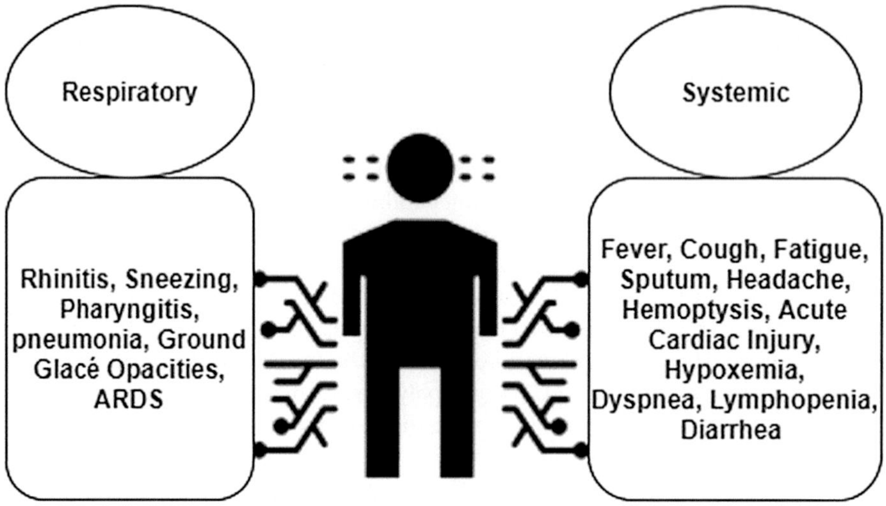

Figure 5.2 The respiratory and systemic disorders of SARS-CoV-2 infection.

prevent transmission, the virus continued to spread rapidly, with the number of daily new cases of COVID-19 outside China exceeding for the first time the cases recorded within China on February 26, 2020. As of Wednesday, March 11, 114 countries around the world had been exposed to the virus, bringing the total number of cases to 126,000, with approximately 4,300 deaths. This led the WHO to declare COVID-19 a global pandemic. The last time it made such a statement was in 2009 with the H1N1 pandemic. To date (January 2021), over 85 million cases have been diagnosed worldwide with more than 1.85 million deaths. It is noteworthy that the cases have increased from 32 million in September 2020 because of the so-called second wave of the pandemic (WHO, 2021).

PREVALENCE OF THE DISEASE

Prevalence estimates are exploding as not only the cases but also the availability of diagnostic tests multiplies. Children and adolescents seem to be just as likely to get the new virus as adults, although symptomatic cases are rarer (ECRIN, 2020). Regarding the distribution of the disease by age group, at the beginning of the pandemic, the incidence of COVID-19 was clearly higher among the elderly. However, during June–August 2020, there was a change in the age distribution curve as the incidence of COVID-19 appeared to be higher in people aged 20–29, who accounted for 20% of all confirmed cases in a study published by the CDC in autumn 2020. A similar age change occurred in Europe, where the mean age of COVID-19 cases decreased from 54 years in January–May to 39 years in June–July, during which persons aged 20–29 years accounted for the largest percentage of cases (19.5%) (Xinhua, 2020).

Basic Reproduction Number (R0)

The R0 is a transmissibility measure, which indicates the theoretically expected number of secondary cases from each given case during an epidemic transmission period. An R0 $>$ 1 is consistent with the spread of the epidemic. Considering the transmission period of the epidemic,

R0 was estimated at 2–5, with the average ranging from 1.4–5.7. As expected, R0 has decreased since the outbreak of the pandemic in China and areas of Europe following the implementation of disease control measures (Xinhua, 2020).

MORTALITY RATE

One of the most important parameters highlighting the severity of the COVID-19 disease is mortality. Countries around the world have reported very different mortality rates, namely the number of COVID-19-associated deaths divided by the number of confirmed cases. According to the Center for Systems Science and Engineering at Johns Hopkins University, mortality on September 26, 2020, ranged from 0.2–0.4% in countries such as Qatar, Sri Lanka, and others, reaching up to 10.5% in Mexico or 11.7% in Italy. The differences in mortality can be caused by differences in the number of people tested. It is known that with more tests, more people are identified with milder symptoms and therefore the prevalence of the disease increases. The data collected so far on the number of cases and the evolution of the pandemic differ from country to country, as most of them cannot provide testing to many people and therefore there is a lack of reliable data on the prevalence of the virus in a representative random sample of the general population. For example, mortality is higher in population groups with underlying diseases, immunosuppression, or other risk factors such as age. Therefore, a country with a larger percentage of its population falling into these groups will also have a higher number of accidental cases and deaths. The COVID-19 pandemic is pressing health systems around the world. The booming demand for health facilities, sanitary ware, technology equipment, and health workers threaten to leave some health systems exposed and unable to function effectively in the face of the new threat. Many other factors remain unknown (Johns Hopkins Coronavirus Resource Center, 2021).

VULNERABLE GROUPS

The most common health conditions associated with more severe morbidity or mortality rate among adult patients with COVID-19 include arterial hypertension, diabetes mellitus, cardiovascular and coronary disease, chronic respiratory conditions, chronic kidney failure, immunocompromised status, cancer, smoking, obesity, and pregnancy (Brandt et al., 2020; ECDC, 2020a). Among children and adolescents, pre-existing medical conditions have also been associated with a higher risk of severe disease and admission to the ICU (Rajapakse & Dixit, 2020). According to a European multi-center cohort study, the most common conditions among patients in the COVID-19 ICU were chronic pulmonary conditions, cancer, neurological diseases, congenital heart disease, chromosomal abnormalities, and chronic kidney failure. A higher rate of hospitalization and admission to the ICU has also been documented among women (Brandt et al., 2020).

PATHOGENESIS

In its mechanism, the pathogenesis of COVID-19 is still weak. The common laboratory findings during hospitalization include lymphopenia and pneumonia, with usual bilateral changes as pulmonary glass in computed tomography (Zhu et al., 2020). Bilateral alveolar lesions were seen in biological lung, liver, and cardiac tissue biopsies from fatal events, using bilateral fibromyxoid cell secretions and lymphocyte-dominated interstitial mono-inflammatory infiltrations (Xu et al., 2020). SARS and MERS clinical signs are the same. Interestingly, clinical and historic findings in the upper and lower respiratory tract are closely linked to humans in animal models with a SARS-CoV-2 infection. In the first step, exudative inflammation showed that after a week, diffuse inflammation and necrosis, alveolar hurt, and proliferation resulted (Chan et al., 2020). As a result, COVID-19 is predicted to lead to incremental respiratory collapse leading to alveolar damage and death. The nucleus, brain, and kidney ACE-2, which are related to SARS-CoV-2, have a large pattern of high expression in type II alveolar cells, both in the lungs and the gastrointestinal tract. COVID-19 can destroy tissues and organs outside the pulmonary system as illustrated in Figure 5.3 (Steardo et al., 2020).

The global expertise in the care of patients with COVID-19 with ARDS is booming by adopting mechanical processes and the ventilation of respiratory organs (Pan et al., 2020). In the last two decades, the variance in ARDS has risen. In an explanatory endeavor, subgroups of people with various biological, behavioral, psychiatric, and attentive characteristics have been established (Fan et al., 2018). An increased hospital burden on COVID-19 patients and healthcare staff, also with inadequate services to rescue ARDS patients, led to the revelation that the variability results in all medical characteristics of patients with COVID-19. The findings were presented with heterogeneity. Phenotypic heterogeneity is an important principle, but it may be overused or abused by certain principles, which may adversely affect the efficiency of ventilation management. Given the importance of lung defense in ARDS, ventilation techniques in this area have been explored in recent studies addressing the phenotypic heterogeneity of COVID-19 ARDS patients (Gattinoni et al., 2020). We highly advocate the implementation of evidence-driven management (Phua et al., 2020) based on clinical physiology and supported by current results, with a clear evidence base that can drive a transition from the existing patient care paradigm.

Diagnosis

The SARS-CoV-2 genome was sequenced at the start of the outbreak and complete sequence data have been published that have allowed accurate diagnostic methods of COVID-19 to be established (Zhu et al., 2020). The WHO has published SARS-CoV-2 N, E, S, and RdRP viral protocols for ERC screening (RT-PCR). If other respiratory diseases are suspected, all patients that are associated with the case definition should be screened for COVID-19 (Corman et al., 2020). Samples of RNA, if COVID-19 is accused of triggering mainly the deficiency of upper airway, are extracted from the nasal lavage.

These samples should be collected and shipped at 2–8°C immediately within one to five days for the authorized laboratory. In rectal, semen, and saliva swabs, the COVID-19 virus was contained but not in urine (To et al., 2020). In addition to molecular research, sequencing observations can also be used as an aid in the identification of mutations in the viral genome, and improvements in molecular testing can also be carried out (World Health Organization, 2020). Moreover, other serological experiments are carried out but must be checked as a counterpart to the RT-PCR test.

PHARMACOEPIDEMIOLOGY

Rapid COVID-19 epidemiological shifts pose a significant challenge to drugs and vaccines developed for this disease. At the beginning of the pandemic, many efforts were put into repurposing

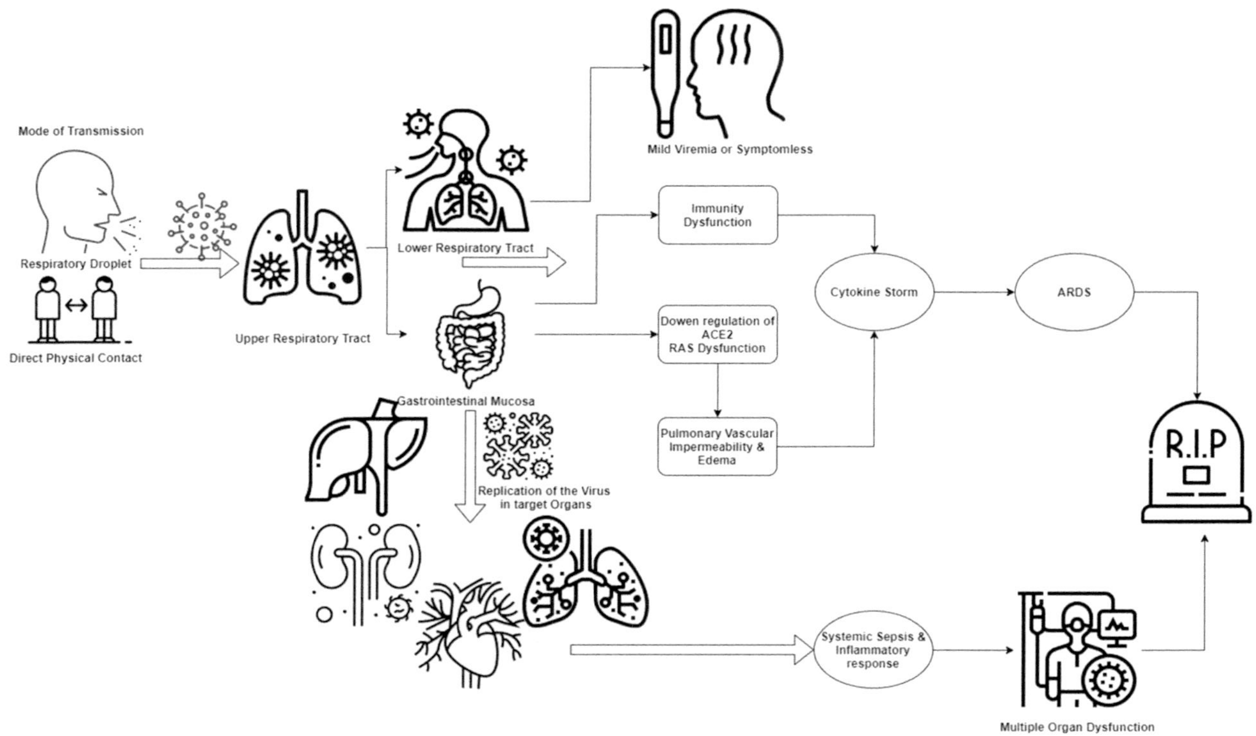

Figure 5.3 Suggested pathogenesis of COVID-19. ACE-2, angiotensin-converting enzyme-2; RAS, renin–angiotensin system; ARDS, acute respiratory distress syndrome.

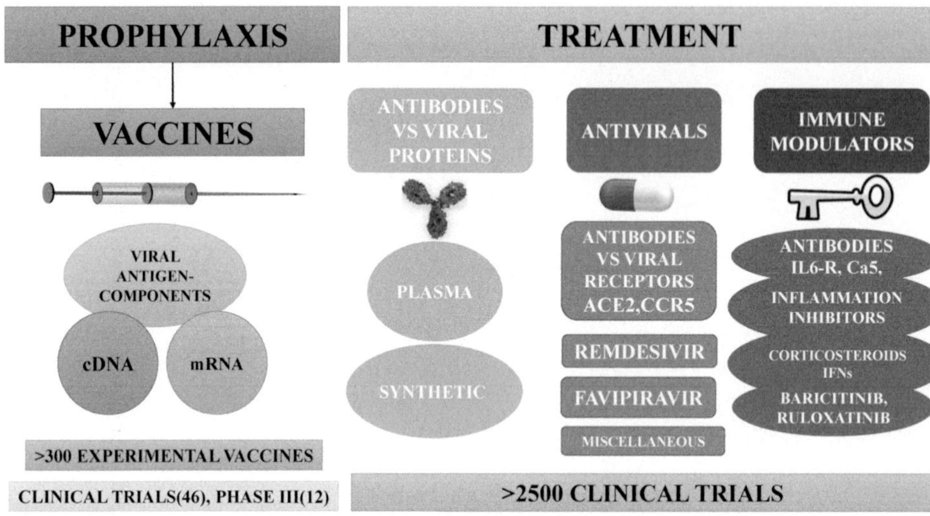

Figure 5.4 An overview of COVID-19 vaccines and drugs at the end of 2020.

existing regimens and optimizing symptomatic treatment of the disease. Drug development efforts were initiated with a focus on antiviral agents, monoclonal antibodies, and vaccines (Sahebnasagh et al., 2020). Studying the use and effects of drugs in large populations resulted in a relatively rapid assessment of their beneficial – if any – and adverse effects (Coma et al., 2020). While the landscape of COVID-19 treatment is continually changing, this section attempts to provide a critical outline of milestones in the field. An overview of the COVID-19 pharmacological landscape as of early 2021 is shown in Figure 5.4. The therapeutic approach is divided between prophylaxis and treatment. Prophylaxis is based on vaccines. As of December 2020, over 300 vaccines were developed; 46 vaccines have been in clinical trials and 12 of them have made it to phase III. At the same time, regulatory bodies in different countries have provided emergency or provisional use authorization (EUA) to the vaccines of Pfizer–BioNTech, Moderna, Sinopharm, and the Gamaleya Institute (ECDC, 2020b; Weber, 2021). The vaccines of Pfizer–BioNTech and Moderna are based on viral messenger RNA (m RNA), a novel technology that accelerated their development. The BBIBP-CorV vaccine of Sinopharm consists of inactivated viral vectors, while the Gam-COVID-Vac of the Gamaleya Institute consists of a viral two-vector vaccine based on two human adenoviruses encoding the SARS-CoV-2 spike protein (CDC, 2020). These vaccines have shown promising results in terms of mitigating the risk of developing severe infection. According to existing studies, it may be possible to contract and transmit the virus after vaccination, while evidence regarding pregnant women and children is not available to date. The special storing requirements of each vaccine in combination with the need for massive manufacturing have generated several challenges in terms of transportation and timely vaccination of the population. While prioritization of vulnerable or age groups is still debated, efforts to administer the vaccine to more than 70% of the population – a milestone associated with herd immunity – are expected to last for months (Sahebnasagh et al., 2020).

In this timeframe, drugs in combination with preventive measures are expected to play an important role in decreasing COVID-19 mortality. Available drugs include antiviral agents, antibiotics, immunomodulatory agents, anticoagulants, and corticosteroids. Since the onset of the pandemic, treatment algorithms have been repeatedly modified. Certain regimens such as hydroxychloroquine would gain traction only to be proved ineffective a few months later (Chou et al., 2020; ECDC, 2020b). Remdesivir, an RNA polymerase inhibitor, has been assessed as capable of increasing the odds of clinical improvement for inpatients. However, both the WHO and research teams around the world have expressed concerns about its efficacy. Recently, its partial and delayed interaction with the RNA polymerase of SARS-CoV–2, has been associated with its outcomes (Beigel et al., 2020; Dyer, 2020).

Monoclonal antibodies have also been expected to change the tide in the battle against COVID-19. However, their clinical spectrum appears narrower than expected. Most of them are beneficial if they are administered to patients fulfilling certain criteria in a timely manner (Office of the Commissioner, 2020). Convalescent plasma (CP) has also caused a great deal of controversy. RCTs have proven its association with lower mortality or decreased viral load. However, disparities in terms of efficacy have been pointed out considering the inability of physicians to assess the content of a CP unit in antibodies against SARS-CoV-2 in most cases (Casadevall et al., 2020; Janssen et al., 2020). At the same time, controversy concerns widely used drugs that seem to increase COVID-19 morbidity and mortality. Proton pump inhibitors (PPI) and other antacid regimens were associated with a higher risk of infection and worse clinical outcomes early in 2020 (S. W. Lee et al., 2021; Lelie & Taghavi, 2020). Similar concerns have been announced regarding over-the-counter NSAIDs (Sahebnasagh et al., 2020). So far, the pharmacology of COVID-19 has overlapped with epidemiology and health policy, considering the denial of certain countries to submit vaccines developed in their land for assessment in other countries' regulatory bodies. With a stalemate of evidence on hand, human challenge studies have gained attention. These studies are based on the intentional infection of participants. They can provide a powerful scientific method for the testing of vaccines and drugs requiring small numbers of participants – usually not exceeding 100 people. Nonetheless, this type of study faces ethical and regulatory obstacles due to the exposure of the participants and third-party individuals to a potentially lethal pathogen (Cornwall, 2020).

Aspects of Prevention

The National Research Center (NIH) of the United States defines prevention as an action aimed at reducing the likelihood of disease (NIH, 2020). In ancient times, discourses of the Hippocratic Collection emphasized the superiority of prevention over (laborious) treatment (Borysiewicz, 2009). In the middle of the 20th century, the definition of health by the WHO reinforced this perception by highlighting psychosocial well-being as opposed to the absence of disease (Sartorius, 2006). In 2001, Geoffrey Rose distinguished two basic prevention strategies: the high-risk strategy (focused on vulnerable groups/high-risk individuals) and the risk-sharing strategy for the entire population (shift distribution of risk) (Rose, 2001). In both cases, the individual preventive interventions are structured in three levels: primary, secondary, and tertiary prevention (Kisling & M Das, 2020).

Primary prevention involves interventions before the disease develops. It is based on the breakdown of the causal sequence of genetic and environmental factors that lead to the disease. Change in lifestyle (lifestyle modification) in combination with training and information can prevent the development of infectious and non-infectious diseases. The use of personal protective measures and the education and empowerment of the population in matters of personal hygiene are examples of primary prevention in the context of COVID-19 (IWH, 2015; Wall, 2001). Secondary prevention refers to the early detection of a developing but non-clinically manifest disease or health problem. The purpose of secondary prevention is to make the prognosis of the disease more favorable when it occurs. Early diagnosis of atrial fibrillation, for example, and prophylaxis can prevent the onset of a stroke. In the case of COVID-19, the WHO's "test, test, test" strategy aiming for the early detection of asymptomatic carriers is a secondary prevention intervention. Tertiary prevention prevents the recurrence of a disease that has occurred in the past, such as a stroke or myocardial infarction. At this level of prevention, emphasis is shifted toward rehabilitating and reintegrating patients into their family, work, and social environment. In the case of COVID-19, this level of prevention corresponds to the return of patients, whether hospitalized or not, to their daily activity after the symptoms have subsided and the detection tests for the virus are negative (IWH, 2015; Kisling & M Das, 2020).

Prevention strategies globally have been unequally distributed between communicable and non-communicable diseases (NCDs) before the pandemic. In low and middle-income countries (LMICs), infections were prevalent because of their low vaccination coverage and correspondingly high mortality rates. In the western world, programs to prevent and reduce communicable diseases such as AIDS or seasonal flu coexisted with interventions aimed at the multilevel prevention of coronary heart disease, cancer, and stroke, among others (WHO, 2002).

The pandemic shifted the focus of preventive interventions to COVID-19 worldwide and created two dilemmas. The first dilemma pertains to whether imposing horizontal universal traffic ban measures should be preferred over the adoption of more targeted interventions. In the first phase of the pandemic, the first strategy seemed more effective. The earlier it was adopted, the lower COVID-19 prevalence and mortality were. The second dilemma comprises the concomitant losses of those prevention strategies. The success of horizontal measures in reducing cases has been overshadowed by poor prevention of non-communicable diseases. In contrast, the critical epidemiological picture of countries that have adopted less stringent measures, such as Sweden, is – up to an extent – counteracted by more adequate prevention of other diseases (Nakatani, 2016; Nussbaumer-Streit et al., 2020).

Prior to the pandemic, the balance fluctuated between prevention and, most commonly, effective treatment. A myocardial infarction indicated the failure of prevention, which could be compensated by timely angioplasty (Nakatani, 2016). The pandemic has shown the superiority of prevention because of the lack of effective symptomatic or, ideally, causal treatment. Therefore, the existing guidelines emphasize preventive interventions. This is critically relevant regarding the previously listed vulnerable groups (Nussbaumer-Streit et al., 2020). It is worth emphasizing that the development and implementation of prevention strategies are based on the cooperation of healthcare workers, the public, and the state (Rose, 2001).

The following are recommended for medical staff (Chou et al., 2020; Mullins et al., 2020; Nussbaumer-Streit et al., 2020; L. C. Poon et al., 2020, 2020; Liona C. Poon et al., 2020, p. 201): provision and/or posting of educational material (brochures, posters, etc.) in the waiting areas; organization of a sorting area and the provision of the necessary personal protection measures to those who work there; taking a brief history of patients arriving for an examination to rule out suspicious symptoms; patients who have been exposed to the virus and either remain asymptomatic or have mild symptoms should delay their scheduled visit by 14 days; reduction of the number of patients in the outpatient clinics and isolation of those with suspicious symptoms; and healthcare personnel with possible exposure to the virus should minimize contact with patients. In cases of exposure of health personnel without protection measures, isolation for seven days is recommended. The seasonal flu vaccination is also recommended (Donzelli, 2018).

In classical epidemiology, the paradox of prevention is defined as the disease of a larger number of people at low or intermediate risk in proportion to those at high risk (Rose, 2001). In many countries, this phenomenon has been observed in the second wave of the COVID-19 pandemic, when many young or middle-aged people acquired the virus after the relaxation of the sanitary measures (Gostin & Salmon, 2020). Young people have been red-flagged as super-spreaders on many occasions, however, their familiarity with social media and sources of information contribute to their awareness. This is also the case of vulnerable groups, who are more vigilant and have more frequent communication with healthcare professionals because of their underlying conditions (Gostin & Salmon, 2020; Schwartz, 2020; WHO, 2020c). Further studies toward this end will be of particular interest.

Future Insights

The COVID-19 that began as an outbreak in China in December 2019 has quickly transmitted globally, therefore, in early 2020, the WHO announced the infection as a pandemic. Vulnerable health systems in several countries have significant obstacles to providing primary healthcare for such an epidemic. Now, the danger confronting the world requires developing rapid and effective measures to safeguard susceptible populations for transmission. For such a purpose, the WHO has sped up research in diagnostics, vaccines, and therapeutics (Agrawal et al., 2020).

Serious measures to limit COVID-19 spread are needed to address the ongoing outbreak. Special concerns and efforts should be there to safeguard vulnerable populations such as children, healthcare professionals, and the elderly. Technical guidelines regarding COVID-19 should be disseminated for healthcare staff, population health practitioners, and researchers (Jin et al., 2020). The premature mortality of the COVID-19 outbreak mainly targeted the elderly, perhaps poor immunity allowing rapid progress of the virus (Li et al., 2020; Wang et al., 2020). Public facilities and services should routinely provide disinfectants for cleaning hands. Direct contact with contaminated and wet items should be regarded in handling the virus, particularly samples of urine and feces, which could be another route of spread (Assiri et al., 2013; N. Lee et al., 2003).

Many countries have adopted serious prevention and control interventions such as screening travelers to control more virus transmission (Carlos et al., 2020). Epidemiological modifications in the coronavirus should be monitored, considering possible modes of transmission and subclinical conditions, as well as the adaptation, mutation, and virus transmission between humans and potential intermediate reservoirs. There remains a need for more investigations to figure out more and accurate facts about those who have been tested, positivity, and the variation of such rates. Limited cases among children have been reported either for the scarcity of testing or lack of susceptibility. Of those who have been tested, who have developed severe illness and who have tested positive but showed no clinical symptoms? Addressing such questions precisely would provide a structure for further specific and comprehensive population health interventions to be adopted.

CONCLUSIONS

COVID-19 is an arising human coronavirus like earlier SARS and MERS outbreaks. The pandemic potential of COVID-19 is still adding a significant burden to health worldwide. Following China's outbreak of COVID-19, SARS-CoV-2 has gained global concern as a critical infection of the respiratory tract. Bats are mostly the reservoir for coronaviruses. The primary route of transmission of COVID-19 is via inhaling respiratory droplets and direct or indirect physical contact, and the infection's average incubation period has been estimated to be around five days. The high-risk factors causing deaths from SARS-CoV-2 are comorbid conditions and old age. There is not a complete understanding regarding the pathogenesis of COVID-19, however, the infection shows that it resembles SARS in some aspects, while it varies in others, such as excessive mucus secretion in the lungs of severely ill patients.

To control viral transmission, governments worldwide have adopted containment policies as well as declaring emergency responses. Yet, considering the existing data, the viral transmission potential went beyond estimates and there is no specific antiviral therapeutics available, however, vaccines are now being marketed for the public. This chapter detailed the current understanding of COVID-19 and introduced the existing measures. There is an urgent need to build more solutions for effectively controlling such an emerging critical viral infection. The findings of the current review should inform more investigations and health strategies to get ready for future COVID-19 outbreaks.

REFERENCES

Agrawal, S., Goel, A. D., & Gupta, N. (2020). Emerging prophylaxis strategies against COVID-19. *Monaldi Archives for Chest Disease = Archivio Monaldi Per Le Malattie Del Torace, 90*(1). https://doi.org/10.4081/monaldi.2020.1289

Assiri, A., Al-Tawfiq, J. A., Al-Rabeeah, A. A., Al-Rabiah, F. A., Al-Hajjar, S., Al-Barrak, A., Flemban, H., Al-Nassir, W. N., Balkhy, H. H., Al-Hakeem, R. F., Makhdoom, H. Q., Zumla, A. I., & Memish, Z. A. (2013). Epidemiological, demographic, and clinical characteristics of 47 cases of Middle East respiratory syndrome coronavirus disease from Saudi Arabia: A descriptive study. *Lancet. Infectious Diseases, 13*(9), 752–761. https://doi.org/10.1016/S1473-3099(13)70204-4

Beigel, J. H., Tomashek, K. M., Dodd, L. E., Mehta, A. K., Zingman, B. S., Kalil, A. C., Hohmann, E., Chu, H. Y., Luetkemeyer, A., Kline, S., Lopez de Castilla, D., Finberg, R. W., Dierberg, K., Tapson, V., Hsieh, L., Patterson, T. F., Paredes, R., Sweeney, D. A., Short, W. R., … Lane, H. C. (2020). Remdesivir for the treatment of Covid-19: Final report. *New England Journal of Medicine, 383*(19), 1813–1826. https://doi.org/10.1056/NEJMoa2007764

Borysiewicz, L. (2009). Prevention is better than cure. *Clinical Medicine, 9*(6), 572–583. https://doi.org/10.7861/clinmedicine.9-6-572

Bourgonje, A. R., Abdulle, A. E., Timens, W., Hillebrands, J.-L., Navis, G. J., Gordijn, S. J., Bolling, M. C., Dijkstra, G., Voors, A. A., Osterhaus, A. D., van der Voort, P. H., Mulder, D. J., & van Goor, H. (2020). Angiotensin-converting enzyme 2 (ACE2), SARS-CoV-2 and the pathophysiology of coronavirus disease 2019 (COVID-19). *Journal of Pathology, 251*(3), 228–248. https://doi.org/10.1002/path.5471

Brandt, J. S., Hill, J., Reddy, A., Schuster, M., Patrick, H. S., Rosen, T., Sauer, M. V., Boyle, C., & Ananth, C. V. (2020). Epidemiology of coronavirus disease 2019 in pregnancy: Risk factors and associations with adverse maternal and neonatal outcomes. *American Journal of Obstetrics and Gynecology, 224*(4), 389.e1–e9. https://doi.org/10.1016/j.ajog.2020.09.043

Carlos, W. G., Dela Cruz, C. S., Cao, B., Pasnick, S., & Jamil, S. (2020). Novel Wuhan (2019-nCoV) coronavirus. *American Journal of Respiratory and Critical Care Medicine, 201*(4), P7–P8. https://doi.org/10.1164/rccm.2014P7

Casadevall, A., Grossman, B. J., Henderson, J. P., Joyner, M. J., Shoham, S., Pirofski, L., & Paneth, N. (2020). The assessment of convalescent plasma efficacy against COVID-19. *Med, 1*(1), 66–77. https://doi.org/10.1016/j.medj.2020.11.002

CDC. (2020, February 11). *COVID-19 and Your Health*. Centers for Disease Control and Prevention. https://www.cdc.gov/coronavirus/2019-ncov/vaccines/different-vaccines.html

Chan, J. F.-W., Zhang, A. J., Yuan, S., Poon, V. K.-M., Chan, C. C.-S., Lee, A. C.-Y., Chan, W.-M., Fan, Z., Tsoi, H.-W., Wen, L., Liang, R., Cao, J., Chen, Y., Tang, K., Luo, C., Cai, J.-P., Kok, K.-H., Chu, H., Chan, K.-H., … Yuen, K.-Y. (2020). Simulation of the clinical and pathological manifestations of coronavirus disease 2019 (COVID-19) in a golden Syrian hamster model: Implications for disease pathogenesis and transmissibility. *Clinical Infectious Diseases, 71*(9), 2428–2446. https://doi.org/10.1093/cid/ciaa325

Chou, R., Dana, T., Jungbauer, R., Weeks, C., & McDonagh, M. S. (2020). Masks for prevention of respiratory virus infections, including SARS-CoV-2, in health care and community settings. *Annals of Internal Medicine, 173*(7), 542–555. https://doi.org/10.7326/M20-3213

Coma, E., Mora, N., Méndez, L., Benítez, M., Hermosilla, E., Fàbregas, M., Fina, F., Mercadé, A., Flayeh, S., Guiriguet, C., Balló, E., Martinez Leon, N., Mas, A., Cordomí, S., Lejardi, Y., & Medina, M. (2020). Primary care in the time of COVID-19: Monitoring the effect of the pandemic and the lockdown measures on 34 quality of care indicators calculated for 288 primary care practices covering about 6 million people in Catalonia. *BMC Family Practice, 21*(1), 208. https://doi.org/10.1186/s12875-020-01278-8

Corman, V. M., Landt, O., Kaiser, M., Molenkamp, R., Meijer, A., Chu, D. K., Bleicker, T., Brünink, S., Schneider, J., Schmidt, M. L., Mulders, D. G., Haagmans, B. L., van der Veer, B., van den Brink, S., Wijsman, L., Goderski, G., Romette, J.-L., Ellis, J., Zambon, M., … Drosten, C. (2020). Detection of 2019 novel coronavirus (2019-nCoV) by real-time RT-PCR. *Eurosurveillance, 25*(3). https://doi.org/10.2807/1560-7917.ES.2020.25.3.2000045

Cornwall, W. (2020). New challenges emerge for planned human challenge trials. *Science, 370*(6521), 1150–1150. https://doi.org/10.1126/science.370.6521.1150

Devaux, C. A., Rolain, J.-M., & Raoult, D. (2020). ACE2 receptor polymorphism: Susceptibility to SARS-CoV-2, hypertension, multi-organ failure, and COVID-19 disease outcome. *Journal of Microbiology, Immunology, and Infection = Wei Mian Yu Gan Ran Za Zhi, 53*(3), 425–435. https://doi.org/10.1016/j.jmii.2020.04.015

Donzelli, A. (2018). Influenza vaccinations for all pregnant women? Better evidence is needed. *International Journal of Environmental Research and Public Health, 15*(9). https://doi.org/10.3390/ijerph15092034

Dyer, O. (2020). Covid-19: Remdesivir has little or no impact on survival, WHO trial shows. *BMJ, 371*, m4057. https://doi.org/10.1136/bmj.m4057

ECDC. (2020a, November 16). *Risk Factors and Risk Groups*. European Centre for Disease Prevention and Control. https://www.ecdc.europa.eu/en/covid-19/latest-evidence/epidemiology

ECDC. (2020b, December 9). *Vaccines and Treatment of COVID-19*. European Centre for Disease Prevention and Control. https://www.ecdc.europa.eu/en/covid-19/latest-evidence/vaccines-and-treatment

ECRIN. (2020, August 12). *COVID-19 Literature Reviews*. ECRIN. https://ecrin.org/covid-19-literature-reviews

Fan, E., Brodie, D., & Slutsky, A. S. (2018). Acute respiratory distress syndrome: Advances in diagnosis and treatment. *JAMA, 319*(7), 698–710. https://doi.org/10.1001/jama.2017.21907

Gattinoni, L., Chiumello, D., Caironi, P., Busana, M., Romitti, F., Brazzi, L., & Camporota, L. (2020). COVID-19 pneumonia: Different respiratory treatments for different phenotypes? *Intensive Care Medicine, 46*(6), 1099–1102. https://doi.org/10.1007/s00134-020-06033-2

Gorbalenya, A. E., Baker, S. C., Baric, R. S., de Groot, R. J., Drosten, C., Gulyaeva, A. A., Haagmans, B. L., Lauber, C., Leontovich, A. M., Neuman, B. W., Penzar, D., Perlman, S., Poon, L. L. M., Samborskiy, D., Sidorov, I. A., Sola, I., & Ziebuhr, J. (2020). Severe acute respiratory syndrome-related coronavirus: The species and its viruses: A statement of the coronavirus study group. *BioRxiv*, 2020.02.07.937862. https://doi.org/10.1101/2020.02.07.937862

Gostin, L. O., & Salmon, D. A. (2020). The dual epidemics of COVID-19 and influenza: Vaccine acceptance, coverage, and mandates. *JAMA, 324*(4), 335. https://doi.org/10.1001/jama.2020.10802

Hoffmann, M., Kleine-Weber, H., Schroeder, S., Krüger, N., Herrler, T., Erichsen, S., Schiergens, T. S., Herrler, G., Wu, N.-H., Nitsche, A., Müller, M. A., Drosten, C., & Pöhlmann, S. (2020). SARS-CoV-2 cell entry depends on ACE2 and TMPRSS2 and is blocked by a clinically proven protease inhibitor. *Cell, 181*(2), 271–280.e8. https://doi.org/10.1016/j.cell.2020.02.052

IWH. (2015, April). *Primary, Secondary and Tertiary Prevention*. https://www.iwh.on.ca/what-researchers-mean-by/primary-secondary-and-tertiary-prevention

Janssen, M., Schäkel, U., Djuka Fokou, C., Krisam, J., Stermann, J., Kriegsmann, K., Haberbosch, I., Novotny, J. P., Weber, S., Vehreschild, M., Bornhäuser, M., Bullinger, L., Schmitt, M., Liebregts, T., Dreger, P., Lorenz, H.-M., Plaszczyca, A., Bartenschlager, R., Müller, B., … Müller-Tidow, C. (2020). A randomized open label phase-II clinical trial with or without infusion of plasma from subjects after convalescence of SARS-CoV-2 infection in high-risk patients with confirmed severe SARS-CoV-2 disease (RECOVER): A structured summary of a study protocol for a randomised controlled trial. *Trials, 21*(1), 828. https://doi.org/10.1186/s13063-020-04735-y

Jin, Y.-H., Cai, L., Cheng, Z.-S., Cheng, H., Deng, T., Fan, Y.-P., Fang, C., Huang, D., Huang, L.-Q., Huang, Q., Han, Y., Hu, B., Hu, F., Li, B.-H., Li, Y.-R., Liang, K., Lin, L.-K., Luo, L.-S., Ma, J., … Wang, X.-H. (2020). A rapid advice guideline for the diagnosis and treatment of 2019 novel coronavirus (2019-nCoV) infected pneumonia (standard version). *Military Medical Research*, *7*. https://doi.org/10.1186/s40779-020-0233-6

Johns Hopkins Coronavirus Resource Center. (2021). *Mortality Analyses*. Johns Hopkins Coronavirus Resource Center. https://coronavirus.jhu.edu/data/mortality

Kisling, L. A., & Das, J. M. (2020). Prevention strategies. In *StatPearls*. StatPearls Publishing. http://www.ncbi.nlm.nih.gov/books/NBK537222/

Kupferschmidt, K., & Cohen, J. (2020). Race to find COVID-19 treatments accelerates. *Science*, *367*(6485), 1412–1413. https://doi.org/10.1126/science.367.6485.1412

Lee, N., Hui, D., Wu, A., Chan, P., Cameron, P., Joynt, G. M., Ahuja, A., Yung, M. Y., Leung, C. B., To, K. F., Lui, S. F., Szeto, C. C., Chung, S., & Sung, J. J. Y. (2003). A major outbreak of severe acute respiratory syndrome in Hong Kong. *The New England Journal of Medicine*, *348*(20), 1986–1994. https://doi.org/10.1056/NEJMoa030685

Lee, S. W., Ha, E. K., Yeniova, A. Ö., Moon, S. Y., Kim, S. Y., Koh, H. Y., Yang, J. M., Jeong, S. J., Moon, S. J., Cho, J. Y., Yoo, I. K., & Yon, D. K. (2021). Severe clinical outcomes of COVID-19 associated with proton pump inhibitors: A nationwide cohort study with propensity score matching. *Gut*, *70*(1), 76–84. https://doi.org/10.1136/gutjnl-2020-322248

van der Lelie, D., & Taghavi, S. (2020). COVID-19 and the gut microbiome: More than a gut feeling. *MSystems*, *5*(4), e00453–20. https://doi.org/10.1128/mSystems.00453-20

Li, Q., Guan, X., Wu, P., Wang, X., Zhou, L., Tong, Y., Ren, R., Leung, K. S. M., Lau, E. H. Y., Wong, J. Y., Xing, X., Xiang, N., Wu, Y., Li, C., Chen, Q., Li, D., Liu, T., Zhao, J., Liu, M., … Feng, Z. (2020). Early transmission dynamics in Wuhan, China, of novel coronavirus-infected pneumonia. *New England Journal of Medicine*, *382*(13), 1199–1207. https://doi.org/10.1056/NEJMoa2001316

Mullins, E., Evans, D., Viner, R. M., O'Brien, P., & Morris, E. (2020). Coronavirus in pregnancy and delivery: Rapid review. *Ultrasound in Obstetrics & Gynecology: The Official Journal of the International Society of Ultrasound in Obstetrics and Gynecology*, *55*(5), 586–592. https://doi.org/10.1002/uog.22014

Nakatani, H. (2016). Global strategies for the prevention and control of infectious diseases and non-communicable diseases. *Journal of Epidemiology*, *26*(4), 171–178. https://doi.org/10.2188/jea.JE20160010

NIH. (2020, February 18). *Prevention Research Defined*. Office of Disease Prevention. https://prevention.nih.gov/about-odp/prevention-research-defined

Nussbaumer-Streit, B., Mayr, V., Dobrescu, A. I., Chapman, A., Persad, E., Klerings, I., Wagner, G., Siebert, U., Christof, C., Zachariah, C., & Gartlehner, G. (2020). Quarantine alone or in combination with other public health measures to control COVID-19: A rapid review. *Cochrane Database of Systematic Reviews*, *4*. https://doi.org/10.1002/14651858.CD013574

Office of the Commissioner. (2020, November 23). *Coronavirus (COVID-19) Update: FDA Authorizes Monoclonal Antibodies for Treatment of COVID-19*. FDA. https://www.fda.gov/news-events/press-announcements/coronavirus-covid-19-update-fda-authorizes-monoclonal-antibodies-treatment-covid-19

Pan, C., Chen, L., Lu, C., Zhang, W., Xia, J.-A., Sklar, M. C., Du, B., Brochard, L., & Qiu, H. (2020). Lung recruitability in COVID-19-associated acute respiratory distress syndrome: A single-center observational study. *American Journal of Respiratory and Critical Care Medicine*, *201*(10), 1294–1297. https://doi.org/10.1164/rccm.202003-0527LE

Phua, J., Weng, L., Ling, L., Egi, M., Lim, C.-M., Divatia, J. V., Shrestha, B. R., Arabi, Y. M., Ng, J., Gomersall, C. D., Nishimura, M., Koh, Y., Du, B., & Asian Critical Care Clinical Trials Group. (2020). Intensive care management of coronavirus disease 2019 (COVID-19): Challenges and recommendations. *Lancet. Respiratory Medicine*, *8*(5), 506–517. https://doi.org/10.1016/S2213-2600(20)30161-2

Pongpirul, W. A., Wiboonchutikul, S., Charoenpong, L., Panitantum, N., Vachiraphan, A., Uttayamakul, S., Pongpirul, K., Manosuthi, W., & Prasithsirikul, W. (2020). Clinical course and potential predictive factors for pneumonia of adult patients with Coronavirus Disease 2019 (COVID-19): A retrospective observational analysis of 193 confirmed cases in Thailand. *PLOS Neglected Tropical Diseases*, *14*(10), e0008806. https://doi.org/10.1371/journal.pntd.0008806

Poon, L. C., Yang, H., Lee, J. C. S., Copel, J. A., Leung, T. Y., Zhang, Y., Chen, D., & Prefumo, F. (2020). ISUOG Interim Guidance on 2019 novel coronavirus infection during pregnancy and puerperium: Information for healthcare professionals. *Ultrasound in Obstetrics & Gynecology, 55*(5), 700–708. https://doi.org/10.1002/uog.22013

Poon, L. C., Yang, H., Kapur, A., Melamed, N., Dao, B., Divakar, H., McIntyre, H. D., Kihara, A. B., Ayres-de-Campos, D., Ferrazzi, E. M., Renzo, G. C. D., & Hod, M. (2020). Global interim guidance on coronavirus disease 2019 (COVID-19) during pregnancy and puerperium from FIGO and allied partners: Information for healthcare professionals. *International Journal of Gynecology & Obstetrics, 149*(3), 273–286. https://doi.org/10.1002/ijgo.13156

Rajapakse, N., & Dixit, D. (2020). Human and novel coronavirus infections in children: A review. *Paediatrics and International Child Health, 41*(1), 36–55. https://doi.org/10.1080/20469047.2020.1781356

Rose, G. (2001). Sick individuals and sick populations. *International Journal of Epidemiology, 30*(3), 427–432. https://doi.org/10.1093/ije/30.3.427

Sahebnasagh, A., Avan, R., Saghafi, F., Mojtahedzadeh, M., Sadremomtaz, A., Arasteh, O., Tanzifi, A., Faramarzi, F., Negarandeh, R., Safdari, M., Khataminia, M., Rezai Ghaleno, H., Habtemariam, S., & Khoshi, A. (2020). Pharmacological treatments of COVID-19. *Pharmacological Reports*, 1–33. https://doi.org/10.1007/s43440-020-00152-9

Sartorius, N. (2006). The Meanings of Health and its Promotion. *Croatian Medical Journal, 47*(4), 662–664.

Schwartz, D. A. (2020). An analysis of 38 pregnant women with COVID-19, their newborn infants, and maternal-fetal transmission of SARS-CoV-2: Maternal coronavirus infections and pregnancy outcomes. *Archives of Pathology & Laboratory Medicine, 144*(7), 799–805. https://doi.org/10.5858/arpa.2020-0901-SA

Steardo, L., Steardo, L., Zorec, R., & Verkhratsky, A. (2020). Neuroinfection may contribute to pathophysiology and clinical manifestations of COVID-19. *Acta Physiologica, 229*(3), e13473. https://doi.org/10.1111/apha.13473

To, K. K.-W., Tsang, O. T.-Y., Leung, W.-S., Tam, A. R., Wu, T.-C., Lung, D. C., Yip, C. C.-Y., Cai, J.-P., Chan, J. M.-C., Chik, T. S.-H., Lau, D. P.-L., Choi, C. Y.-C., Chen, L.-L., Chan, W.-M., Chan, K.-H., Ip, J. D., Ng, A. C.-K., Poon, R. W.-S., Luo, C.-T., … Yuen, K.-Y. (2020). Temporal profiles of viral load in posterior oropharyngeal saliva samples and serum antibody responses during infection by SARS-CoV-2: An observational cohort study. *The Lancet Infectious Diseases, 20*(5), 565–574. https://doi.org/10.1016/S1473-3099(20)30196-1

Wall, S. (2001). Cancer epidemiology: Principles and methods. *Statistics in Medicine, 20*(5), 821–822. https://doi.org/10.1002/sim.759

Walls, A. C., Park, Y.-J., Tortorici, M. A., Wall, A., McGuire, A. T., & Veesler, D. (2020). Structure, function, and antigenicity of the SARS-CoV-2 spike glycoprotein. *Cell, 181*(2), 281–292.e6. https://doi.org/10.1016/j.cell.2020.02.058

Wang, W., Tang, J., & Wei, F. (2020). Updated understanding of the outbreak of 2019 novel coronavirus (2019-nCoV) in Wuhan, China. *Journal of Medical Virology, 92*(4), 441–447. https://doi.org/10.1002/jmv.25689

Weber, S. (2021, January 12). *What to Know about the COVID-19 Vaccine*. https://www.uchicagomedicine.org/forefront/coronavirus-disease-covid-19/what-to-know-about-the-covid-19-vaccine

WHO. (2002). *WHO Strategy for Prevention and Control of Chronic Respiratory Diseases*. World Health Organization. https://www.who.int/respiratory/publications/crd_strategy/en/

WHO. (2020a, January 30). *IHR Emergency Committee on Novel Coronavirus (2019-nCoV)*. https://www.who.int/director-general/speeches/detail/who-director-general-s-statement-on-ihr-emergency-committee-on-novel-coronavirus-(2019-ncov)

WHO. (2020b, February 11). *WHO Director-General's Remarks at the Media Briefing on 2019-nCoV on 11 February 2020*. https://www.who.int/director-general/speeches/detail/who-director-general-s-remarks-at-the-media-briefing-on-2019-ncov-on-11-february-2020

WHO. (2020c, August 14). *Coronavirus Disease (COVID-19): Food Safety and Nutrition*. https://www.who.int/news-room/q-a-detail/coronavirus-disease-covid-19-food-safety-and-nutrition

WHO. (2021, January 4). *WHO Coronavirus Disease (COVID-19) Dashboard*. https://covid19.who.int

Wiersinga, W. J., Rhodes, A., Cheng, A. C., Peacock, S. J., & Prescott, H. C. (2020). Pathophysiology, transmission, diagnosis, and treatment of coronavirus disease 2019 (COVID-19): A review. *JAMA, 324*(8), 782–793. https://doi.org/10.1001/jama.2020.12839

World Health Organization. (2020). Laboratory testing for coronavirus disease (COVID-19) in suspected human cases: Interim guidance, 19 March 2020 (WHO/COVID-19/laboratory/2020.5). Article WHO/COVID-19/laboratory/2020.5. https://apps.who.int/iris/handle/10665/331501

Worldometer. (2021, May 1). *Coronavirus Graphs: Worldwide Cases and Deaths: Worldometer.* https://www.worldometers.info/coronavirus/worldwide-graphs/

Wrapp, D., Wang, N., Corbett, K. S., Goldsmith, J. A., Hsieh, C.-L., Abiona, O., Graham, B. S., & McLellan, J. S. (2020). Cryo-EM structure of the 2019-nCoV spike in the prefusion conformation. *Science, 367*(6483), 1260–1263. https://doi.org/10.1126/science.abb2507

Wu, A., Peng, Y., Huang, B., Ding, X., Wang, X., Niu, P., Meng, J., Zhu, Z., Zhang, Z., Wang, J., Sheng, J., Quan, L., Xia, Z., Tan, W., Cheng, G., & Jiang, T. (2020). Genome composition and divergence of the novel coronavirus (2019-nCoV) originating in China. *Cell Host & Microbe, 27*(3), 325–328. https://doi.org/10.1016/j.chom.2020.02.001

Xie, M., & Chen, Q. (2020). Insight into 2019 novel coronavirus: An updated interim review and lessons from SARS-CoV and MERS-CoV. *International Journal of Infectious Diseases, 94*, 119–124. https://doi.org/10.1016/j.ijid.2020.03.071

Xinhua. (2020, April 6). *Timeline of China releasing information on COVID-19 and advancing international cooperation.* http://en.nhc.gov.cn/2020-04/06/c_78861.htm

Xu, Z., Shi, L., Wang, Y., Zhang, J., Huang, L., Zhang, C., Liu, S., Zhao, P., Liu, H., Zhu, L., Tai, Y., Bai, C., Gao, T., Song, J., Xia, P., Dong, J., Zhao, J., & Wang, F.-S. (2020). Pathological findings of COVID-19 associated with acute respiratory distress syndrome. *Lancet Respiratory Medicine, 8*(4), 420–422. https://doi.org/10.1016/S2213-2600(20)30076-X

Zhou, P., Yang, X.-L., Wang, X.-G., Hu, B., Zhang, L., Zhang, W., Si, H.-R., Zhu, Y., Li, B., Huang, C.-L., Chen, H.-D., Chen, J., Luo, Y., Guo, H., Jiang, R.-D., Liu, M.-Q., Chen, Y., Shen, X.-R., Wang, X., … Shi, Z.-L. (2020). A pneumonia outbreak associated with a new coronavirus of probable bat origin. *Nature, 579*(7798), 270–273. https://doi.org/10.1038/s41586-020-2012-7

Zhu, N., Zhang, D., Wang, W., Li, X., Yang, B., Song, J., Zhao, X., Huang, B., Shi, W., Lu, R., Niu, P., Zhan, F., Ma, X., Wang, D., Xu, W., Wu, G., Gao, G. F., & Tan, W. (2020). A novel coronavirus from patients with pneumonia in China, 2019. *New England Journal of Medicine, 382*(8), 727–733. https://doi.org/10.1056/NEJMoa2001017

Chapter 6

Challenges and Innovations in Mathematical Modelling of COVID-19

Swarnali Sharma and Malay Banerjee*

CONTENTS

INTRODUCTION

Coronavirus disease 2019 (COVID-19), the highly infectious disease caused by severe acute respiratory syndrome coronavirus 2 (SARS-CoV-2), has had a catastrophic effect on the world's demographics, resulting in more than 3.8 million deaths worldwide, emerging as the most consequential global health crisis. After the first outbreak of COVID-19 in Wuhan, Hubei Province, China, in late December 2019 (Hui et al. 2020), SARS-CoV-2 rapidly spread across the world in a short span of time, compelling the World Health Organization (WHO) to declare it as a global pandemic on 11 March 2020. Since being declared a global pandemic, COVID-19 has ravaged many countries worldwide and has overwhelmed many healthcare systems. Among these countries, the alarming epidemic situations are in the United States (39,146,646 total cases, 646,258 deaths), India (32,649,947 total cases, 437,370 deaths), Brazil (20,728,605 total cases, 579,010 deaths), Russia (6,863,541 total cases, 180,840 deaths), France (6,711,268 total cases, 114,083 deaths), the UK (6,698,486 total cases, 132,376 deaths), Iran (4,895,448 total cases, 105,901 deaths), Spain (4,831,809 total cases, 84,000 deaths), Italy (4,524,292 total cases, 129,056 deaths), and Germany (3,934,117 total cases, 92,597 deaths), as of 28 August 2021 (Worldometer).

The COVID-19 virus spreads primarily through droplets of saliva or discharge from the nose, which enter a person's body through various contact routes such as mouth, eyes, or nose, causing a mild to moderate respiratory illness, like the common cold, which includes dry cough, fever, sore throat, loss of sense of smell and taste, headache, shortness of breath, and so on, while

DOI: 10.1201/9781003178514-8

developing serious illness or even death in cases of older people and those with underlying medical problems like cardiovascular disease, diabetes, chronic respiratory disease, and cancer. Due to the absence of a definitive treatment modality like appropriate/effective medicine or vaccines in the initial stages of the outbreak, physical distancing, wearing masks, washing hands, and so on have been accepted globally as the most efficient strategies for reducing the severity and spread of the virus and gaining control over it at some extent (Nouvellet et al. 2021). So, governments of most countries decided to lockdown from the mid or end of March 2020, resulting in a drop in the number of infected people. As this complete lockdown has also resulted in the loss of livelihoods, which has had a rippling effect on the global economy, all countries have taken some policies towards unlocking from mid-May 2020.

Although substantial progress in medical support has led to more control of the continuing spread of the virus, the emergence of mutant variants of the virus means many countries are experiencing a second or third wave of outbreaks of this viral illness. Among the several variants of SARS-CoV-2, only a few are considered variants of concern by the WHO such as alpha (the first variant of concern described in the UK in late December 2020), beta (first reported in South Africa in December 2020), gamma (first reported in Brazil in early January 2021), and delta (first reported in India in December 2020). The active vaccination campaign started in late December 2020 with the expectation of a decrease in the mortality rate, resulting in 32.9% of the world population with at least one dose of a COVID-19 vaccination, and 24.8% being fully vaccinated (OurWorldinData). Since the number of vaccines remains insufficient, the vaccination strategy adopted in many countries consists of the priority vaccination of more vulnerable elderly people and the more exposed groups of the population, such as medical workers. Despite the unprecedented speed of vaccine development against the prevention of COVID-19 and robust global mass vaccination efforts, the emergence of these new SARS-CoV-2 variants threatens to overturn the significant progress made so far in limiting the spread of this viral illness (Figure 6.1).

The global problem of the outbreak of COVID-19 has attracted the interest of researchers of different areas including mathematical modellers. Mathematical modelling based on systems of differential equations may provide a simple but comprehensive mechanism for the dynamics of COVID-19 transmission. Several modelling studies have already been performed for the COVID-19 outbreak (Giordano et al. 2020, Kucharski et al. 2020, Quilty et al. 2020, Tang et al. 2020a, Tang et al. 2020b, Yuan et al. 2020). In Lin et al. (2020), the authors suggested a conceptual model for a coronavirus disease started at the end of 2019, which effectively captured the timeline of the COVID-19 outbreak. A mathematical model for reproducing the stage-based transmissibility of a novel coronavirus was proposed and analysed by Chen et al. (2020). Wu et al. (2020) developed a susceptible exposed infectious recovered model (SEIR) based on the reported data from 31 December 2019 to 28 January 2020 to clarify the transmission dynamics and projected national and global spread of the disease. They also calculated the basic reproduction number at around 2.68 for COVID-19. Tang et al. (2020a) proposed a compartmental deterministic model that would combine the clinical development of the disease, the epidemiological status of the patient, and measures for intervention. Researchers also found that the value of controlled reproduction number may be as high as 6.47, and that method of intervention including intensive contact tracing followed by quarantine and isolation would effectively minimize COVID-19 cases (Tang et al. 2020b). For the basic reproductive number (R_0), Read et al. (2020) reported a value of 3.1 based on the data fitting of an SEIR model using an assumption of Poisson-distributed daily time increments. S. Zhao et al. (2020) estimated the mean R_0 for 2019-nCoV in the early phase of the outbreak ranging from 3.3 to 5.5 (likely to be belowfivebut above three with a rising rate of reported cases), which appeared slightly higher than those of SARS-CoV (R_0: 2–5) (Chen 2020). A report by

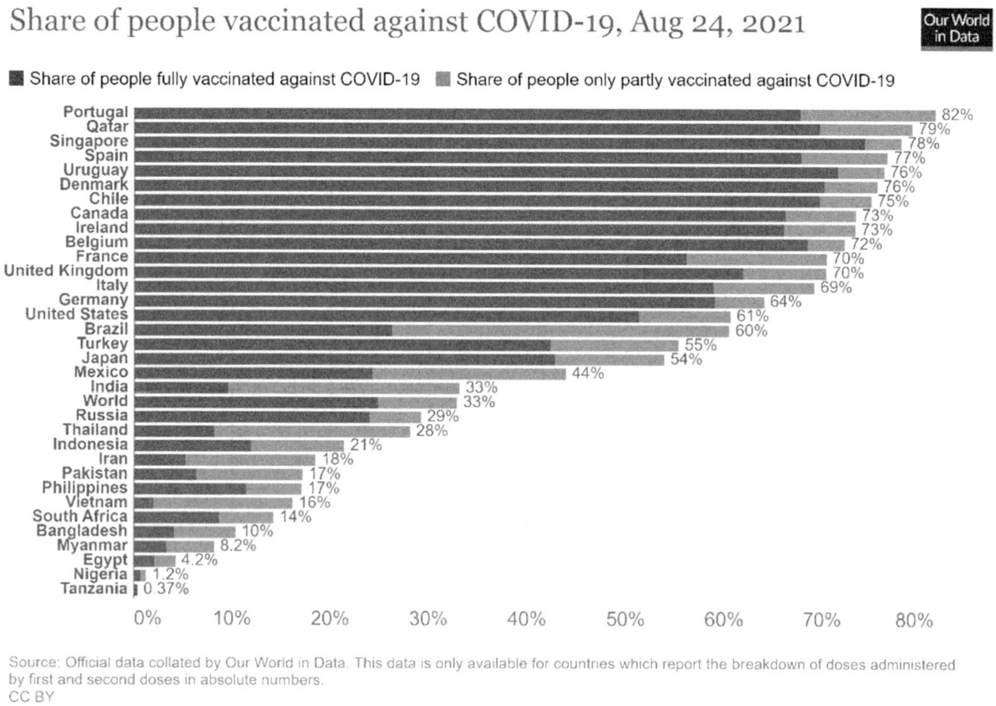

Figure 6.1 Percentage of fully vaccinated and partially vaccinated population worldwide.

Cambridge University has indicated that India's countrywide three-week lockdown would not be adequate to prevent a resurgence of the new coronavirus epidemic that could bounce back in months and cause several thousands of infections (Singh and Adhikari 2020). They suggested that two or three lockdowns can extend the slowdown longer with five-day breaks in between or a single 49-day lockdown. Data-driven mathematical modelling plays a key role in disease prevention, planning for future outbreaks, and determining the effectiveness of control. Several data-driven modelling experiments have been performed in various regions (Tang et al. 2020). In de León et al. (2020), a compartmental mathematical model was developed to understand the outbreak of COVID-19 in Mexico. This data-driven analysis would let us compare how different the outbreak would be in the two studied regions. In Rojas et al. (2020), the authors estimated the value of R_0, which helped them to predict that in the city of Cali, the outbreak under the current intervention of isolation and quarantine would last for five to six months and would need around 3500 beds on a given day during the peak of the outbreak. There are other relevant works where the basic reproduction number is estimated for different countries (Belgaid et al. 2020, Dolbeault and Turinici 2020, Kochańczyk et al. 2020, Krantz et al. 2020, Shim and Chowell 2020, Sinha 2020, Srivastava and Chowell 2020). The most common mathematical formulations which represent the individual transition in a community between "compartments" describe the situation of individual infections with significant insight. Ram and Schaposnik (2021) had presented a modified age-structured SIR model based on known patterns of social contact and distancing measures within Washington, USA, with the findings that population age distribution has a significant effect on disease spread and mortality rate, and contribute to the efficacy of age-specific contact and treatment measures.

Mathematical models can be a profoundly helpful tool to make public health decisions and ensure optimal use of resources to reduce the morbidity and mortality associated with the COVID-19 pandemic, but only if they are rigorously evaluated and validated and their projections are robust and reliable. The main challenge faced during the mathematical modelling of the COVID-19 outbreak and making decisions based on the model predictions is the lack of data availability. The modellers include different compartments like exposed, asymptomatic infected, symptomatic infected, quarantined, hospitalized, recovered, and so on to make their models more realistic from an epidemiological point of view, while the country-wise or state-wise daily infected and daily death are the only available data for the disease. Therefore, the researchers do not have sufficient data for the different compartments, resulting in the failure of the validation of the models. Parameter estimation also fails due to this lack of data. Because of infrastructural inefficiency in highly populated countries like India, COVID tests are only done for symptomatic patients. As a result, there are major parts of the population in those countries that are asymptomatic and are never tested though they may be infected, questioning the reliability of the daily infected data. The quality of data on infections, deaths, tests, and other factors are often limited by under detection or inconsistent detection of cases, reporting delays and poor documentation, all of which affect the quality of any model output and its predictions. Models may capture aspects of epidemics effectively while considering other factors, such as the accuracy of diagnostic tests, whether immunity will wane, if reinfection could occur, whether social distancing and wearing masks are maintained properly, and population characteristics such as age distribution, percentage of older adults with comorbidities, and risk factors. Models should also seek to use the best possible data for local predictions as it is unlikely that epidemics will follow identical paths in all regions of the world due to the different localized issues (for example the level of immunity) for different regions.

In this chapter, we have tried to construct some mathematical models containing different compartments while incorporating the factors of COVID-19 disease progression mechanisms to overcome the challenges of disease modelling to some extent. These compartmental models for disease progression segregate a population into groups depending on each individual's infectious state and related population sizes with respect to time. First, we have discussed a single group multi-compartmental model that initially consists of six compartments, namely susceptible, exposed, infected, quarantined, hospitalized, and recovered. We have divided the exposed compartment into two subcompartments (denoted by E_1 and E_2) depending on their infectiousness and also divided the infected class into two subcompartments, namely, asymptomatic (I_a) and symptomatic (I_s). Interesting and significant contributions of our work are the consideration of the time-dependent rate of infection over various periods of time. This variation is adopted into the model in order to capture the effect of lockdown, social distancing, and so on, which plays a crucial role in the mechanism of disease transmission. We have also divided susceptible, exposed, and infected classes into two subclasses each based on their classification or behaviour which is directly responsible for the alteration of the rate of disease spread to incorporate the effect of the unlocking period or the post-lockdown period resulting in an increase of disease transmission. The classification or division into two different groups may be due to the different age groups, different implementation of distancing measures, proper and improper use of face masks, and so on. Next, we estimated the parameters of focal interest using MATLAB® and fitted our first and second model simulations with those best-fitted parameter values based on the available data of daily reported cases and cumulative cases of some countries like Germany, Spain, Israel, which indicates a good agreement of our model outcomes with the reported cases. This also depicts the fact that the nature of disease transmission is different for different countries depending on the protective measures and policies taken by the government, different age distribution of the population, lack of consciousness, and many others. Next, we considered different vaccination strategies and determined the outcome of the vaccination campaign depending on the distribution of vaccinated individuals between the groups.

MATHEMATICAL MODEL

Simple epidemic models with a homogeneous population are mainly divided into two groups: the model with demography and the model without demography. These two types of models are developed, analysed, and validated with empirical data for a wide range of epidemic diseases and consist of multiple compartments. The number of different compartments required to be considered is determined by the nature and spreading pattern of the disease. However, consideration of demographic terms is justified once the spreading pattern and various demographic components are well known. For example, now we have a rough estimate of the average number of people suffering from the common flu in different countries, we can find an estimate for the rate of transfer of healthy individuals to the susceptible compartment every year (Flahault et al.1994). This kind of information is beyond our knowledge as of now and hence consideration of demographic parameters in the context of COVID-19 is a debatable issue. Here, we consider two ordinary differential equation models with multiple compartments without demography, one for a single group and another for two groups with epidemic progression. All the parameters involved with the models are assumed to be constant except the rate of infection which is varied over time to take care of lockdown restriction and step-by-step relaxation of lockdown restrictions during unlocking periods. Without considering any particular functional form for the rate of infection, we have estimated the parameter over different time intervals.

Single Group Multi-Compartment Model

We have considered a dynamic SEIQR type model for the COVID-19 disease progression. Basically, the model consists of susceptible (S), exposed (E), infected (I), quarantined (Q), hospitalized (H), and recovered (R) class. In the context of COVID-19, the exposed class is divided into two subclasses, namely non-infectious (E_1) and infectious (E_2) and the infected class is divided into two subclasses, namely asymptomatic (I_a) and symptomatic (I_s), where $N = S + E_1 + E_2 + I_a + I_s + Q + H + R$ and N is not fixed since deceased individuals are not considered in the model explicitly. The system of differential equations that will model the dynamics of coronavirus spread is as follows:

$$\frac{dS}{dt} = -\frac{\beta S}{N}\left(I_s + q_1 I_a + q_2 E_2 + q_3 Q + q_4 H\right), \tag{2.1a}$$

$$\frac{dE_1}{dt} = \frac{\beta S}{N}\left(I_s + q_1 I_a + q_2 E_2 + q_3 Q + q_4 H\right) - \mu_1 E_1, \tag{2.1b}$$

$$\frac{dE_2}{dt} = \mu_1 E_1 - \mu_2 E_2, \tag{2.1c}$$

$$\frac{dI_a}{dt} = (1-\gamma)\mu_2 E_2 - \eta_1 I_a, \tag{2.1d}$$

$$\frac{dI_s}{dt} = \gamma \mu_2 E_2 - (\sigma_1 + \zeta_1 + \eta_2 + \zeta_2) I_s, \tag{2.1e}$$

$$\frac{dQ}{dt} = \zeta_1 I_s - (\xi + \eta_3)Q, \tag{2.1f}$$

$$\frac{dH}{dt} = \zeta_2 + \xi - (\sigma_2 + \eta_4)H, \tag{2.1g}$$

$$\frac{dR}{dt} = \eta_1 I_a + \eta_2 I_s + \eta_3 Q + \eta_4 H. \tag{2.1h}$$

Simulation results for model (2.1)

We have fitted the parameters $\beta, q_1, q_2, q_3, q_4, \mu_1, \mu_2, \sigma, \eta_1, \sigma_1, \eta_3$ for the range of the values given in Table 6.1 and took $\zeta_1, \zeta_2, \xi, \sigma_2, \eta_4$ fixed as given in Table 6.1. We estimated those values for three different time intervals (1–30th day, 31–42nd day, 43–95th day) (Sharma et al. 2020). We have considered the initial values of the parameters as given in Table 6.1. We have chosen the time interval and end values of different compartments from the fittings over the previous time intervals. Here, we have considered $\frac{\beta S}{N}\left(I_s + q_1 I_a + q_2 E_2 + q_3 Q + q_4 H\right)$ as the daily reported case and the sum of this part over the desired time interval is considered as the cumulative number of infected cases.

The optimization of parameters to describe the outbreak of COVID-19 in Germany was fitted by minimizing the sum of squared errors (SSE), in such a way that the solutions obtained by the model approximate the reported cumulative number of infected cases. We applied three searches to minimize the SSE function: by using a gradient-based method first, followed by a step of minimization with a gradient-free method, again followed by a third step of a gradient-based method. MATLAB based nonlinear least-square solver *fmincon* and *patternsearch* are used to fit simulated and observed day-wise cumulative number of infected cases for three different time intervals. Detailed descriptions of this method and its implementation can be found in Kelley (1999), Caccavo (2020), and de León et al. (2020).

As there is no uniformity of the daily reported cases, perhaps due to irregular reporting, we have used seven-day moving average as daily data instead of daily raw data for our model simulation. The model (2.1) is simulated with best-fitted parameter values (Sharma et al. 2020) as mentioned previously and the simulation result against the seven-day moving average for daily reported data is presented in Figure 6.2 for 15 February 2020 to 19 May 2020. In this case of Figure 6.2(a), the values of β are constants over three different ranges of days: 3.98 for the first 30 days, 1.77 for the next 12 days, and 1.05 for the rest of the period, whereas in Figure 6.2(b), the value of β is constant at 3.98 for the first 30 days, and then monotone, decreasing over a range 12days from 3.98 to 1.05, and then remaining constant at 1.05 for the rest of the period. The number of days for which $\beta(t)$ remains constant and then starts decaying is adjusted in such a way that the outcome matches well with both the cumulative and daily data. Accordingly, the slope of decaying $\beta(t)$, the day up to which it decays and the lower value of $\beta(t)$ are chosen. The numerical simulation and fitting with the data are carried out with the objective that the simulation result should be pretty close to the cumulative number of reported cases. We can claim that our attempt is successful as the cumulative number of reported cases for Germany on 15 May 2020 obtained from the simulation taking three constant values of β for three different time periods is 180,788 and the reported data (see [3]) shows it is equal to 182,250, whereas in this case, the choice of $\beta(t)$, as for Figure 6.2(b), the cumulative number of reported cases obtained from the

TABLE 6.1 DESCRIPTION OF PARAMETERS INVOLVED WITH THE MODEL (2.1).

Parameter	Interpretation	Value	Unit
β	Rate of infection per unit of time by the symptomatic infected	varying	day^{-1}
q_1	Reduction factor of infectivity by the I_a class compared with the I_s class	0.05–0.34	–
q_2	Reduction factor of infectivity by the E class compared with the I_s class	0.05–0.34	–
q_3	Reduction factor of infectivity by the Q class compared with the I_s class	0.05–0.34	–
q_4	Reduction factor of infectivity by the H class compared with the $I_s$class	0.05–0.34	–
μ_1	Rate at which individuals of E_1 class become infectious exposed	0.25–0.33	day^{-1}
μ_2	Rate at which individuals of E_2 class become infected	0.5–1	day^{-1}
γ	Fraction of infectious exposed population E_2 that becomes symptomatic infected $(0 < \gamma < 1)$	0–1	–
η_1	Rate of recovery of the asymptomatic infected individuals without any medical intervention	0.1–0.9	day^{-1}
η_2	Rate of recovery of the symptomatic infected individuals without any medical intervention	0.1	day^{-1}
η_3	Rate of recovery from the infection after being quarantined	0.05–0.1	day^{-1}
η_4	Rate of transfer of hospitalized individuals to recovered class	0.05	day^{-1}
σ_1	Rate of mortality due to the infection for the individuals of infected class with symptom	0.05–0.1	day^{-1}
σ_2	Rate of mortality of hospitalized individuals	0.07	day^{-1}
ξ	Rate of hospitalization of the quarantined individuals	0.14	day^{-1}
ζ_1	Rate at which the symptomatic infected individuals are quarantined	0.07	day^{-1}
ζ_2	Rate of hospitalization of the symptomatic infected individuals	0.14	day^{-1}

Sources: The range of parameter values is obtained from de Leon et al. (2020), Rojas et al. (2020), Dolbeault and Turinici (2020), and Kochańczyk et al. (2020).

simulation is equal to 180,808, indicating that both the simulated values are close to the reported data with the relative percentage error less than 1% (precisely equal to 0.79%).

Two Group Multi-Compartment Model

To incorporate the effect of the unlocking period/post-lockdown period (viz, the reluctance of the population in following the regular measures like wearing masks, washing hands, maintaining social distancing), we have divided the susceptible population (S), exposed population (consists with infected but not infectious (E_1) and infected as well as infectious (E_2)), asymptomatic infective (I_a), and symptomatic infective (I_s) of the ordinary differential equation model

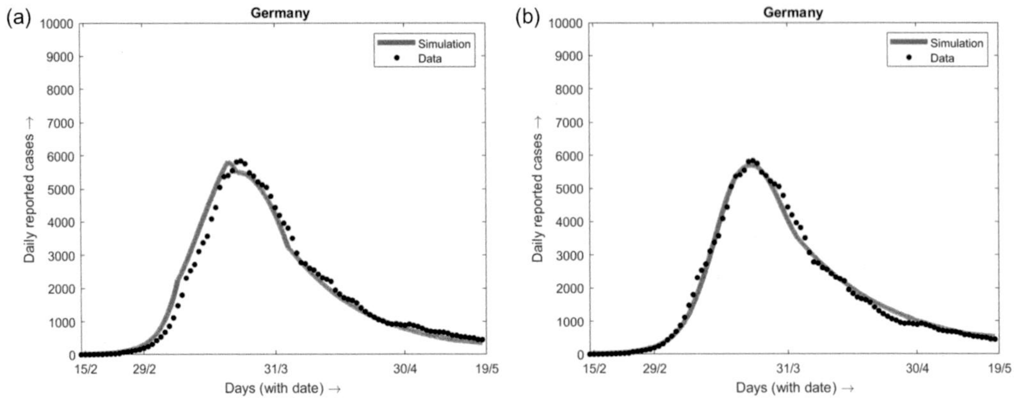

Figure 6.2 Simulation results and daily reported cases (seven-day moving average) (a) for $\beta(t)$ with three constant values for three different time periods and (b) for $\beta(t)$with monotonic value. Greycurves are an indication of our model simulation whereas the black dots indicate the daily reported cases.

(2.1) into two subclasses, namely $S_1, S_2, E_{11}, E_{21}, E_{12}, E_{22}, I_{a1}, I_{a2}, I_{s1}, I_{s2}$ respectively, based on their classification or behaviour which is directly responsible for the alteration of the rate of disease spread. The classification or division into two different groups may be due to the different age groups, different implementations of distancing measures, proper and improper use of face masks, and so on, all related to human behaviours. The total population size can be written as $N = S_1 + S_2 + E_{11} + E_{21} + E_{12} + E_{22} + I_{a1} + I_{a_2} + I_{s1} + I_{s2} + Q + H + R$ and N is not fixed since the deceased compartment is not included in the model. The differential equations representing the extended model formulation are given as follows:

$$\frac{dS_1}{dt} = -\frac{S_1}{N}\left[\beta_{11}\left(I_{s1} + q_{11}I_{a1} + q_{12}E_{12}\right) + \beta_{12}\left(I_{s2} + q_{21}I_{a2} + q_{22}E_{22}\right) + \beta_Q Q + \beta_H H\right], \quad (2.2a)$$

$$\frac{dS_2}{dt} = -\frac{S_2}{N}\left[\beta_{21}\left(I_{s1} + q_{31}I_{a1} + q_{32}E_{12}\right) + \beta_{22}\left(I_{s2} + q_{41}I_{a2} + q_{42}E_{22}\right) + \beta_Q Q + \beta_H H\right], \quad (2.2b)$$

$$\frac{dE_{11}}{dt} = \frac{S_1}{N}\left[\beta_{11}\left(I_{s1} + q_{11}I_{a1} + q_{12}E_{12}\right) + \beta_{12}\left(I_{s2} + q_{21}I_{a2} + q_{22}E_{22}\right) + \beta_Q Q + \beta_H H\right] - \mu_{11}E_{11}, \quad (2.2c)$$

$$\frac{dE_{21}}{dt} = \frac{S_2}{N}\left[\beta_{21}\left(I_{s1} + q_{31}I_{a1} + q_{32}E_{12}\right) + \beta_{22}\left(I_{s2} + q_{41}I_{a2} + q_{42}E_{22}\right) + \beta_Q Q + \beta_H H\right] - \mu_{21}E_{21}, \quad (2.2d)$$

$$\frac{dE_{12}}{dt} = \mu_{11}E_{11} - \mu_{12}E_{12}, \quad (2.2e)$$

$$\frac{dE_{22}}{dt} = \mu_{21}E_{21} - \mu_{22}E_{22}, \quad (2.2f)$$

$$\frac{dI_{a1}}{dt} = (1 - \gamma_1)\mu_{12}E_{12} - \eta_{11}I_{a1}, \quad (2.2g)$$

$$\frac{dI_{a2}}{dt} = (1 - \gamma_2)\mu_{22}E_{22} - \eta_{21}I_{a2}, \quad (2.2h)$$

$$\frac{dI_{s1}}{dt} = \gamma_1 \mu_{12} E_{12} - (\sigma_{11} + \zeta_{11} + \eta_{12} + \zeta_{12}) I_{s1}, \quad (2.2i)$$

$$\frac{dI_{s2}}{dt} = \gamma_2 \mu_{22} E_{22} - (\sigma_{21} + \zeta_{21} + \eta_{22} + \zeta_{22}) I_{s2}, \quad (2.2j)$$

$$\frac{dQ}{dt} = \zeta_{11} I_{s1} + \zeta_{21} I_{s2} - (\xi + \eta_3) Q, \quad (2.2k)$$

$$\frac{dH}{dt} = \zeta_{12} I_{s1} + \zeta_{22} I_{s2} + \xi Q - (\sigma_2 + \eta_4) H, \quad (2.2l)$$

$$\frac{dR}{dt} = \eta_{11} I_{a1} + \eta_{21} I_{a2} + \eta_{12} I_{s2} + \eta_{22} I_{s2} + \eta_3 Q + \eta_4 H. \quad (2.2m)$$

Here β_{11}, β_{21} and β_{12}, β_{22} are rates of infection per unit of time by the symptomatic infected I_{s1}, I_{s2} respectively, β_Q, β_J are rates of infection per unit of time by the quarantined and hospitalized population (Q, H) respectively, q_{11}, q_{31}; q_{12}, q_{32}; q_{21}, q_{41}; q_{22}, q_{41} are the reduction factor of infectivity by I_{a1}, E_{12}, I_{a2} and E_{22} respectively compared to I_{s1} and I_{s2} and satisfy the restriction $0 \le q_{ij} < 1,\ i, j = 1, 2, 3, 4$. μ_{11} and μ_{21} are the rates at which E_{11} and E_{21} progress to the infectious exposed compartments E_{12} and E_{22} respectively. The infectious exposed individuals leave the respective classes at rates μ_{12} and μ_{22}. The parameters γ_j, σ_{j1}, ζ_{j1}, ζ_{j2} and η_{j2} (j = 1, 2) have a similar interpretation as that of $\gamma, \sigma_1, \zeta_1, \zeta_2$ and η_2 as described in Table 6.1 for model (2.1). Here, $\sigma_{11}, \sigma_{21}, \xi$ and σ_2 are the disease-related death rates for the compartments I_{s1}, I_{s2}, Q, and H respectively.

Simulation Results for Model (2.2)

Here, we are interested in understanding the usefulness of the model (2.2) for the unlocking period or post-lockdown period when people are engaging with social contact gradually with restrictions like using masks, maintaining social distances, washing hands, and so on. It is very obvious that all the population are not equally serious about following the restrictions and guidelines, resulting in the gradual increase of cases that could be controlled to some extent during the lockdown period. To incorporate this situation, we assume that a fraction of the population is not following the guidelines and another fraction is following the safety and preventive norms properly. Let us define the "coefficient of social interactions" as S_1/N and is denoted by K. If we assume that the 10% of the population is not following the norm then $S_1 / N \equiv K = 0.1$ and hence $S_2 / N = 0.9 = 1 - K$. Initial densities of E_{11} and E_{21} can be distributed with the same proportion to K and $1 - K$ of the value of E_1 on the last day of lockdown. The same procedure is adopted for other components except for Q, H, and R. For simplicity, we also assume that the other parameters involved with the two-group model are equal to the values of the corresponding parameter involved with the model (2.1) (Sharma et al. 2020).

Currently available data for the unlocking period/post-lockdown period indicates a significant increase in daily reported cases in Italy, with a full-scale second wave of the epidemic in Spain and Israel. Based upon the recently available data for Spain, we have fitted our second model with the daily reported cases for Spain where the second wave in the epidemic has been noticed and has the best-fitted value of K as 0.3 for which our model simulation has a good

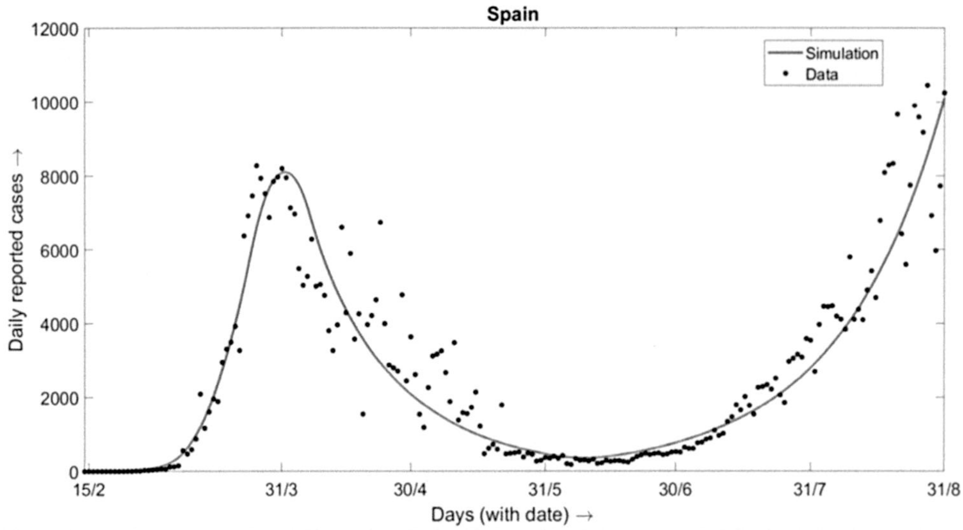

Figure 6.3 Numerical simulation result of epidemic progression for Spain with model (2.2). The values of the coefficients β_{ij} are as follows: $\beta_{11} = 3.7, \beta_{22} = 1.126, \beta_{12} = \beta_{21} = 2.413$. The values of other parameters are given in the appendix. The value of K after lockdown changes to 0.3.

agreement with the real data for daily reported cases. The fitting with data for Spain is presented in Figure 6.3. The choices of different parameters involved with the model (2.2) are the same as discussed in the previous section (Sharma et al. 2020). Another example of the validation of our model (2.2) is presented in Figure 6.4 based on the daily reported cases of Israel where the second wave of the pandemic is going on (Volpert et al. 2021).

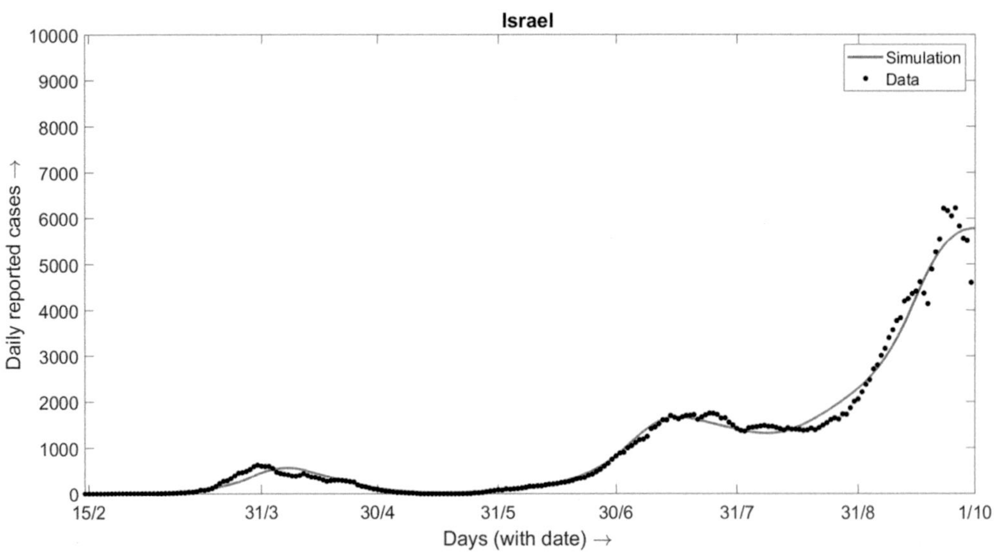

Figure 6.4 Numerical simulation result of epidemic progression for Israel with model (2.2). The values of the coefficients β_{ij} are as follows: $\beta_{11} = 2.91, \beta_{22} = 0.3, \beta_{12} = \beta_{21} = 1.17$. The values of other parameters are given in the appendix. The value of K after lockdown changes from 0.1 to 0.3.

The detailed calculations for the basic reproduction number, the final size of the epidemic, and other relevant epidemic characteristics for the models (2.1) and (2.2) are available in Sharma et al. (2020). The way we have derived the basic reproduction number as well as the effective reproduction number for the model (2.2) can easily be extended for a model of a similar type consisting of more than two groups.

MATHEMATICAL MODEL FOR VACCINATION

The mathematical models for the vaccination of COVID-19 open up a new direction of mathematical modelling as the vaccine is not available regularly and has not reached the required number of vaccines. It is a well-known fact in epidemiology that the vaccination of entire populations or susceptible individuals is not required in most epidemic diseases. As a result, the mathematical modelling and related control theoretical approach are utilized to determine the proportion of the population required to be vaccinated, assuming that enough vaccines are available. In the case of the vaccines for COVID-19, availability is neither regular nor adequate. As a result, some batches of vaccines are available for administration from time to time and hence the optimal allocation policy is the main question to address. The usual epidemic model with vaccination will not work and hence we have proposed and analysed a simple model which is based upon a two-group SI type epidemic model (Brauer and Castillo-Chavez 2012). The most effective model is quite complicated in nature and its validation demands a sophisticated data set that is not easily available as of now.

We have considered that the susceptible and infected individuals are divided into two groups, denoted by (S_1, I_1) and (S_2, I_2). Individuals of two groups, belonging to the susceptible compartment, who are getting the vaccine, are denoted by V_1 and V_2 respectively. Primarily, we can assume that the vaccinated individuals cannot be infective anymore and hence will have no role to play with further progression of the epidemic. Based upon this assumption, we can describe the simplest form of the model as follows:

$$\frac{dS_1}{dt} = -(\beta_{11}I_1 + \beta_{12}I_2)\frac{S_1 - V_1}{N}, \tag{3.1a}$$

$$\frac{dS_2}{dt} = -(\beta_{21}I_1 + \beta_{22}I_2)\frac{S_2 - V_2}{N}, \tag{3.1b}$$

$$\frac{dI_1}{dt} = (\beta_{11}I_1 + \beta_{12}I_2)\frac{S_1 - V_1}{N} - \sigma_1 I_1, \tag{3.1c}$$

$$\frac{dI_2}{dt} = -(\beta_{21}I_1 + \beta_{22}I_2)\frac{S_2 - V_2}{N} - \sigma_2 I_2, \tag{3.1d}$$

where $\beta_{ij}, i, j = 1,2$ is the rate of infection transmitted from infected individuals of j-th group to the susceptible individual belonging to i-th group, $\sigma_j, j = 1,2$ is the clearance rate of infected individuals, which are the sums of recovery as well as disease-related death. Here, N is the size of the total population. Even with this simple formulation, it is quite tedious to determine the estimates for the final size of the epidemic, the maximum number of daily infected, the total number of infected individuals during an outbreak, and the time to the maximum number of infected. With the help of some approximation techniques, we have obtained these measures for the model (Anita et al. 2021). There could be various characteristics for consideration of two groups but primarily we can assume that one group can get the infection and/or spread the infection rapidly compared with the individuals belonging to another group. One simple example is: one group of people are wearing the mask properly and maintaining social distancing, and the other group consists of individuals violating these norms. Our mathematical findings and related numerical simulations, with a hypothetical parameter set, clearly indicate that a significantly higher proportion of people, who are prone to get and spread the infection quickly, are required to be vaccinated to control the epidemic outbreak. However, the percentage of the total population that is required to be vaccinated depends upon the distribution of the people into two groups.

We mentioned earlier that the required number of vaccines is not available at this time and hence the model can be modified to a system of differential equations defined over some disjoint time intervals. As a simplest case, we assume that a total of V number of vaccines is administrated at the time point $t=t_1$. Then we can consider the following system of equations:

$$\frac{dS_1}{dt}=-(\beta_{11}I_1+\beta_{12}I_2)\frac{S_1}{N}, \tag{3.2a}$$

$$\frac{dS_2}{dt}=-(\beta_{21}I_1+\beta_{22}I_2)\frac{S_2}{N}, \tag{3.2b}$$

$$\frac{dI_1}{dt}=(\beta_{11}I_1+\beta_{12}I_2)\frac{S_1}{N}-\sigma_1 I_1, \tag{3.2c}$$

$$\frac{dI_2}{dt}=(\beta_{21}I_1+\beta_{22}I_2)\frac{S_2}{N}-\sigma_2 I_2, \tag{3.2d}$$

defined for $t \le t_1$. Then the number of susceptible at time t_1+0 can be defined as

$$S_1(t_1+0)=S_1(t_1)-\kappa V, S_2(t_1+0)=S_2(t_1)-(1-\kappa)V$$

where $0<\kappa<1$, the proportion of vaccinated into two groups are κ and $(1-\kappa)$ respectively. It is worthy to mention here that the values of infected individuals remain unaltered and hence

$$I_1(t_1+0)=I_1(t_1), I_2(t_1+0)=I_2(t_1).$$

Based upon these newly defined $S_1(t_1+0)$ and $S_2(t_1+0)$, we have to consider the previous model for $t>t_1$. In case of successive vaccination drives at the time points say $t_2, t_3, t_4, \ldots$, then we need to redefine the values of S_1 and S_2 at the instances of time t_2+0, t_3+0, t_4+0 etc. At this point, another important scenario arises: (i) whether the number of available vaccines is the same or not and (ii) whether they are distributed into two groups in the same ratio or not. If not, then we have to adopt the notations V_n and σ_n instead of V and σ respectively. Based upon this type of modelling approach, we have obtained the basic characteristics of epidemic spread in Volpert et al. (2021). The most effective as well as the most challenging modelling approach will be the implementation of this setup into a multi-compartment model as we have discussed in the previous section and with more than two groups. Consideration of two groups is originated from a simple but realistic assumption. The most effective formalism will be to divide the entire population based upon their age-specific risk of getting infected and taking care of the clinical history of individuals (details of co-morbidity).

DISCUSSIONS

The main challenge in modelling epidemic diseases like COVID-19 is the lack of appropriate information about the various possible routes of disease transmission and its propagation through different channels. Social gatherings without appropriate protection can be responsible for quick transmission of the disease and travelling by trains and aeroplanes is another probable place for rapid disease transmission. However, the nature and pattern of disease spread through social gatherings and travelling by aeroplane are somehow different. To be specific, the social gathering of people at a particular place can be responsible for disease spread if there are asymptomatic individuals and people present there are not obeying the protective measures like wearing masks. However, travel by aeroplane from one country to another followed by a weak protection mechanism may be responsible for the spread of new variants of the virus at the destination country. During June 2021, all travellers arriving at Heathrow airport are mandated for at least ten days of hotel quarantine in the vicinity of the airport followed by an RT-PCR test before starting the journey to their destination within the UK. However, these measures are rarely observed in several developing countries. In order to answer the question of whether this measure is useful to control the disease spread partially or not, we need a data set that is rarely available from easily accessible sources. Theoretically, this kind of measure can regulate the disease spread –there is no doubt about it. Based upon this point, one can raise the question of whether such kind of mandatory quarantine may not be required for people who are completely vaccinated. Again, we have arrived at another challenging issue of getting appropriate data for the number of people who tested positive during or at the end of mandatory quarantine having two doses of vaccination, a single dose of the vaccine, and without vaccination. A multi-scale modelling approach is required to be adopted to build up an effective model to understand the effectiveness of quarantine measures at the airport. The multi-scale model is important to take care of the size of total passengers travelling through various international airports across the country and the flights connecting different countries.

For largely populated countries like India, we find different trends for the rate of disease spread at various states, to be specific, at different cities. Collecting the necessary data, building up an appropriate model for different states, and summing up the results to match the data for the entire country are challenging issues. Population density, availability and preparedness of healthcare facilities, weather, heterogeneity of residents with respect to their financial status, and many other factors vary significantly from one state to another in India (Figure 6.5 shows

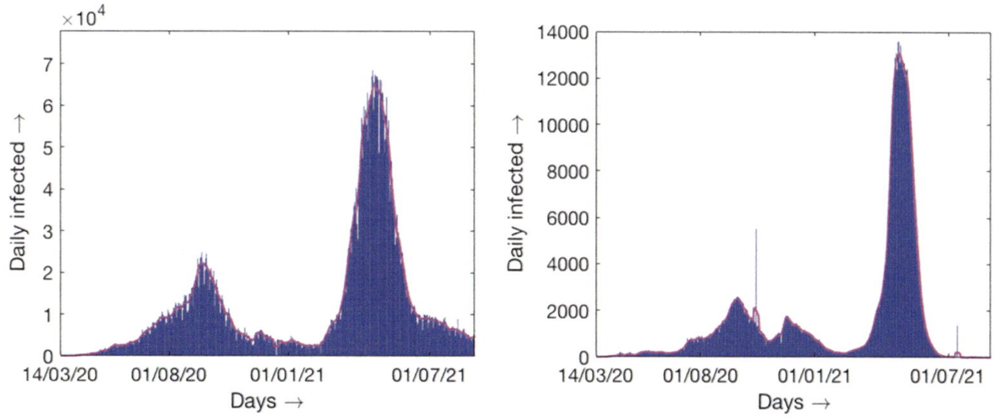

Figure 6.5 Daily reported cases of COVID-19 infected (blue) and seven-day moving average (magenta) for two states in India, Maharashtra (left) and Madhya Pradesh (right). Data source: https://github.com/covid19india/api.

significant variation in the number of daily reported cases of COVID-19 infection in two neighbouring states of India). Most of these factors have some silent role to shape the disease propagation pattern. It is quite difficult to identify the people from different age groups, work profile, infection from COVID-19, and how they are treated in the hours of need. Here, the phrase "treatment" includes their isolation/quarantine, availability of medicine, and daily needs.

Consideration of a single model for largely populated countries often leads to erroneous conclusions as we can see distinctively different trends of disease progression at different parts of the country. To be specific, if we consider the daily reported cases of COVID-19 infection in Maharashtra and Madhya Pradesh (two states of India), from 14th March 2020 to 27th August 2021, we can observe that the peaks of successive outbreaks at these two neighbouring states have appeared at different times. Further, in Maharashtra, we can identify two peaks during the first wave and the second wave respectively. But we find two consecutive peaks of more or less the same heights at Madhya Pradesh during the first wave. Here, the first wave is required to be identified with the help of basic reproduction numbers. Apart from mathematical identification, one may be interested to know the reason behind such kind of trends, which is beyond the scope of this chapter. Based upon other relevant data-based information, like number of daily testing, number of recoveries, number of COVID related deaths, we can calculate various parameters like test positivity rate, rate of infection, mortality rate, and so on. Once we compare these parameters among different states of India, we can reveal a huge variation in their measures with respect to the magnitude as well as time frame. Some detailed discussion on this matter is available in Banerjee et al. (2021). This observation clearly indicates the necessity of multi-scale models to understand basic patterns of disease spread in the countries where we find various types of environmental and behavioural patterns across the entire population of the country. It is needless to say, the spreading pattern and intensity of COVID-19 are largely influenced by human behaviour.

The duration of effectiveness of the vaccine and the possibility of vaccinated individuals becoming susceptible after a finite duration of time lead to another interesting problem that will be worth investigating. In order to develop an appropriate data-driven model, an enormous amount of effort is required to collect individual-based information about the duration of the efficacy of the vaccine. It is reasonable to assume that the duration of the efficacy of the vaccine varies significantly from one individual to another and it is solely determined by the immune response. One possible way out is to measure the antibody on a regular basis –theoretically, it is encouraging but cost-effectiveness is the main burden to carry out this exercise, even for a small group of the people. Consideration of an immuno-epidemiological model will be the suitable choice for an affirmative answer but the outcomes solely depend upon the parameterization of the relevant functional forms involved with the model (Banerjee et al. 2020, Bocharev et al. 2018).

REFERENCES

Anita, S., Banerjee, M., Ghosh, S., Volpert, V. (2021). Vaccination in a two group epidemic model. *Applied Mathematics Letters*, **119**: 107197.

Banerjee, M., Tokarev, A., Volpert, V. (2020). Immuno-epidemiological model of two-stage epidemic growth. *Mathematical Modelling of Natural Phenomena*, **15**: 27.

Banerjee, M., Ghosh, S., Volpert, V. (2021). *Epidemic Progression in a Heterogeneously Distributed Population.* Bentham Publications.

Belgaid, Y., et al. (2020). Analysis of a model for coronavirus spread. *Mathematics*, **8**(5): 820.

Bocharov, G., Volpert, V., Ludewig, B., Meyerhans, A. (2018). *Mathematical Immunology of Virus Infection*. Springer International Publishing, Switzerland.

Brauer, F., Castillo-Chavez, C. (2012). *Mathematical Models in Population Biology and Epidemiology*. Springer, New York.

Caccavo, D. (2020). Chinese and Italian COVID-19 outbreaks can be correctly described by a modified SIRD model. doi: 10.1101/2020.03.19.20039388.

Chen, J. (2020). Pathogenicity and transmissibility of 2019-nCoV—a quick overview and comparison with other emerging viruses. *Microbes and Infection*, **22**(2): 69–71.

Chen, T.-M., et al. (2020). A mathematical model for simulating the phase-based transmissibility of a novel coronavirus. *Infectious Diseases of Poverty*, **9**(1): 1–8.

de León, U. A.-P., et al. (2020). An SEIARD epidemic model for COVID-19 in Mexico: Mathematical analysis and state-level forecast. *Chaos, Solitons & Fractals*, **140**: 110–165.

Dolbeault, J. and G. Turinici (2020). Heterogeneous social interactions and the COVID-19 lockdown outcome in a multi-group SEIR model. *Mathematical Modelling of Natural Phenomena*, **15**: 36.

Flahault, A., Dequen, S., Valleron, A.J. (1994). A mathematical model for the European spread of influenza. *European Journal of Epidemiology*, **10**: 471–474.

Giordano, G., et al. (2020). Modelling the COVID-19 epidemic and implementation of population-wide interventions in Italy. *Nature Medicine*, **26**(6): 855–860.

Hui, D. S., et al. (2020). The continuing 2019-nCoV epidemic threat of novel coronaviruses to global health—The latest 2019 novel coronavirus outbreak in Wuhan, China. *International Journal of Infectious Diseases*, **91**: 264–266.

Kelley, C. (1999). *Iterative Methods for Optimization*. SIAM, Philadelphia.

Kochańczyk, M., et al. (2020). Dynamics of COVID-19 pandemic at constant and time-dependent contact rates. *Mathematical Modelling of Natural Phenomena*, **15**: 28.

Krantz, S. G., et al. (2020). True epidemic growth construction through harmonic analysis. *Journal of Theoretical Biology*, **494**: 110243.

Kucharski, A. J., et al. (2020). Early dynamics of transmission and control of COVID-19: A mathematical modelling study. *The Lancet Infectious Diseases*, **20**(5): 553–558.

Li, Q., Guan, X., Wu, P., Wang, X., Zhou, L., Tong, Y., Ren, R., Leung, K. S. M., Lau, E. H. Y., Wong, J. Y., Xing, X., Xiang, N., Wu, Y., Li, C., Chen, Q., Li, D., Liu, T., Zhao, J., Liu, M., Feng, Z. (2020). Early transmission dynamics in Wuhan, China, of novel coronavirus-infected pneumonia. *The New England Journal of Medicine*, **382**(13): 1199–1207. https://doi.org/10.1056/NEJMoa2001316.

Lin, Q., et al. (2020). A conceptual model for the coronavirus disease 2019 (COVID-19) outbreak in Wuhan, China with individual reaction and governmental action. *International Journal of Infectious Diseases*, **93**: 211–216.

Nouvellet, P., et al. (2021). Reduction in mobility and COVID-19 transmission. *Nature Communications*, **12**(1): 1–9.

Quilty, B. J., et al. (2020). Effectiveness of airport screening at detecting travellers infected with novel coronavirus (2019-nCoV). *Eurosurveillance*, **25**(5): 2000080.

Ram, V., Schaposnik, L. P. (2021). A modified age-structured SIR model for COVID-19 type viruses. *Scientific Reports*, **11**(1): 1–15.

Read, J. M., et al. (2020). Novel coronavirus 2019-nCoV: Early estimation of epidemiological parameters and epidemic predictions. *Philosophical Transactions of The Royal Society B Biological Sciences*, **19**: 376.

Rojas, J. H.et al. (2020), Mathematical modeling & the transmission dynamics of SARS-CoV-2 in Cali, Colombia: Implications to a 2020 Outbreak & public health preparedness, *medRxiv*. https://doi.org/10.1101/2020.05.06.20093526.

Sharma, S., Volpert, V., Banerjee, M. (2020). Extended SEIQR type model for COVID-19 epidemic and data analysis. *Mathematical Biosciences and Engineering*, **17**(6): 7562–7604.

Shim, E., Chowell, G. (2020). Regional variability in time-varying transmission potential of COVID-19 in South Korea. doi: 10.1101/2020.07.21.20158923.

Singh, R., Adhikari, R. (2020). Age-structured impact of social distancing on the COVID-19 epidemic in India. *arXiv preprint arXiv:2003.12055*.

Sinha, S. (2020). Epidemiological dynamics of the COVID-19 pandemic in India: An interim assessment. *Statistics and its Application*, **18**: 333–350.

Srivastava, A., Chowell, G. (2020). Understanding spatial heterogeneity of COVID-19 pandemic using shape analysis of growth rate curves. doi: 10.1101/2020.05.25.20112433.

Tang, B., et al. (2020a). An updated estimation of the risk of transmission of the novel coronavirus (2019-nCov). *Infectious Disease Modelling*, **5**: 248–255.

Tang, B., et al. (2020b). Estimation of the transmission risk of the 2019-nCoV and its implication for public health interventions. *Journal of Clinical Medicine*, **9**(2): 462.

Volpert, V., Banerjee, M., Petrovskii, S. (2020). On a quarantine model of coronavirus infection and data analysis. *Mathematical Modelling of Natural Phenomena*, **15**, 24.

Volpert, V., et al. (2021). Epidemic progression and vaccination in a heterogeneous population. Application to the covid-19 epidemic. *Ecological Complexity*: 100940.

World Health Organization, Coronavirus disease 2019. cited March 15, 2020. Available from: https://www.who.int/health-topics/coronavirus.

World Health Organization (2020). *Population-based Age-stratified Seroepidemiological Investigation Protocol for Covid-19 Virus Infection*. World Health Organization

Worldometer. Available from: https://www.worldometers.info/coronavirus.

Wu, J. T., et al. (2020). Nowcasting and forecasting the potential domestic and international spread of the 2019-nCoV outbreak originating in Wuhan, China: A modelling study. *The Lancet*, **395**(10225): 689–697.

Yuan, J., et al. (2020). Monitoring transmissibility and mortality of COVID-19 in Europe. *International Journal of Infectious Diseases*, **95**: 311–315.

Zhao, S., et al. (2020). Preliminary estimation of the basic reproduction number of novel coronavirus (2019-nCoV) in China, from 2019 to 2020: A data-driven analysis in the early phase of the outbreak. *International Journal of Infectious Diseases*, **92**: 214–217.

Chapter 7

Immuno-Pathologic Basis of COVID-19 and the Management of Mild and Moderate Cases

Debdeep Dasgupta*, Srijan Goswami, and Chiranjeeb Dey

CONTENTS

INTRODUCTION

In December 2019, a cluster of communicable severe acute respiratory illness (SARI) cases caused by a novel Coronavirus was reported for the first time in the Hubei province of China. On 11 February 2020, the World Health Organization (WHO) and the International Committee for Taxonomy of Viruses officially named the disease and the causative organism as COVID-19 and SARS-CoV-2, respectively. In March 2020, COVID-19 was officially declared a public health emergency of global concern. COVID-19 caused by SARS-CoV-2 shows important phases of illness, first, the initial viral response phase, and second, the inflammatory response phase. COVID-19 is an influenza-like illness (ILI) characterized by general symptoms like fever, cough, malaise, myalgia, headache, and loss of taste and smell. Severe symptoms of COVID-19 include shortness of breath with a marked decrease in oxygen saturation, pneumonia leading to acute respiratory distress syndrome (ARDS), sepsis, septic shock, multisystem organ failure (MSOF), and death (WHO, 2020a, b, c).

SARS-CoV-2 is an enveloped coronavirus having positive-sense single-stranded RNA (+ssRNA) as the genetic material. It has four membrane proteins out of which the spike (S) protein is of major concern from a pathophysiological perspective. The spike protein helps SARS-CoV-2 attach to the membrane of the host cell by a specialized receptor angiotensin converting enzyme-2 (ACE-2) receptor. The virus colonizes the nasopharynx from which it spreads by respiratory droplets and

DOI: 10.1201/9781003178514-9

aerosols. The virus that contains droplets is produced by speaking, coughing, or sneezing. After exposure, the mean incubation period is about five days, which can be extended up to 14 days (Kumar and Al Khodor, 2020). The shedding of viral particles begins ~two to three days before the onset of symptoms until five days after the appearance of symptoms. The infected individual may be completely symptomatic or may show serious clinical symptoms. Patients have fever, cough, myalgia, headache, anosmia, dysgeusia, and diarrhea. Severe patients may present with COVID pneumonia with hypoxia and thrombotic episodes. Extrapulmonary manifestations affect nearly every organ, for example, cardiac complications include thrombosis, myocardial infarction, myocarditis, and arrhythmias. Neurologic complications can include myoclonus, seizures, delirium, and encephalitis. Renal damage is common, with about one-third of patients who require mechanical ventilation also requiring renal dialysis. Finally, death can occur due to ARDS and multiorgan failure (WHO, 2014, 2020a, c, d).

IMMUNO-PATHOLOGIC BASIS OF COVID-19

Immunopathophysiology: The Initial Viral Response Stage

SARS-CoV-2, the virus causing COVID-19, is transmitted through aerosols or respiratory droplets from one person to another. As COVID-19 is a disease of the respiratory system, SARS-CoV-2 enters the upper respiratory tract and attaches itself to nasal epithelial cells. The attachment of SARS-CoV-2 with nasal and respiratory epithelial cells is mediated by the binding of spike proteins of the virus with the ACE-2-TMPRSS-2 complex of the host cells. TMPRSS-2 cleaves the spike protein, thus initiating the binding of the S1 subunit to the ACE-2 receptor and S2 subunit mediated membrane fusion followed by clathrin-mediated endocytosis resulting in the release of viral contents (WHO, 2020a; Yuki et al., 2020; Kumar and Al Khodor, 2020; Parasher, 2021; Cevik et al., 2020). The viral component undergoes replication followed by the formation of negative-strand RNA. From the newly synthesized negative-strand RNA, the strands of positive-sense RNA and corresponding proteins are synthesized. Transportation of newly formed viral particles in Golgi vesicles toward the cell membrane takes place and finally the viral particles are released by the process of exocytosis (see Chapter 2). The new viral particles produced perform two activities, some invade and infect the adjacent epithelial cells while others act as fresh infective material for community transmission via respiratory droplets. SARS-CoV-2 migrates from the nasal epithelium to the upper airway respiratory tract, subsequently giving rise to symptoms like fever, dry cough, malaise, and a sore throat. In the majority of cases, the immune response of an individual's body prevents the progress of the virus and halts the spread of the infection. In about one-fifth of infected patients, the disease may progress to involve the lower respiratory tract and will develop severe symptoms. The virus invades and enters the type II pneumocytes of the alveolus. ACE-2 receptors that bind the spike protein of SARS-CoV-2, help to gain entry into type II Pneumocytes. The virus-infected cells release a wide range of specific chemicals known as cytokines and inflammatory markers in uncontrolled amounts at the site of inflammation (the cytokine storm). These cytokines attract inflammatory cells like neutrophil, and they also attract CD8+ cytotoxic T cells and CD4+ helper T cells. Epithelial cells, dendritic cells, and alveolar macrophages act as innate immune cells to fight against viruses until adaptive immunity is induced. The virus-infected cells can be phagocytosed by dendritic cells and macrophages. The antigen-presenting cells move to drain lymph

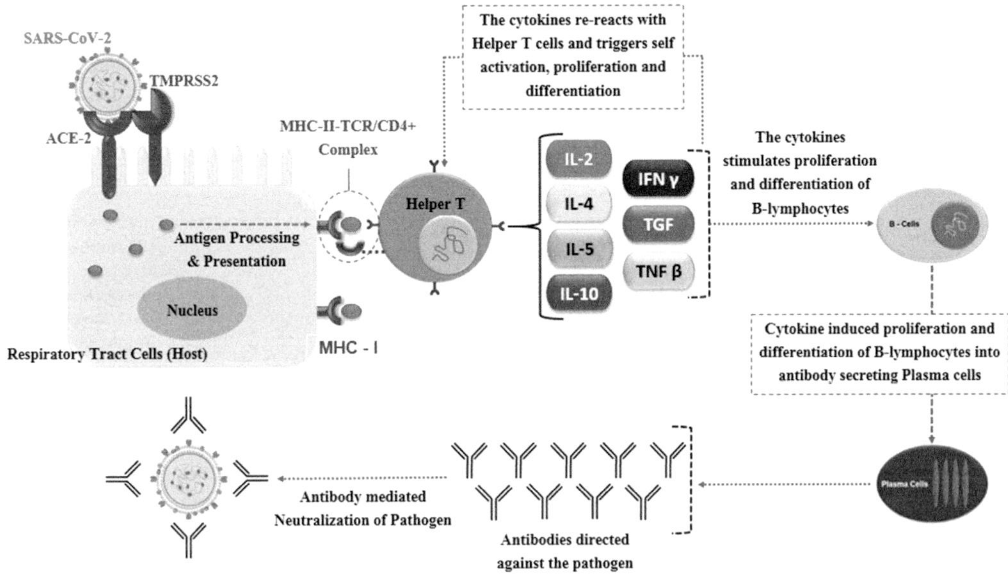

Figure 7.1 Schematic representation of immunological events elicited by CD4+ helper T cells.

nodes to present viral antigens to T cells and B cells. CD4+ helper T cells activate B cells which are responsible for the production of viral-specific antibodies. Figure 7.1 provides a schematic representation of immunological events elicited by CD4+ helper T cells. The SARS-CoV-2 antigens present in the host cell cytoplasm are processed and presented to the helper T cells and cytotoxic T cells through MHC class II and MHC class I surface molecules, respectively. When the antigen is presented through MHC class II surface molecules, it binds with CD4+ molecule and TCR present on the surface of helper T cells, thus forming an MHC II-TCR/CD4+ complex. This interaction triggers the formation and release of cytokines (like IL-2, IL-4, IL-5, IL-10, IFN-γ, TGF, TNF, etc.). These cytokines stimulate the proliferation and differentiation of B lymphocytes into antibody-secreting plasma cells. These antibodies are directed against SARS-CoV-2 protein antigens. Also, the same group of cytokines re-reacts with helper T cells and thus initiate self-activation, proliferation, and differentiation. Activation of CD8+ T cells initiates the cell-mediated killing of virus-infected cells. Figure 7.2 provides a schematic representation of immunological events elicited by CD8+ cytotoxic T cells. When the antigen is presented through MHC class I surface molecules, it binds with the CD8+ molecule and TCR present on the surface of cytotoxic T cells, thus forming an MHC I-TCR/CD8+ complex. This interaction triggers the formation and release of cytokines (like IL-22, IL-4, TGF-α, TNF-α, TNF-β, etc.). These cytokines not only stimulate the B lymphocytes but also re-stimulate other cytotoxic T cells for self-activation, differentiation, and proliferation. The cytotoxic T cells attack and destroy the cells infected with the same pathogen (in this case, SARS-CoV-2) in the future. Granulocyte monocyte-colony stimulating factor (GM-CSF) is produced by T cells which helps in the differentiation of innate immune cells and augment T cell function (Oliveira et al., 2020). These sequences of events continue for a prolonged period of time and in an uncontrolled manner, which results in tissue damage. In adaptive immunity, T cells play a major role as they not only

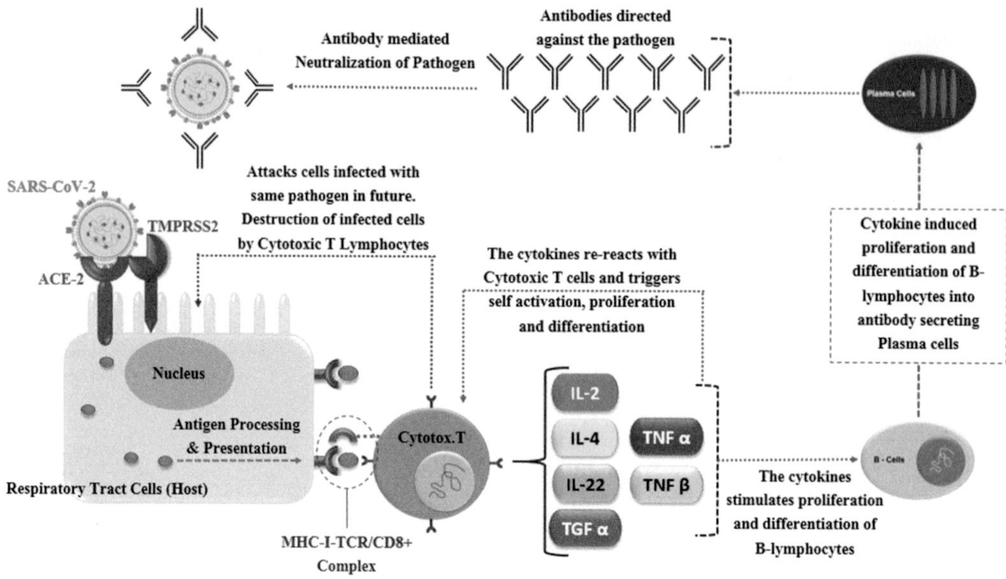

Figure 7.2 Schematic representation of immunological events elicited by CD8+ cytotoxic T cells.

kill the virus-infected cells but also contribute to lung injury. CD14–CD16 inflammatory monocyte subsets are found in COVID-19. These inflammatory cells have a high expression of IL-6 and thus contribute to systemic inflammation (WHO, 2020a; Yuki et al., 2020; Kumar and Al Khodor, 2020; Parasher, 2021; Cevik et al., 2020; Abbas et al., 2016; Dutta et al., 2020).

Immunopathophysiology: The Inflammatory Response (Cytokine Storm) Stage

In immunocompetent individuals, SARS-CoV-2 infection leads to hypercytokinemia, an unregulated hyperinflammatory response that results from the systemic spread of a localized inflammatory response to viral or bacterial infection. Increased proliferation, differentiation, and activation of T-lymphocytes, NK-cells, macrophages, elevated secretion of pro-inflammatory cytokines, and chemokines are indicative of a potentially fatal condition, the cytokine storm. In the initial stages of hypercytokinemia, the rise in the concentration of tumor necrosis factor and interleukin-1β (acute response cytokines) and interleukin-8 and monocyte chemoattractant protein-1 (chemotactic cytokines) leads to an increase in the concentration of interleukin-6 (IL-6). Interleukin-6 promotes inflammatory processes by binding to membrane-bound or soluble IL-6 receptors (mIL-6R [cis-signaling] or sIL-6R [trans-signaling]), creating interaction with glycoprotein-130 (gp-130) and through the JAK-STAT pathway regulates the concentration of IL-6, MCP-1, and GM-CSF. The serum concentration of ferritin, complement, C-reactive protein, and coagulation factors are increased due to the acute phase reaction triggered by IL-6 and associated inflammatory mediators. The reduction in the rate of viral clearance during this stage is related to a decrease in cytotoxic T lymphocyte count, a decrease in total lymphocyte count, and an abnormal rise in serum cytokine levels induced by IL-6. Leakage from blood vessels and

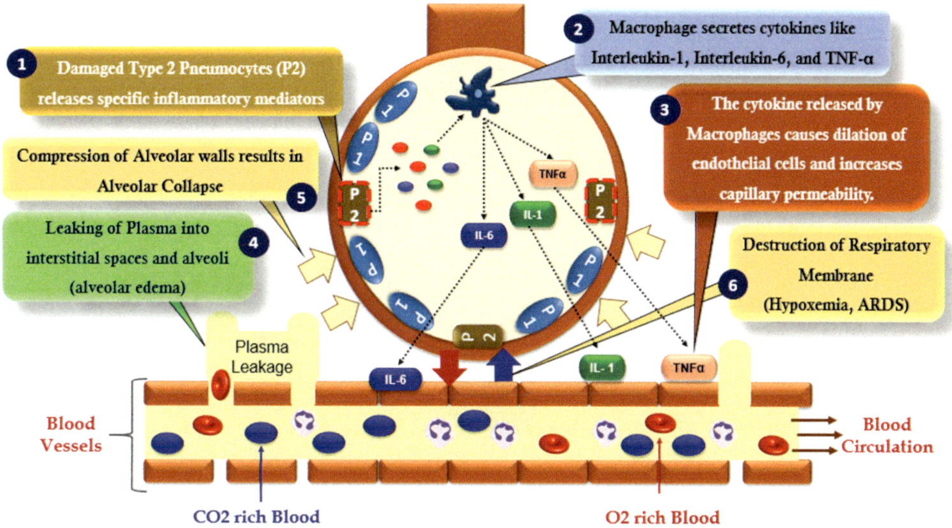

Figure 7.3 Schematic representation of major events at the inflammatory response (cytokine storm) stage leading to the destruction of the respiratory membrane, which results in hypoxemia and acute respiratory distress syndrome (ARDS).

complement and coagulation pathway activation caused by IL-6 may lead to severe cytokine release syndrome (CRS) or diffuse intravascular coagulation (DIC). An increased level of IL-6 may cause cardiac dysfunction, endothelial dysfunction, hypotension, and blood clotting disorders (Price et al., 2020; Weirsinga et al., 2020; Fajgenbaum and June, 2020) (Figure 7.3).

Activation of non-resident macrophages of the lungs (monocyte-derived macrophages) and increased secretion of IL-1β are characteristic features of SARS-CoV-2 infection. These events together are responsible for severe damage (tissue injury, endothelial damage, and ARDS) associated with cytokine storms. The damage to pulmonary microvasculature and respiratory membranes (see Chapter 3) is caused by abnormally elevated levels of IL-6, IL-8, IL-1β, tumor necrosis factor-α. GM-CSF, CCL2, CCL3. CCL5, CXCL8, CXCL9, CXCL10, and reactive oxygen species (ROS) lead to vascular leakage, alveolar edema, hypoxia, pulmonary fibrosis, and death. In severe COVID-19 patients, blood analysis revealed abnormally increased levels of interferon-γ, IL-1, IL-6, IL-12, and transforming growth factor-β, IL-8, CCL2, CXCL-9, and CXCL10 (Price et al., 2020; Dutta et al., 2020; Fajgenbaum and June, 2020) (Figure 7.4).

The levels of IL-2, IL-7, IL-10, GSCF, IP-10, MCP1, MIP1a, and TNF-α in the blood of severely ill COVID-19 patients were also elevated. In short, the aberrant release of multiple cytokines appears to trigger a cytokine storm that produces immunopathogenic damage to tissues and organs, even while the immune response seeks to suppress and eradicate the virus (Wiersinga et al., 2020). Thus, it can be mentioned that the cytokine storm involves an immune response that causes collateral damage that may be greater than the immediate benefit of the immune response. Figure 7.5 and Table 7.1 represent specific organs involved and respective signs and symptoms of a systemic cytokine storm. Further studies should be done to find out the detailed pathogenesis of COVID-19 and cytokine storms (Wiersinga et al., 2020; Price et al., 2020; Dutta et al., 2020; Fajgenbaum and June, 2020; WHO, 2020a; Yuki et al., 2020; Kumar and Al Khodor, 2020; Parasher, 2021; Cevik et al., 2020; Abbas et al., 2016; Oliveira et al, 2020).

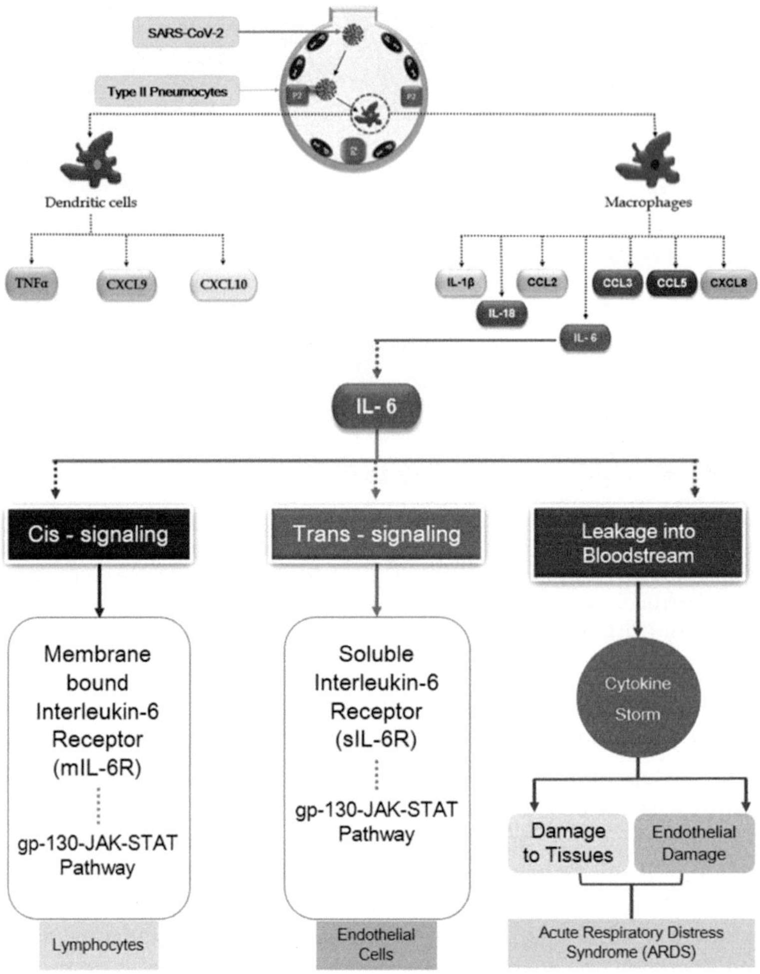

Figure 7.4 Interleukin-6 promotes inflammatory responses mediated by binding to membrane-bound or soluble IL-6 receptors (mIL-6R [cis-signaling] or sIL-6R [trans-signaling]), creating interaction with glycoprotein-130 (gp-130) and through the JAK-STAT pathway regulates the concentration of IL-6, MCP-1, and GM-CSF.

Immunopathophysiology: Thrombosis and Pulmonary Embolism

Thrombosis refers to the formation of blood clots inside a blood vessel; the clot formed is termed a thrombus. Thrombus prevents the normal circulation of blood to concerned organs. The formation of blood clot or coagulation is the body's first line of defense against bleeding. Embolism, also known as thromboembolism, represents blockage in one of the arteries of the body due to a blood clot that has broken off from another location in the body (embolus) and traveled through the bloodstream to lodge in a small blood vessel (Cecil et al., 2012; Kumar et al., 2014; Hall, 2015; McPhee et al., 2021).

The blockage may limit or stop blood flow. A clot that adheres to a vessel wall is called a thrombus, whereas an intravascular clot that floats in the blood is termed an embolus. Thus, a detached

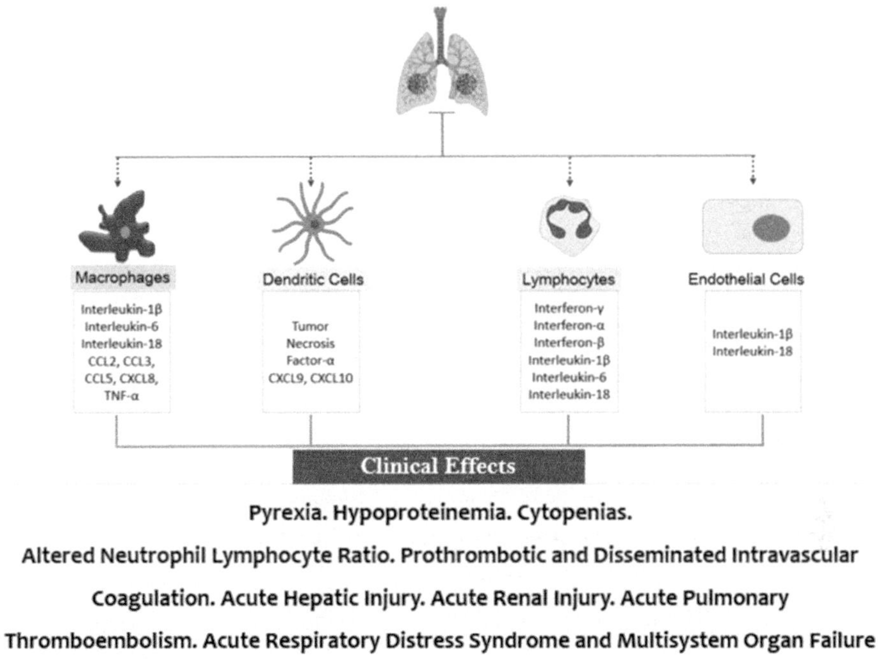

Figure 7.5 Clinical effects of cytokines released by cells of the immune system as a result of a systemic cytokine storm.

thrombus becomes an embolus. Pulmonary embolism is a blockage in one of the pulmonary arteries in your lungs (Cecil et al., 2012; Kumar et al., 2014; Hall, 2015; McPhee et al., 2021).

It is evident from several studies that there is a definite association between COVID-19 and a hypercoagulable state and venous and arterial thrombosis. Both pulmonary embolism and thrombosis can occur in moderate to severe disease with a higher incidence of pulmonary embolism. The probable idea of the association is represented in Figure 7.6 but the exact pathophysiology is not well known and is under investigation. Endothelial cells have ACE-2 receptors on their cell membrane. SARS-CoV-2 binds with those receptors. Thus, endothelial cells are infected and local inflammation at the endothelial cells commences, which results in endothelial dysfunction. As a result of this endothelial level inflammation, there is increased production of tissue factors and amplification of the coagulation cascade resulting in increased fibrin production and coagulation. The endothelial inflammation causes increased production of plasminogen activator inhibitors (PAI-1). Thus, plasminogen to plasmin formation is hampered and fibrinolysis is reduced. Endothelial inflammation causes damage to the endothelial surface and the deposition of complement C5b-9, which is also produced due to inflammation (Price et al., 2020). Thus, coagulation cascade is activated. Apart from endothelial inflammation, hypoxemia also plays a role in thrombosis. As a result of hypoxemia activation of cytokines, tissue factors, Plasminogen Activator Inhibitor 1 (PAI-1) takes place which finally leads to thrombosis. Hypoxia also causes vasoconstriction and stimulates thrombosis. Multiple mechanisms trigger the phenomenon of thrombosis but which mechanism plays the key role is yet to be discovered. Because of the thrombotic phenomenon, the treatment protocol for COVID-19 recommends the use of various

TABLE 7.1 SPECIFIC ORGAN INVOLVED AND RESPECTIVE SIGNS AND SYMPTOMS OF SYSTEMIC CYTOKINE STORM

S. No	Organ Involved	Signs and Symptoms
1.	Brain and nervous system	Confusion. Delirium. Aphasia. Seizures.
2.	Lungs	Pneumonitis. Pulmonary edema. Dyspnea. Hypoxemia. Acute respiratory distress syndrome.
3.	Liver	Hepatomegaly. Elevated liver enzymes. Increased Hepcidin. Hypoalbuminemia. Liver injury. Cholestasis. Liver failure.
4.	Kidneys	Acute renal dysfunction. Renal failure.
5.	Vascular and lymphatic system	Cytopenia. Anemia. Leukocytosis. Coagulopathy. Hyperferritinemia. Increase in other acute phase reactants (e.g., CRP, D-dimer.). Increased cytokines and growth factor. Endothelial damage and vascular permeability. Capillary leak syndrome. Vasodilatory shock. Spontaneous hemorrhage. Lymphadenopathy.
6.	Heart	Hypotension. Tachycardia. Cardiomyopathy.
7.	Rheumatologic system	Vasculitis. Arthritis. Arthralgia.
8.	Gastrointestinal system	Nausea. Vomiting. Diarrhea. Ascites.
9.	Skin	Rashes. Edema.
10.	Constitutional symptoms	Fever. Anorexia. Fatigue.

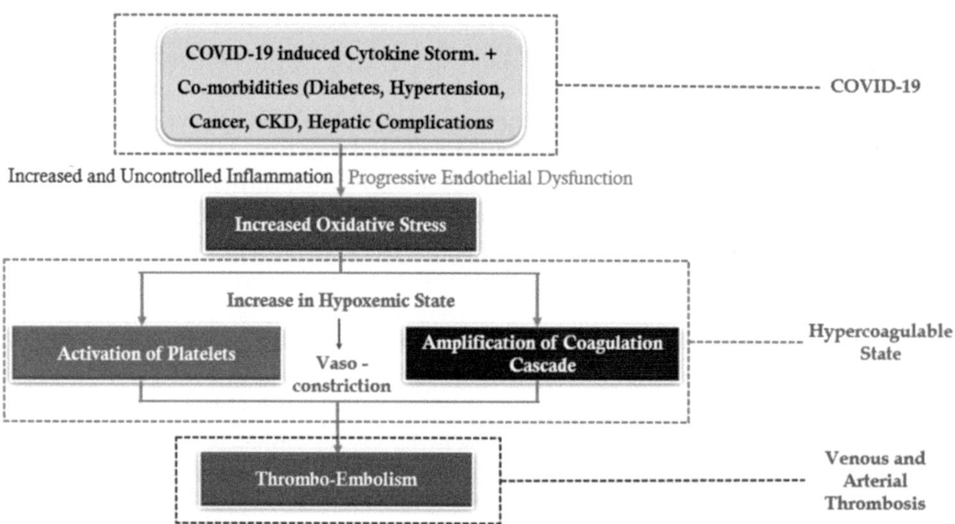

Figure 7.6 The probable idea of an association between COVID-19 and a hypercoagulable state and venous and arterial thrombosis.

anticoagulants at different stages of the disease (Wiersinga et al., 2020; Price et al., 2020; Dutta et al., 2020; Fajgenbaum and June, 2020; WHO, 2020a; Yuki et al., 2020; Kumar and Al Khodor, 2020; Parasher, 2021; Cevik et al., 2020; Abbas et al., 2016; Oliveira et al., 2020).

GENERAL MANAGEMENT OF MILD AND MODERATE COVID-19 CASES

This section points out the treatment strategies available for mild and moderate COVID-19 patients, the risk factors associated with treatment modules, and the aspects associated with caring for COVID-19 patients in a home setting. The presenting signs and symptoms for COVID-19 may vary from individual to individual. These include most prominent symptoms like fever (83–99%), cough (59–82%), fatigue (44–70%), anorexia (40–84%), shortness of breath (31–40%), and myalgia (11–35%), and less common symptoms like soreness of throat, nasopharyngeal congestion, gastrointestinal troubles, and loss of taste and smell (WHO COVID-19 Clinical Management, 2021). Older people and individuals having underlying immunosuppressed conditions may show uncommon symptoms like severe tiredness, reduced mobility, loss of appetite, no fever, encephalopathy, lack of wakefulness, diarrhea, and delirium. Adverse events during pregnancy and physiological adaptations like shortness of breath, fever, gastrointestinal complications, and tiredness may converge with symptoms of COVID-19 in pregnant women. The symptomatic patient meeting the case definition criteria (given by the World Health Organization) and without hypoxia and pneumonia is classified as a mild-COVID-19 case. While managing the mild-COVID-19 cases, first ensure whether the presenting symptoms are because of other infections or not (irrespective of respiratory symptoms) because co-infection is a common event. Second, the patient is to be isolated and generally does not require hospitalization. Routine antibiotic therapies are not recommended. General care treatment may include the administration of antipyretic drugs to keep any fever under control, and adequate hydration, nutrition, and rest are ensured. Constant monitoring of the patient is necessary so that if the patient deteriorates, appropriate steps can be taken (WHO, 2020e, 2021). Moderate COVID-19 cases can be defined as symptomatic patients having met the case definition (given by the World Health Organization), with clinical signs of pneumonia (not severe pneumonia; refer to Chapter 1 for case definitions). The patient is diagnosed for the presence of any infectious or non-infectious health conditions where the signs and symptoms may coincide with the signs and symptoms of COVID-19. Following isolation, symptomatic management is provided as needed for the patient. The administration of routine antibiotic therapy is not recommended until and unless there are indications of secondary bacterial infections along with COVID-19. Constant monitoring of any patient over 60 years of age and having underlying co-morbid conditions (diabetes, hypertension, obesity, cardiac disease, chronic pulmonary complications, chronic kidney disease, cancer, and other immunosuppressive states) is to be ensured as there may be a risk for the sudden and rapid deterioration of the patient (WHO, 2020e, 2021).

HOME ISOLATION OF MILD AND MODERATE COVID-19 PATIENTS

COVID-19 patients (adults and children) who do not require hospitalization or in situations where hospital care is not available (because of insufficiency) then home isolation with proper infection control precautions may be performed. The decision for home isolation of a person is to be made based on the detailed assessment of the patient, detailed assessment of the home where the patient will be kept, and availability of trained caregivers and healthcare professionals. The infection prevention and control (IPC) recommendations like hand and respiratory hygiene measures, environmental cleaning, adequate ventilation, and restricted movement in and out of the home are to be strictly maintained. Checking of patients by caregivers should be performed at regular intervals regarding the warning signs of disease severity like dizziness, confusion, shortness of breath, tachypnea, pain and a constricted feeling in the chest, and signs of dehydration. Pregnant or recently pregnant women suspected of COVID-19 may be kept under home isolation if there is no risk of rapid and severe deterioration of health conditions. Pregnant women with underlying co-morbidities, pre-existing pregnancy-related complications, and/or an immunosuppressive state should be isolated at a healthcare facility with an emergency response team and settings. The decision for home isolation should be made based on a complete evaluation of patient conditions, the situation at home, vulnerable family members at home, and the availability of caregivers and healthcare professionals. Home isolation should be discontinued when it is clinically confirmed that they are no longer infectious. Anyone who was in contact with the isolated patient (like family members and caregivers) should be quarantined at home and get their health status monitored for 14 days from the last day of possible contact (WHO Headquarters, 2020; WHO, 2020e, f, 2021).

REFERENCES

Abbas, A., Lichtman, A., & Pillai, S. (2016). *Cellular and molecular immunology* (9th ed.). Elsevier.

Cecil, R. L., In Goldman, L., & In Schafer, A. I. (2012). *Goldman's Cecil medicine*. Elsevier.

Cevik, M., Kuppalli, K., Kindrachuk, J., & Peiris, M. (2020). Virology, transmission, and pathogenesis of SARS-CoV-2. *BMJ, 371*, m3862. https://doi.org/10.1136/bmj.m3862

Dutta, J., Goswami, S., & Mitra, A. (2020). *COVID-19 and emerging environmental trends* (1st ed.). CRC Press.

Fajgenbaum, D. C., & June, C. H. (2020). Cytokine storm. *New England Journal of Medicine, 383*(23), 2255–2273.

Hall, J. (2015). *Guyton and hall textbook of medical physiology* (13th ed.). Elsevier Saunders.

Kumar, M., & Al Khodor, S. (2020). Pathophysiology and treatment strategies for COVID-19. *Journal of Translational Medicine, 18*(1), 1–9.

Kumar, V., Abbas, A., & Aster, J. (2014). *Robbins & Cotran pathologic basis of disease* (9th ed.). Elsevier.

McPhee, S. J., Papadakis, M. A., & Rabow, M. W. (2021). *Current medical diagnosis & treatment 2021* (60th ed.). McGraw-Hill Medical.

Oliveira, T. L., Melo, I. S., Cardoso-Sousa, L., Santos, I. A., El Zoghbi, M. B., Shimoura, C. G., ... & Sabino-Silva, R. (2020). Pathophysiology of SARS-CoV-2 in lung of diabetic patients. *Frontiers in Physiology, 11*, 1506.

Parasher, A. (2021). COVID-19: Current understanding of its pathophysiology, clinical presentation and treatment. *Postgraduate Medical Journal, 97*(1147), 312–320.

Price, L. C., McCabe, C., Garfield, B., & Wort, S. J. (2020). Thrombosis and COVID-19 pneumonia: The clot thickens! *European Respiratory Journal, 56*(1), 2001608. https://doi.org/10.1183/13993003.01608-2020

WHO. (2014). Infection prevention and control of epidemic- and pandemic-prone acute respiratory infections in health care; 2014. Geneva: World Health Organization https://apps.who.int/iris/bitstream/handle/10665/112656/9789241507134_eng.pdf?sequence=1

WHO. (2020a, January 30) Modes of transmission of virus causing COVID –19 IMPLICATIONS for IPC precautions recommendations; 2020. Retrieved from https://www.who.int/news-room/commentaries/detail/modes-of-transmission-of-virus-causing-covid-19-implications-for-ipc-precaution-recommendations on 22nd June 2020.

WHO. (2020b, January 30). Naming the coronavirus disease (COVID-19) and the virus that causes it; 2020. Retrieved from https://www.who.int/emergencies/diseases/novel-coronavirus-2019/technical-guidance/naming-the-coronavirus-disease-(covid-2019)-and-the-virus-thatcauses-it on 24th June 2020.

WHO. (2020c, January 30). Pneumonia of unknown cause: China. Retrieved May 27, 2021, from https://www.who.int/csr/don/05-january-2020-pneumonia-of-unkown-cause-china/en/

WHO. (2020d). Report of the WHO-China Joint Mission on Coronavirus Disease 2019 (COVID-19) 16–24 February 2020 [Internet]. Geneva: World Health Organization; 2020 Available from: https://www.who.int/docs/default-source/coronaviruse/who-china-joint-mission-on-covid-19-final-report.pdf.

WHO. (2020e, August 13). Homecare for Patients with suspected or confirmed COVID-19 and management of their contacts. *Interim Guidance*. https://www.who.int/publications/i/item/home-care-for-patients-with-suspected-novel-coronavirus-(ncov)-infection-presenting-with-mild-symptoms-and-management-of-contact.

WHO. (2020f, August 7). Public health surveillance for COVID-19: interim guidance, 7 August 2020. Retrieved March 7, 2022, from https://apps.who.int/iris/handle/10665/333752

WHO. (2021 25 January). COVID-19 clinical management: Living guidance. https://www.who.int/publications/i/item/WHO-2019nCoV-clinical-2021-1

WHO Headquarters. (2020, June 17). *Criteria for Releasing COVID-19 Patients from Isolation*. World Health Organization. Retrieved March 7, 2022, from https://www.who.int/publications/i/item/criteria-for-releasing-covid-19-patients-from-isolation

Wiersinga, W. J., Rhodes, A., Cheng, A. C., Peacock, S. J., & Prescott, H. C. (2020). Pathophysiology, transmission, diagnosis, and treatment of coronavirus disease 2019 (COVID-19): A review. *JAMA*, *324*(8), 782–793.

Yuki, K., Fujiogi, M., & Koutsogiannaki, S. (2020). COVID-19 pathophysiology: A review. *Clinical Immunology*, *215*, 108427.

Chapter 8

Diagnosis of COVID-19 Using Clinical Examination, Immunoassays, and Molecular Diagnostic Techniques

Srijan Goswami* and Ushmita Gupta Bakshi

CONTENTS

INTRODUCTION

Diagnosis is the art of identifying a clinical condition from its signs and symptoms. A sign is the effect of a disease that can be observed by someone else, for example, coughing, sneezing, rise in body temperate, and so on. Whereas symptoms are effects experienced only by the person who has the condition, for example, headache, the feeling of tightness in the chest, muscular pain, severe weakness, and so on. According to the World Health Organization, cases of COVID–19 are identified by three methods: molecular tests, antigen tests, and antibody tests. It takes around five to six days for symptoms to manifest. Molecular techniques and antigen tests are used to detect an active SARS-CoV-2 infection while antibody tests are used to detect past infections. A molecular technique like an RT-PCR test detects active SARS-CoV-2 infection by targeting the viral genetic material, it amplifies a small quantity of viral genome sample until it reaches the adequate amount. Antigen tests detect an active SARS-CoV-2 infection by specifically binding to target viral proteins. Any past infections are detected by the antibody test due to the antibodies that the patient develops in response to infection. The management of individual patients and maintaining public health safety are the two fundamental reasons that make laboratory diagnosis of SARS-CoV-2 important. Laboratory diagnostic procedures may be used to ensure active

DOI: 10.1201/9781003178514-10

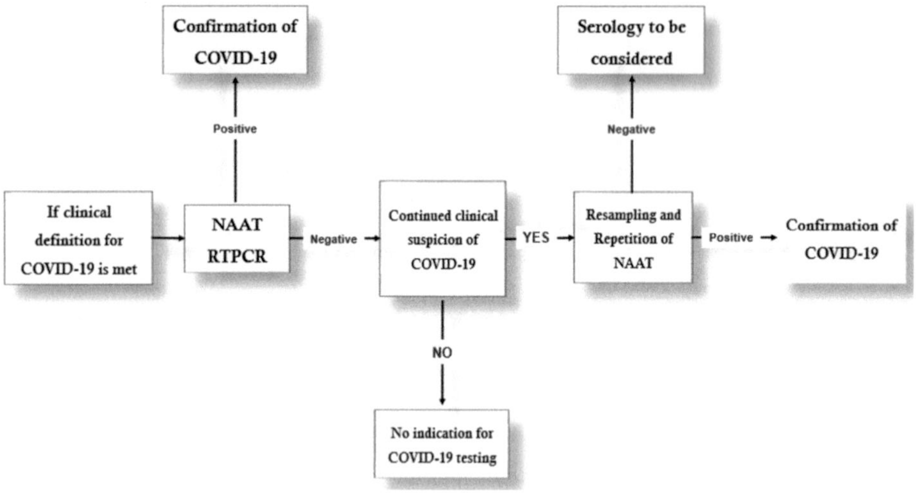

Figure 8.1 The general strategy or pathway for the selection of COVID-19 diagnostic procedures as per the World Health Organization's guidelines.

infection in clinically suspected patients or they can be used to learn about past infections. Instances may arise where the signs and symptoms overlap with other non-COVID illnesses, in such scenarios, differential diagnosis becomes very important. It is to be understood that a positive test for pathogens other than SARS-CoV-2 does not rule out the possibility of SARS-CoV-2 infection. Also, a positive test for SARS-CoV-2 does not mean the complete absence of other co-infections. In several COVID-19 patients, respiratory co-infections were documented that were caused by viruses, bacteria, or fungi. Laboratory diagnosis for associated pathogens may be performed if needed (World Health Organization: Geneva, 2020).

This chapter provides a concise idea about situations based on which SARS-CoV-2 test to be considered, different diagnostic tests for SARS-CoV-2, and common laboratory abnormalities associated with COVID-19 (Figure 8.1).

PRELIMINARY PHYSICAL EXAMINATION AND TRIAGE

The clinical assessment of patients admitted with a possible influenza-like illness (ILI) should begin with a thorough investigation of their vital signs through physical examination. First, check whether the patient is hypertensive (having elevated blood pressure) or hypotensive (having low blood pressure). These values are important because abnormal blood pressure is considered a risk factor for individuals as this may lead to a progressive deterioration of health. After blood pressure, the heart rate of the patient is checked, and observations are made as to whether there is tachycardia (value greater than equal to 100 beats per minute) or not. If the patient is tachycardic, then that could be a potential sign of underlying hypoxemia. After heart rate, the respiratory rate of the individual should be checked. The clinician should notice whether the individual is tachypnic or bradypnic. Heavy and rapid breathing is called tachypnea – this can be called an increased respiratory rate. A respiratory rate greater than 22 breaths per minute is considered a tachypnic state. The body temperature is checked orally to check if the patient is showing signs of fever (temperature greater than or equal to 100.4°F) (Healthcare Workers, 2020a; World Health Organization: Geneva, 2020; Patient Assessment, 2020). After preliminary vital signs are recorded, a physical examination of the individual is performed by the clinician. These sequences of preliminary assessment help the concerned medical team perform triage. In medicine, the word "triage" refers to "the assignment of degrees of urgency to illnesses to decide the order of treatment of a large number of patients or casualties". First auscultation of the lungs is performed and the sounds generated are studied minutely. COVID-19 caused by the SARS-CoV-2 virus is known to cause lung damage and acute lung injury (potentially pneumonia), making auscultation of the lungs very important. Depending on the case, the clinician might hear one of the following lung sounds (Healthcare Workers, 2020a; World Health Organization: Geneva, 2020; Patient Assessment, 2020; Stuart et al., 2018):

- The clinician may hear higher-pitched breath sounds called bronchial breath sounds, which may be indicative of consolidation (potential pneumonia).
- The clinician may auscultate for any wheezing or bronchoconstriction and any kind of mucus plugging. The wheezing could be indicative that there could either be some type of mucus plugging or severe bronchoconstriction and not a lot of air is getting in or out.
- The clinician may also look for a type of sound called crackles. Crackles are categorized as "fine" or "coarse" and may indicate alveolar edema – there might be some fluid that is accumulating within the lungs (potential pneumonia).
- The clinician may also hear a sound called rhonchi, which could be indicative of severe mucus secretions within the airways.

Also, if indicated, some special tests like egophony or bronchophony may be performed. So, while auscultating the lungs, the presence of sounds like bronchial breath sounds, wheezing, crackles, rhonchi, egophony, or bronchophony might increase our suspicion of COVID-19 (Healthcare Workers, 2020a; World Health Organization: Geneva, 2020; Patient Assessment, 2020).

DIFFERENT TYPES OF DIAGNOSTIC TESTS FOR COVID-19

Molecular diagnostic tests, antigen detection tests, and antibody detection tests are three fundamental methods used for the identification of SARS-CoV-2 infection in suspected patients. Active infections are detected by molecular diagnostic tests and antigen detection tests while past-resolved infections are detected by antibody detection tests (also known as serological assay). These are laboratory-based diagnostic methods performed at the point of care under research settings. Figure 8.2 provides a simple schematic representation of various strategies implemented for targeting and diagnosing SARS-CoV-2. In addition to the previously mentioned techniques, a few other diagnostic procedures are used such as sample culturing, which is performed to understand the effects of pharmacological substances on the growth rate of the pathogen, and sequencing techniques that are essential in determining the variants (mutation or alteration in the genome) of the pathogen.

The choice of the diagnostic method is completely dependent on the time and course of the infection. For example, antigen-based procedures provide a good result when samples are collected during the initial stages of the disease or at the time when initial symptoms are visible, however, molecular tests are better suited for samples collected at the late stage of the disease (~after two weeks of symptom onset). In individuals meeting the clinical criteria, the nucleic acid amplification test (NAAT), such as RT-PCR, is the major procedure for detecting SARS-CoV-2. If

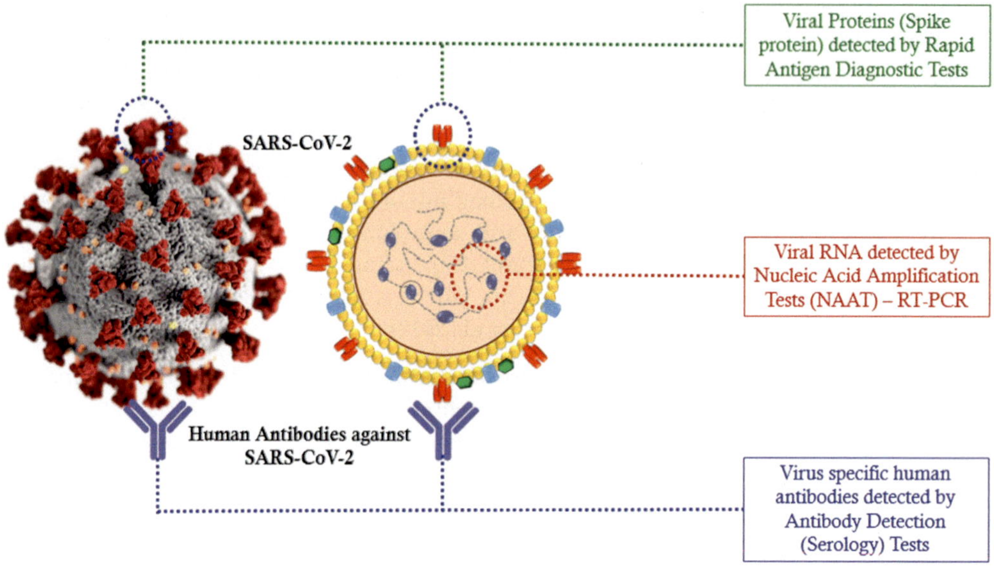

Figure 8.2 Simplified representation of diagnostic strategies for determining COVID-19 cases.

the RT-PCR test is negative and the physical signs and symptoms persist, the test is repeated. If the repeated RT-PCR test is negative and the physical signs and symptoms continue (as per the case definition), the samples are then sent for serological analysis (for confirmation). Let us now understand NAAT, the antigen detection test, and antibody tests separately.

NUCLEIC ACID AMPLIFICATION TESTS

For detecting viral genetic material (in this case, genomic RNA of SARS-CoV-2) molecular diagnostic tests like the reverse transcription-polymerase chain reaction (RT-PCR) test are performed. RT-PCR is a nucleic acid amplification method, which means the genetic material is amplified in amount using this test. High sensitivity and specificity are the reasons for the selection of this diagnostic procedure as compared with other options available. The term sensitivity can be defined as "the percentage of SARS-CoV-2 infected patients who are correctly identified as having SARS-CoV-2 infection" while specificity (less false positives) is defined as "percentage of non-infected individuals who are correctly identified as not having SARS-CoV-2 infection" (Nucleic Acid Amplification Tests (NAATs), 2020; Office of the Commissioner, 2021b; Nucleic Acid Amplification Testing (RT-PCR), 2021).

The sample collection process begins by the insertion of a sterile swab stick inside the nasopharyngeal cavity of the suspected individual through the nostrils and cells with mucus are collected. The test sample collected on the swab is preserved in a vial containing a buffer solution. The buffer solution prevents the sample (in this case, SARS-CoV-2 RNA) from being degraded. The purification of the desired nucleic acid material is a critical step in an RT-PCR test and is performed by trained professionals. Then, using an enzyme called reverse transcriptase (RT), the viral RNA is converted to its complementary DNA sequence (cDNA). This process, known as reverse transcription, is performed because only DNA can be amplified using a polymerase chain reaction and thus the name RT-PCR. For amplification of the test genetic material (SARS-CoV-2 cDNA), ingredients such as primers, fluorescent probes, nucleotides, and enzymes are mixed with the sample genetic material in a vial. The vial is put in an automated RT-PCR machine and the multistep amplification process takes a few hours (~two hours). The first step is the denaturation of the DNA double helix into single strands at 95°C. The second step is annealing where appropriate nucleotides are picked up by the specific primers and the replication process is initiated at 55°C to 65°C. The third step is called extension in which a special thermostable enzyme called Taq polymerase is used for the extension of nucleotides at 72°C. These steps are repeated for around 40 cycles in order to achieve the desired amount of viral genetic material. The primers are tagged with fluorescent dyes that are released after each replication cycle, which are picked up by the sophisticated fluorescence readers. The presence and absence of fluorescence determine the presence or absence of the viral genetic material. Ct value is another factor that is also important in diagnosis. It refers to the PCR cycle at which the amplification of viral genetic material (in this case, SARS-CoV-2) becomes detectable (Nucleic Acid Amplification Tests (NAATs), 2020; Office of the Commissioner, 2021b; Nucleic Acid Amplification Testing (RT-PCR), 2021) (Figure 8.3).

RAPID ANTIGEN DETECTION TESTS

Although being less sensitive than NAATs, rapid antigen tests are used for detecting viral proteins (antigens). These tests are performed in disease stages where the chances of viral load are thought to be high (i.e., ~within seven days after the manifestation of symptoms). There are chances for false negatives as these diagnostic processes may fail to detect a low viral load. Figure 8.4 provides a simple representation of the steps involved in rapid antigen diagnosis (of SARS-CoV-2). In places where there is high community transmission of SARS-CoV-2 and NAAT facilities are not available, rapid antigen tests are performed. If the test result is negative but the suspicious signs and symptoms remain, the individual should be referred to a suspected COVID-19 ward, and if the test result is negative with no suspicious signs and symptoms, the individual is advised to follow infection control guidelines provided for the community. In situations where there is high community transmission of SARS-CoV-2 and there is limited access to NAAT facilities, rapid antigen tests may be performed. If the test is positive for SARS-CoV-2, the individual is to be isolated in a COVID-19 ward based on severity. If the test is negative for SARS-CoV-2 but the signs and symptoms persist, the individual is to be treated as a suspected COVID-19 case. And if the test is negative and concerning signs and symptoms are not present, an RT-PCR test is performed, and based on that result, further decisions are to be made. Figure 8.4 presents the simple representation of this rapid antigen test (Interim Guidance for Antigen Testing for SARS-CoV-2, 2020; Bekliz et al., 2021; Preparedness, 2021)

RAPID ANTIBODY DETECTION TESTS OR SEROLOGICAL ASSAYS

Alveolar macrophages present inside the lungs detect SARS-CoV-2 and perform the process of phagocytosis. Through phagocytosis, the alveolar macrophages engulf SARS-CoV-2 and digest it inside the phagolysosome. The digested protein structures of SARS-CoV-2 (in this case, the portion of spike proteins) are expressed on the MHC-II molecule present on the plasma membrane of the antigen-presenting cells. The presentation of the spike protein antigen by MHC-II

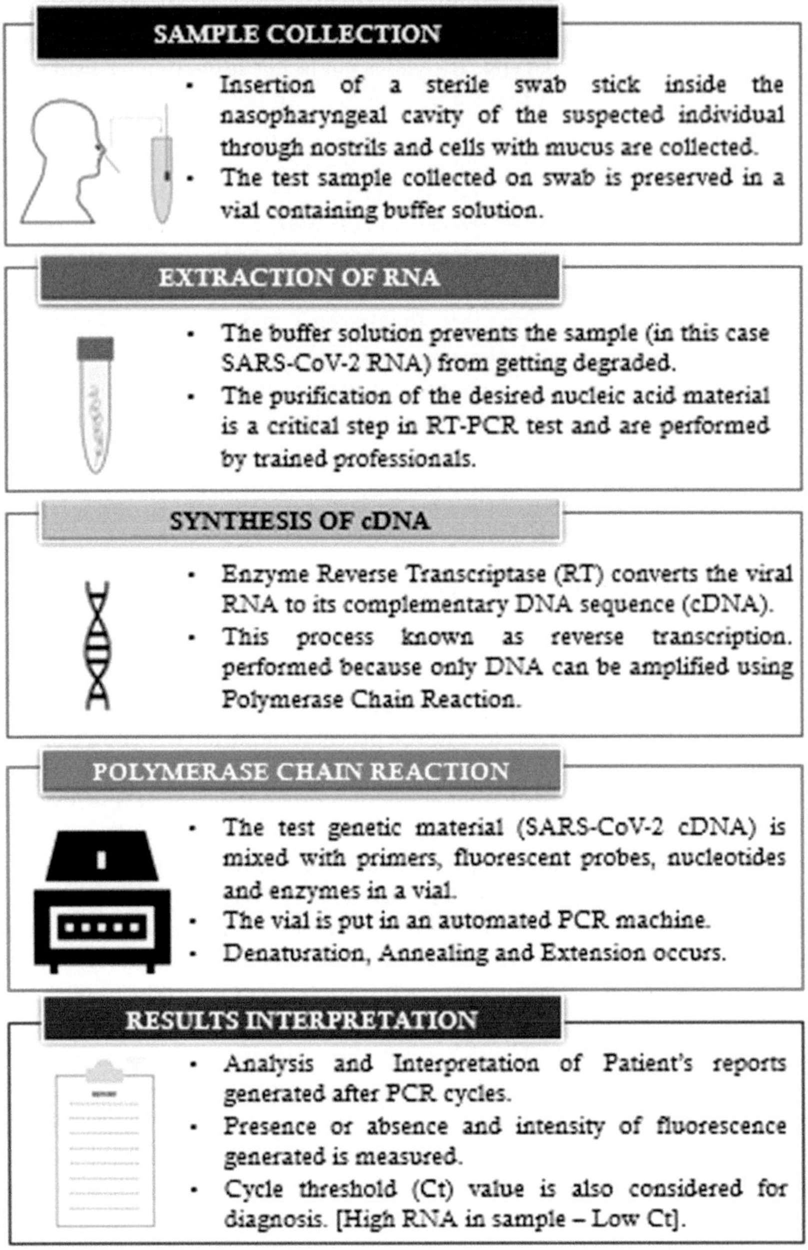

Figure 8.3 Nucleic acid amplification tests (NAATs).

triggers the recruitment of helper T lymphocytes (T_H cells). The T_H cells bind to the spike protein-MHC-II complex with the help of the T-cell receptor (TCR) and CD4+protein molecule. The successful interaction between MHC-II and TCR initiates the synthesis and secretion of a wide range of cytokines. These cytokines not only promote the proliferation and differentiation of B-lymphocytes but also stimulate the plasma cells to secrete antibodies, activate the

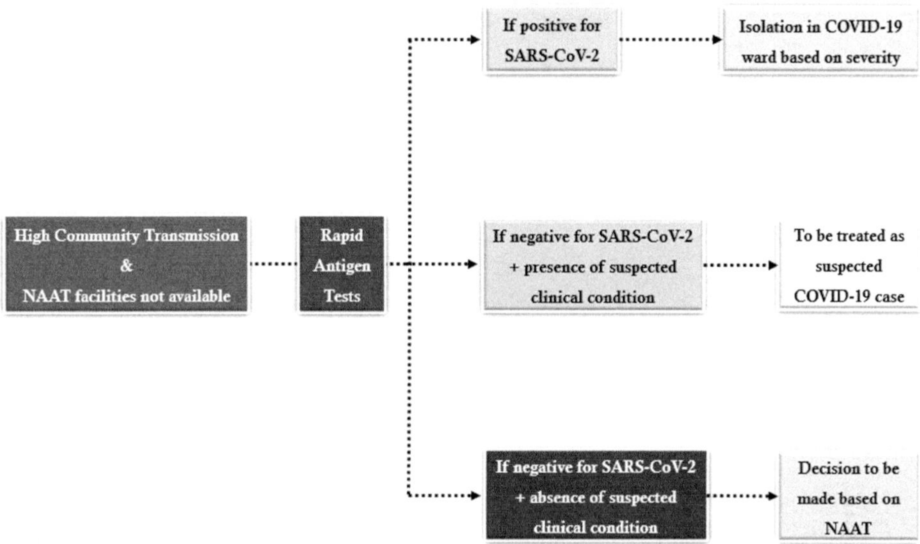

Figure 8.4 General strategies for selecting rapid antigen tests for COVID-19.

complement system, and basically eradicate the threat under concern. This event can be utilized for diagnostic purposes. During the initial stage of infection, the human body produces a specific type of antibody called immunoglobulin M (IgM), which indicates active infection. As the duration of the infection increases, the human body produces another type of antibody called immunoglobulin G (IgG). The presence of IgG either indicates that the patient has recovered from a recent infection, and has some type of immunity, or it may indicate a past infection and that is important when it comes to determining whether the person is immune or not. One of the important aspects is that the production of these antibodies takes time. So, if someone develops symptoms, they might not initially have a positive antibody test. It might take up to a week or more before these antibodies, particularly IgM, are produced. So, that is one of the potential disadvantages. But when serology is combined with RT-PCR, it shows increased sensitivity (CDC, 2020; Center for Devices and Radiological Health, 2021; Uwamino et al., 2021; Kang et al., 2021; Abbasi, 2021).

RAPID IgM/IgG DETECTION

In rapid IgM/IgG detection tests, a small amount of blood sample is collected from the patient. A few drops of the blood sample are put on the marked location on the IgM/IgG test strips, followed by the addition of a test-specific buffer solution. The addition of the buffer solution initiates the lateral movement of the blood sample through the nitrocellulose membrane of the test strip and the subsequent binding with the capture molecule present in the strip. In order for a test to be considered valid, the control mark in the test strip must be positive. Table 8.1 shows this process.

This serological method takes a much longer time as compared with the rapid test and is useful in gathering epidemiological data, as well as helping to develop treatments. ELISA stands for enzyme-linked immunosorbent assay. In this process, a small amount of serum sample is

TABLE 8.1 POSSIBLE COMBINATION OF RESULTS AS OBSERVABLE ON RAPID ANTIGEN TEST KITS

Sample ID	IgM	IgG	Control	Interpretation
Sample 01	No	No	Yes	**Negative result.** The patient does not have active infection
Sample 02	Yes	No	Yes	**Positive result.** The patient has active infection.
Sample 03	No	Yes	Yes	**Positive result.** The patient had past infection and has recovered from the disease and now may also have some degree of immunity.
Sample 04	Yes	No	No	**Invalid test kit.** As the control was not positive, this test strip should be discarded.
Sample 05	No	Yes	No	

collected and put into the microtiter well, then IgG from recovered individuals (primary antibody) is added to it. The idea is that the primary antibody will bind to the spike protein antigen of SARS-CoV-2. After that, a secondary antibody tagged with the specific enzyme is added to the reaction mixture. The enzyme-linked secondary antibody binds to the primary antibody. A chromogenic chemical is added to the reaction mixture that acts as the substrate for the enzyme-linked secondary antibody. This enzyme substrate reaction generates a color that is sensed and analyzed by the ELISA reader. The generation of color means a positive test and the intensity of the color is directly proportional to the concentration of antigens. So these are the serology tests that are combined, in addition to RT-PCR (CDC, 2020; Center for Devices and Radiological Health, 2021; Uwamino et al., 2021; Kang et al., 2021).

NON-SPECIFIC OR SUPPORTIVE LABORATORY DIAGNOSTIC PROCEDURES: ARTERIAL BLOOD GAS AND BIOCHEMICAL ANALYSIS

As a part of a supportive diagnostic procedure, the oxygen saturation percentage (SpO_2) of the patient with ILIs must be monitored. The normal SpO_2 of an individual is around 97 to 100 (of room air). If the SpO_2 level goes below 93% of room air, it might be a sign of concern. When the patient has tested positive through RT-PCR, serology, and physical examination, and SpO2 level decreases to 90% of room air, arterial blood gas (ABG) is performed. Through ABG, conditions like respiratory alkalosis, respiratory acidosis, or metabolic acidosis may be pointed out. In the initial stages, the increase in the respiratory rate (tachypnea) leads to breathing out more CO_2. When excess CO_2 is exhaled, the partial pressure of CO_2 is decreased in blood. Under normal physiological conditions, the following reaction occurs in blood:

$$CO_2 + H_2O \rightarrow \text{Carbonic Acid} \rightarrow \text{Bicarbonate} + \text{Protons}$$

- When the concentration of CO_2 decreases, the reaction shifts to the left, which means the concentration of protons starts decreasing, leading to the rise in pH of the blood. Also, if blood is not getting enough oxygen and the saturation level gets low, leading to a decrease in partial pressure of oxygen in arterial blood, this is a sign of respiratory alkalosis.

- In patients with acute respiratory distress syndrome (ARDS), weakness of the muscles and accumulation of fluid in the lungs becomes prominent, leading to a decrease in clearance of CO_2 from the blood. This may lead to a rise in partial pressure of CO_2 and influences the reaction to shift in a forward direction. The forward reaction increases the number of protons, and thus the pH of the blood decreases. Also, muscular weakness and accumulation of fluid in the lungs block gaseous exchange, thus decreasing the partial pressure of oxygen, leading to hypoxemia.
- In patients having signs of sepsis, the concentration of bicarbonates and partial pressure of CO_2 is drastically affected. During sepsis, the concentration of bicarbonate starts decreasing and the pH of the blood tends to become more acidic. Also, a decrease in the partial pressure of oxygen means the concentration of CO_2 increases in the blood, thus leading to a rise in the partial pressure of CO_2. This condition is termed metabolic acidosis (Bezuidenhout et al., 2021; Visca et al., 2021).

Along with ABG, a wide range of biochemical analyses of body fluids may be performed as supportive diagnostic processes.

- Complete blood count (CBC) and or differential blood count (DBC). This may show whether the patient has thrombocytopenia (low platelets in the blood) or lymphopenia (low levels of lymphocytes in the blood) (Pozdnyakoma et al., 2021; Dhar et al., 2021).
- Comprehensive metabolic panel (CMP). These panel tests help get an idea about electrolytes, glucose level, kidney function, and liver function (Troyer et al., 2020). The patient's liver or kidney can be found to be damaged either directly through the cytopathic effect of the virus or due to multisystem organ failure. Damage to the kidneys leads to decreased urine output, thus increasing the concentration of urea and creatinine in the blood. Also, damage to the liver either due to the cytopathic effect of the virus or due to multisystem organ failure may lead to elevated levels of AST and ALT enzymes (Healthcare Workers, 2020b; O'Shea et al., 2020; Bertolini, 2020).
- Creatine kinase-MB (CK-MB). Due to the cytopathic effect of the virus on the heart or due to multisystem organ failure, cardiac myocytes can be damaged. Elevated levels of CK-MB in the blood are indicative of cardiac myocyte damage (Shi et al., 2020). Also, the levels of troponins may indicate cardiac myocyte damage (Kavsak et al., 2021).
- Procalcitonin (PCT). Increased levels of PCT are found to be associated with a high severity and mortality rate of COVID-19 patients. Serum PCT levels may be used as a prognostic test in this scenario. PCT may also detect superinfections (Hu et al., 2020).
- Coagulation profile. COVID-19 patients have a pronounced hypercoagulability state characterized by impaired endogenous anticoagulation and decreased fibrinolysis (Correa et al., 2020). The most common pattern of coagulopathy observed in patients hospitalized with COVID-19 is characterized by an elevation in fibrinogen and D-dimer levels, and mild prolongation of PTT. This correlates with a parallel rise in the markers of inflammation (Cuker et al., 2021).
- Blood cultures. Studies have shown that blood cultures are only useful in cases of clinical deterioration or suspected hospital-acquired infections. Also, bloodstream infections are very rare for COVID-19 patients, which supports the judicious use of blood cultures in the absence of compelling evidence for bacterial co-infection.
- Inflammatory markers. Studies have shown that patients with severe COVID-19 had significantly higher levels of C-reactive protein (CRP), erythrocyte sedimentation rate (ESR), procalcitonin (PCT), interleukin-6 (IL-6), interleukin-10 (IL-10), interleukin-2R

(IL-2R), serum amyloid A (SAA), and neutrophil-lymphocyte ratio (NLR). The measurement of inflammatory markers could help clinicians rapidly identify the severity level of COVID-19 patients, hence facilitating the early initiation of effective treatment (Mahat et al., 2021; Samprathi and Jayashree, 2021; Zeng et al., 2020).

REFERENCES

Abbasi, J. (2020). Combining rapid PCR and antibody tests improved COVID-19 diagnosis. *JAMA, 324*(14), 1386. https://doi.org/10.1001/jama.2020.19129

Bekliz, M., Adea, K., Essaidi-Laziosi, M., Sacks, J. A., Escadafal, C., Kaiser, L., & Eckerle, I. (2021). SARS-CoV-2 antigen-detecting rapid tests for the delta variant. *The Lancet Microbe*. Published. https://doi.org/10.1016/s2666-5247(21)00302-5

Bertolini, A. (2020, November 1). *Abnormal Liver Function Tests in Patients With COVIDâ-19: Relevance and Potential Pathogenesis*. AASLD. Retrieved November 28, 2021, from https://aasldpubs.onlinelibrary.wiley.com/doi/full/10.1002/hep.31480

Bezuidenhout, M. C., Wiese, O. J., Moodley, D., Maasdorp, E., Davids, M. R., Koegelenberg, C. F., Lalla, U., Khine-Wamono, A. A., Zemlin, A. E., & Allwood, B. W. (2021). Correlating arterial blood gas, acid-base and blood pressure abnormalities with outcomes in COVID-19 intensive care patients. *Annals of Clinical Biochemistry, 58*(2), 95–101. https://doi.org/10.1177/0004563220972539

CDC. (2020, February 11). Using Antibody Tests for COVID-19. Centers for Disease Control and Prevention. Retrieved November 28, 2021, from https://www.cdc.gov/coronavirus/2019-ncov/lab/resources/antibody-tests.html

Center for Devices and Radiological Health. (2021, September 28). *EUA Authorized Serology Test Performance*. U.S. Food and Drug Administration. Retrieved November 28, 2021, from https://www.fda.gov/medical-devices/coronavirus-disease-2019-covid-19-emergency-use-authorizations-medical-devices/eua-authorized-serology-test-performance

Corrêa, T. D., Cordioli, R. L., Campos Guerra, J. C., Caldin Da Silva, B., dos Reis Rodrigues, R., de Souza, G. M., Midega, T. D., Campos, N. S., Carneiro, B. V., Campos, F. N. D., Guimarães, H. P., de Matos, G. F. J., de Aranda, V. F., & Rolim Ferraz, L. J. (2020). Coagulation profile of COVID-19 patients admitted to the ICU: An exploratory study. *PLOS ONE, 15*(12), e0243604. https://doi.org/10.1371/journal.pone.0243604

Cuker, A., Tseng, E. K., Nieuwlaat, R., Angchaisuksiri, P., Blair, C., Dane, K., Davila, J., DeSancho, M. T., Diuguid, D., Griffin, D. O., Kahn, S. R., Klok, F. A., Lee, A. I., Neumann, I., Pai, A., Pai, M., Righini, M., Sanfilippo, K. M., Siegal, D., Skara, M., … Schünemann, H. J. (2021). American society of hematology 2021 guidelines on the use of anticoagulation for thromboprophylaxis in patients with COVID-19. *Blood Advances, 5*(3), 872–888. https://doi.org/10.1182/bloodadvances.2020003763

Dhar, M. S., Marwal, R., Radhakrishnan, Vs, Ponnusamy, K., Jolly, B., Bhoyar, R. C., Sardana, V., Naushin, S., Rophina, M., Mellan, T. A., Mishra, S., Whittaker, C., Fatihi, S., Datta, M., Singh, P., Sharma, U., Ujjainiya, R., Bhatheja, N., Divakar, M. K., Singh, M. K., … Cherian, S. S. (2021). Genomic characterization and epidemiology of an emerging SARS-CoV-2 variant in Delhi, India. *Science (New York, N.Y.), 374*(6570), 995–999. https://doi.org/10.1126/science.abj9932

Healthcare Workers. (2020a, February 11). Centers for Disease Control and Prevention. https://www.cdc.gov/coronavirus/2019-ncov/hcp/non-us-settings/sop-triage-prevent-transmission.html

Healthcare Workers. (2020b, February 11). Centers for Disease Control and Prevention. Retrieved November 28, 2021, from https://www.cdc.gov/coronavirus/2019-ncov/hcp/clinical-care/post-covid-assessment-testing.html

Hu, R., Han, C., Pei, S., Yin, M., & Chen, X. (2020). Procalcitonin levels in COVID-19 patients. *International Journal of Antimicrobial Agents, 56*(2), 106051. https://doi.org/10.1016/j.ijantimicag.2020.106051

Interim Guidance for Antigen Testing for SARS-CoV-2. (2020, February 11). Centers for Disease Control and Prevention. Retrieved November 28, 2021, from https://www.cdc.gov/coronavirus/2019-ncov/lab/resources/antigen-tests-guidelines.html

Kang, K., Huang, L., Ouyang, C., Du, J., Yang, B., Chi, Y., He, S., Ying, L., Chen, G., & Wang, J. (2021). Development, performance evaluation, and clinical application of a Rapid SARS-CoV-2 IgM and IgG Test Kit based on automated fluorescence immunoassay. *Journal of Medical Virology, 93*(5), 2838–2847. https://doi.org/10.1002/jmv.26696

Kavsak, P. A., Hammarsten, O., Worster, A., Smith, S. W., & Apple, F. S. (2021). Cardiac troponin testing in patients with COVID-19: A strategy for testing and reporting results. *Clinical Chemistry, 67*(1), 107–113. https://doi.org/10.1093/clinchem/hvaa225

Mahat, R. K., Panda, S., Rathore, V., Swain, S., Yadav, L., & Sah, S. P. (2021). The dynamics of inflammatory markers in coronavirus disease-2019 (COVID-19) patients: A systematic review and meta-analysis. *Clinical epidemiology and global health, 11*, 100727. https://doi.org/10.1016/j.cegh.2021.100727

Nucleic Acid Amplification Testing (RT-PCR). (2021, July 12). CDC-IDSA. Retrieved November 28, 2021, from https://www.idsociety.org/covid-19-real-time-learning-network/diagnostics/RT-pcr-testing/

Nucleic Acid Amplification Tests (NAATs). (2020, February 11). Centers for Disease Control and Prevention. Retrieved November 28, 2021, from https://www.cdc.gov/coronavirus/2019-ncov/lab/naats.html

Office of the Commissioner. (2021b, September 22). *Coronavirus Disease 2019 Testing Basics*. U.S. Food and Drug Administration. Retrieved November 28, 2021, from https://www.fda.gov/consumers/consumer-updates/coronavirus-disease-2019-testing-basics

O'Shea, P. M., Lee, G. R., Griffin, T. P., Tormey, V., Hayat, A., Costelloe, S. J., Griffin, D. G., Srinivasan, S., O'Kane, M., Burke, C. M., Faul, J., Thompson, C. J., Curley, G., & Tormey, W. P. (2020). COVID-19 in adults: test menu for hospital blood science laboratories. *Irish Journal of Medical Science, 189*(4), 1147–1152. https://doi.org/10.1007/s11845-020-02252-0

Patient Assessment. (2020). *COVID Protocols*. Retrieved November 28, 2021, from https://covidprotocols.org/en/chapters/patient-assessment/

Pozdnyakova, O., Connell, N. T., Battinelli, E. M., Connors, J. M., Fell, G., & Kim, A. S. (2021). Clinical significance of CBC and WBC morphology in the diagnosis and clinical course of COVID-19 infection. *American Journal of Clinical Pathology, 155*(3), 364–375. https://doi.org/10.1093/ajcp/aqaa231

Preparedness, E. (2021, October 6). *Antigen-detection in the Diagnosis of SARS-CoV-2 Infection*. World Health Organization. Retrieved November 28, 2021, from https://www.who.int/publications/i/item/antigen-detection-in-the-diagnosis-of-sars-cov-2infection-using-rapid-immunoassays

Samprathi, M., & Jayashree, M. (2021). Biomarkers in COVID-19: An up-to-date review. *Frontiers in Pediatrics, 8*, 607647. https://doi.org/10.3389/fped.2020.607647

Shi S, Qin M, Shen B, et al. (2020). Association of cardiac injury with mortality in hospitalized patients with COVID-19 in Wuhan, China. *JAMA Cardiology, 5*(7), 802–810. https://doi.org/10.1001/jamacardio.2020.0950

Stuart, R., Penman, I., Strachan, M., & Hobson, R. (2018). *Davidson's Principles and Practice of Medicine* (23rd ed.). Elsevier.

Troyer, E. A., Kohn, J. N., & Hong, S. (2020). Are we facing a crashing wave of neuropsychiatric sequelae of COVID-19? Neuropsychiatric symptoms and potential immunologic mechanisms. *Brain, Behavior, and Immunity, 87*, 34–39. https://doi.org/10.1016/j.bbi.2020.04.027

Uwamino, Y., Wakui, M., Aoki, W., Kurafuji, T., Yanagita, E., Morita, M., Nagata, M., Inose, R., Noguchi, M., Yokota, H., Hasegawa, N., Saya, H., Murata, M., & Keio Donner Project Team (2021). Evaluation of the usability of various rapid antibody tests in the diagnostic application for COVID-19. *Annals of Clinical Biochemistry, 58*(3), 174–180. https://doi.org/10.1177/0004563220984827

Visca, D., Migliori, G. B., Dinh-Xuan, A. T., Centis, R., Belli, S., Vitacca, M., Aliani, M., Zampogna, E., Feci, D., Pignatti, P., Zappa, M., Saderi, L., Sotgiu, G., & Spanevello, A. (2021). The role of blood gas analysis in the post-acute phase of COVID-19 pneumonia. *Archivos de bronconeumologia*. Advance online publication. https://doi.org/10.1016/j.arbres.2021.06.003

World Health Organization. (2020, September). *Diagnostic Testing for SARS-CoV-2: Interim Guidance*. World Health Organization.

Zeng, F., Huang, Y., Guo, Y., Yin, M., Chen, X., Xiao, L., & Deng, G. (2020). Association of inflammatory markers with the severity of COVID-19: A meta-analysis. *International Journal of Infectious Diseases: IJID: Official Publication of the International Society for Infectious Diseases, 96*, 467–474. https://doi.org/10.1016/j.ijid.2020.05.055

Chapter 9

Conventional Pharmacological Strategies, Investigational Drugs, and Immunotherapies for COVID-19

Subhra Bhattacharya*, Srijan Goswami, and Chiranjeeb Dey

CONTENTS

DOI: 10.1201/9781003178514-11

INTRODUCTION

The COVID-19 outbreak caused by SARS-CoV-2 that began in an animal market in Wuhan, Hubei province, China, in December 2019 has created a global health, social, and economic crisis. The virus responsible for the outbreak was initially designated as the 2019 novel coronavirus or 2019-nCoV, later SARS-CoV-2, by the International Committee on Taxonomy of Viruses (ICTV). Subsequently, the disease was named **Co**rona**vi**rus **D**isease of 20**19** or COVID-19 by the World Health Organization (WHO). To date, the contagion has spread to over 222 countries (including UN unrecognized countries), resulting in 259 million cases and 5.17 million deaths (as of November 23, 2021), and has been officially declared a pandemic by the WHO, owing to its extensive and widespread pathogenicity and enhanced mode of infection compared with its counterparts. This has resulted in worldwide lockdown conditions, where international and domestic trades and travels have been called off to avoid further infection and transmission of the disease. As a result, financial losses have triggered an economic crisis, with a possible fall of 5–6% of global trade and reducing global GDP by 2.5% until the first quarter of 2021, as per a World Trade Organization (WTO) report (Wu et al., 2020; Calabrese et al., 2020; Yang, 2020; Booth et al., 2003; Wrapp et al., 2020; Shereen et al., 2020; Chan et al., 2020).

The clinical presentation of SARS-CoV-2 pathogenicity is similar to any other influenza-like illnesses (ILI) and severe acute respiratory illness (SARI). The virus is transmitted from one person to another through respiratory droplets, aerosols, or fomites. There is a possibility of zoonotic transmission, which includes bats, snakes, and pangolins, and reverse zoonosis, which is human to pets (dog, cat). Both are under investigation. The fundamental information available on SARS-CoV-2 is dependent on the scientific literature available on SARS-CoV and MERS-CoV (belonging to the same family). As the virus is highly contagious and there are no evidence-based pharmacological drugs available to treat patients, COVID-19 has proved itself to be a serious challenge. Since there is no proven drug available for COVID-19, several experimental drugs have been authorized to be used as standalone or in combination under emergency use authorization for hospitalized COVID-19 patients. Symptomatic management, hospital intensive care, and supportive interventions are being provided to critically ill patients. Most of the drugs being used under emergency use authorization are not proven for COVID-19 but are based on literature and data available on their previous effects in treating diseases like SARS, MERS, viral hepatitis, influenza, Ebola, and AIDS. Pharmacological agents with anti-inflammatory, antimicrobial, and immunomodulatory properties have the ability to inhibit the viral load at different intervals, including host–pathogen interaction, viral entry into the host cell, replication of the viral genome, and viral polypeptide production. The present chapter deals with the effects of these drugs and their mode of action on molecular targets with respect to SARS-CoV-2 (Wu et al., 2020; Calabrese et al., 2020; Yang, 2020; Booth et al., 2003; Wrapp et al., 2020; Shereen et al., 2020; Chan et al., 2020).

CONVENTIONAL DRUG DESIGNING STRATEGIES FOR COVID-19

In Part 1, we learned about the life cycle of SARS-CoV-2 and the ways COVID-19 develops. Understanding those mechanisms helps in the identification of critical events that can be utilized while designing pharmacological interventions for the treatment of COVID-19 (Wu et al., 2020; Calabrese et al., 2020; Yang, 2020; Booth et al., 2003; Wrapp et al., 2020; Shereen et al.,

2020; Chan et al., 2020; Dutta et al., 2020). This can be achieved through one of the following approaches:

- First, **designing interventions based on receptor binding processes**. The receptor binding process involves components like S1 and S2 subunits of viral spike proteins; the ACE-2 receptor and TMPRSS2 can be used as suitable candidates for drug designing.

  The goal of the clinical trial is to determine whether these investigational pharmacological agents decrease viral load (SARS-CoV-2) early in COVID–19 infection. This may be achieved through the following possibilities.
  - Development of vaccines containing antigens derived from the SARS-CoV-2 spike protein having the ability to boost the recognition capability of immune cells.
  - Development of monoclonal antibodies that bind to the spike protein of SARS-CoV-2 and block the interaction with human cells.
  - Designing drugs that check the spread and pathogenesis of SARS-CoV-2 by inhibiting TMPRSS2 activity.
  - Designing drugs that inhibit the interaction site between ACE-2 and the spike protein.
  - Designing a soluble form of ACE–2 which, when administered in an excess amount, may competitively bind with SARS-CoV-2, thus neutralizing it.
- Second, **designing interventions based on the uncoating, replication, and translation of viral genetic material**. The replication and translation of viral proteins involve multiple components such as viral genomic RNA, viral mRNA, replicase polyproteins, non-structural proteins, and RNA-dependent RNA polymerase (RdRp) that may be used as potential targets for the development of drugs. RdRp is a target of investigational drugs such as remdesivir (Al-Tawfiq et al., 2020) and favipiravir (Qingxian, 2020). Preliminary research has shown both of these agents inhibit RdRp and thus might be useful in the treatment of early and mid-stages of coronavirus disease.
- Third, **designing interventions based on the synthesis of structural proteins and assembly of viral particles**. Chloroquine or hydroxychloroquine (antimalarial agents) are known to show antiviral activity by increasing the pH of host cell lysosomes which in turn inhibits the hydrolytic activity of protease enzymes that are required for the processing of viral glycoprotein during infection. Pharmacological agents belonging to the class of drugs known as the protease inhibitors such as lopinavir-ritonavir (Cai et al., 2020) as well as darunavir-cobicistat (Chen et al., 2020) fall in this category.

To date, there is no specific *medicine* recommended to prevent or *treat* the new Coronavirus. Specific *treatments* are under investigation and will be tested through clinical trials.

DRUGS INHIBITING THE RECEPTOR BINDING PROCESS

SARS-CoV-2 enters the upper respiratory tract through the inhalation of contaminated aerosols or respiratory droplets. Droplets containing SARS-CoV-2 progressively migrate to the lower respiratory tract where they attach with pneumocytes. The attachment of the SARS-CoV-2 spike protein with the host cell is mediated by ACE-2. Other than alveolar pneumocytes, SARS-CoV-2 is known to infect any cell expressing the ACE-2 receptor, which includes the cardiovascular system, gastrointestinal system, renal system, and liver. The investigational drugs that fall under this category are chloroquine, hydroxychloroquine, nitazoxanide, and

TMPRSS2 inhibitors (Wu et al., 2020; Calabrese et al., 2020; Yang, 2020; Wrapp et al., 2020; Shereen et al., 2020; Chan et al., 2020).

Antiviral Agent: Chloroquine and Its Analogs (Viral Entry Inhibitors)

Chloroquine and its analogs belong to the antimalarial group of drugs having multimodal action and are being investigated for their effectiveness in treating malaria and autoimmune disorders. Chloroquine acts by impairing the glycosylation process of ACE-2, restricting its interaction with the spike protein, thus hampering binding. These analogs are known to cause inhibition of protein biosynthesis and enzymatic dysfunction by increasing pH levels. Researchers anticipated that the mechanism of action will be useful in treating COVID-19. Under emergency use authorization, this investigational drug was administered to COVID-19 patients. Clinical trials currently investigating the role of chloroquine in treating COVID-19 patients use doses higher than those recommended for authorized indications. Ongoing scientific evidence shows that chloroquine creates adverse drug reactions such as abnormal electrical activity that affects the heart rhythm (QT-prolongation), liver and kidney damage, nerve cell damage, retinopathy, and hypoglycemia. The clinical data regarding the positive effect of the medicine in the treatment of COVID-19 are limited and inconclusive but there was ample evidence showing serious adverse drug reactions. Because of the serious adverse effects observed in COVID-19 patients receiving the investigational drug, the emergency use authorization on chloroquine was withdrawn by the FDA on June 15, 2020 (EMA, 2020; Office of the Commissioner FDA, 2020; Browning, 2014).

Antiviral Agent: Hydroxychloroquine (Viral Entry Inhibitor)

Hydroxychloroquine is a chloroquine analog having a mode of action resembling chloroquine. These groups of drugs show an immunomodulatory effect by inhibiting certain cellular functions and are thus used as an immunosuppressive treatment in autoimmune disorders. These drugs can create cellular disorientation by entering organelles like lysosomes or endosomes and increasing their pH to damaging levels. Thus, lysosomal and endosomal functions are disrupted. Chloroquine and hydroxychloroquine act as a zinc ionophore that helps zinc enter the cytoplasm of a cell. Also, hydroxychloroquine is known to bind with sialic acid. Some of the possible ways by which hydroxychloroquine may act are as follows:

- First, the host cell membrane possesses a substance called sialic acid that may act as a receptor for the spike protein of coronaviruses. Research shows that hydroxychloroquine binds to sialic acid residues preventing the spike protein of SARS-CoV-2 from binding and essentially preventing the formation of the spike protein–ACE-2 complex. This is another mechanism by which hydroxychloroquine (or chloroquine) can inhibit the SARS-CoV-2 from infecting a host cell (see Figure 9.1).
- Second, lysosomes and endosomes are responsible for the recycling of nutrients and other waste products in and out of a cell. When the spike protein present on the surface of SARS-CoV-2 binds with the ACE-2 receptor on the host's cell membrane, the virus is endocytosed inside the host's cell endosomes. Endosomes traverse through the cytosol and fuse with lysosomes and help in the transfer of the virus. Hydroxychloroquine (or chloroquine analogs) inhibits the process of endocytosis by increasing the pH (see Figure 9.1).

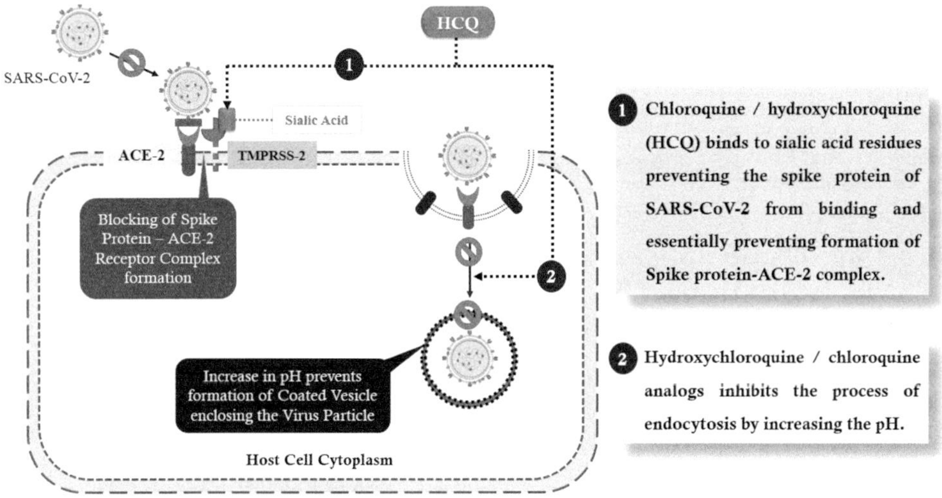

Figure 9.1 Simple representation of the mechanism of action of chloroquine and hydroxychloroquine.

- Third, the drug also acts as a zinc ionophore, meaning it helps transport zinc ions across a lipid membrane in a cell. Without help, zinc bounces off the cell membrane and thus cannot enter a cell. But in the presence of hydroxychloroquine (or chloroquine), zinc binds with it and thus is transported inside the cell. Studies have shown that zinc inhibits coronavirus RNA polymerase activity *in vitro* and block the replication of these viruses in cell culture (see Figure 9.2).

Hydroxychloroquine was assessed using pharmacology based pharmacokinetic (PBPK) modeling on Vero cells against SARS-CoV-2 along with chloroquine. This study revealed that the potency of hydroxychloroquine (EC50 of 0.72 μM) was greater than that of chloroquine (EC50 of 5.47 μM). In addition to this, a similar study conducted in France showed a positive effect against COVID-19 in combination with azithromycin. Like chloroquine, hydroxychloroquine was also administered to COVID-19 patients under emergency use authorization. Clinical trials currently use higher doses of hydroxychloroquine than recommended in the treatment of COVID-19 patients. Ongoing scientific evidence shows that hydroxychloroquine creates adverse drug reactions similar to chloroquine such as abnormal electrical activity that affects the heart rhythm (QT-prolongation), liver and kidney damage, nerve cell damage, retinopathy, and hypoglycemia. The clinical data regarding the positive effect of the medicine in the treatment of COVID-19 are limited and inconclusive but there was ample evidence showing serious adverse drug reactions. Because of the serious adverse effects observed in the COVID-19 patients receiving the investigational drug, the emergency use authorization on chloroquine was withdrawn by the FDA on June 15, 2020 (EMA, 2020; Office of the Commissioner FDA, 2020; Browning, 2014).

Antiviral Agent: Umifenovir (Viral Entry Inhibitor)

Umifenovir, a spike protein-ACE-2 membrane fusion inhibitor is an antiviral agent originally implemented for the management of influenza A, influenza B, hepatitis C virus, hepatitis B virus, and human herpes virus-8 (HHV-8). It blocks membrane fusion. The current data available for

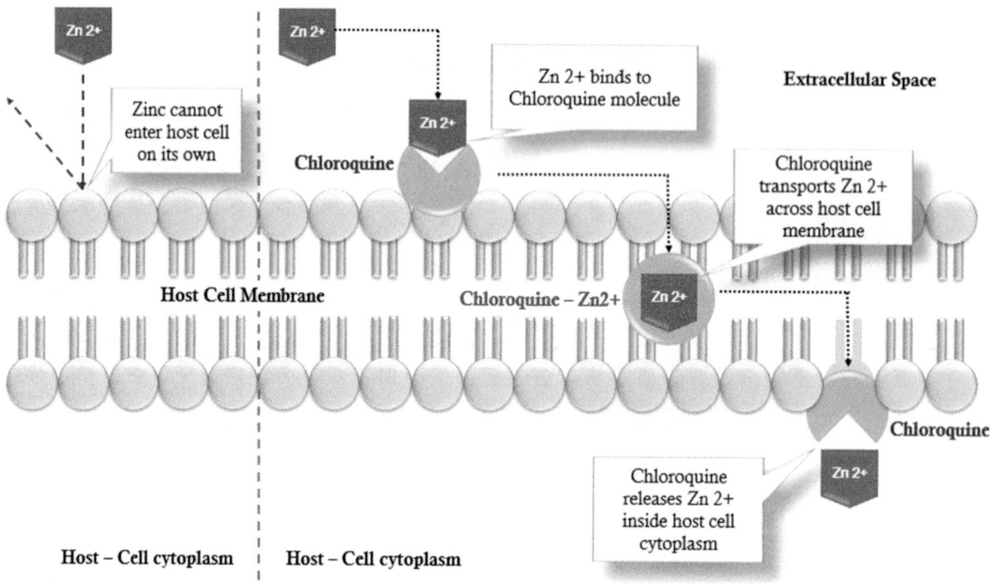

Figure 9.2 Chloroquine and hydroxychloroquine acting as a Zinc ionophore.

the effectiveness of umifenovir for the treatment of COVID-19 is inconclusive. The clinical trials of this experimental drug are in progress (Nojomi et al., 2020; Huang et al., 2021; US National Library of Medicine, 2020a).

DRUGS INHIBITING VIRAL GENOME REPLICATION

Antiviral Agent: Remdesivir (GS-5734 – RdRp Inhibitor)

Originally developed for treating Ebola complications, this experimental antiviral drug is currently undergoing clinical trials for its effectiveness against COVID-19. Remdesivir, the antiviral pro-drug (inactive form of medicine) developed by Gilead Sciences is an adenosine analog. Being an adenosine analog, it mimics natural adenosine in its structure and function and is known to inhibit RNA synthesis. This unapproved drug was initially used to treat COVID-19 patients under emergency use authorization based on data available from *in vitro* and *in vivo* studies against Filoviridae, Paramyxoviridae, and Coronaviridae viruses. Being a pro-drug, remdesivir is metabolized in cells and tissues to become an active nucleoside triphosphate that interferes with RNA polymerase activity of the virus. So, when remdesivir (GS-5734) is administered, it enters target cells and is metabolized into its active form (GS-441524). GS-441524 is an adenosine analog, meaning it is not real adenosine but looks and acts like adenosine. RNA is made up of four types of nucleotide adenine (A), guanine (G), cytosine (C), and uracil (U). As GS-441524 acts like adenosine, the viral RdRp is misdirected and picks up GS-441524 and incorporates it into the viral RNA strand. As the synthesis of viral RNA continues, GS-441524 keeps adding artificial adenosine into the growing chain, thus making it defective. This sequence of events disrupts the formation of normal viral RNA (see Figure 9.3). An important aspect to be considered

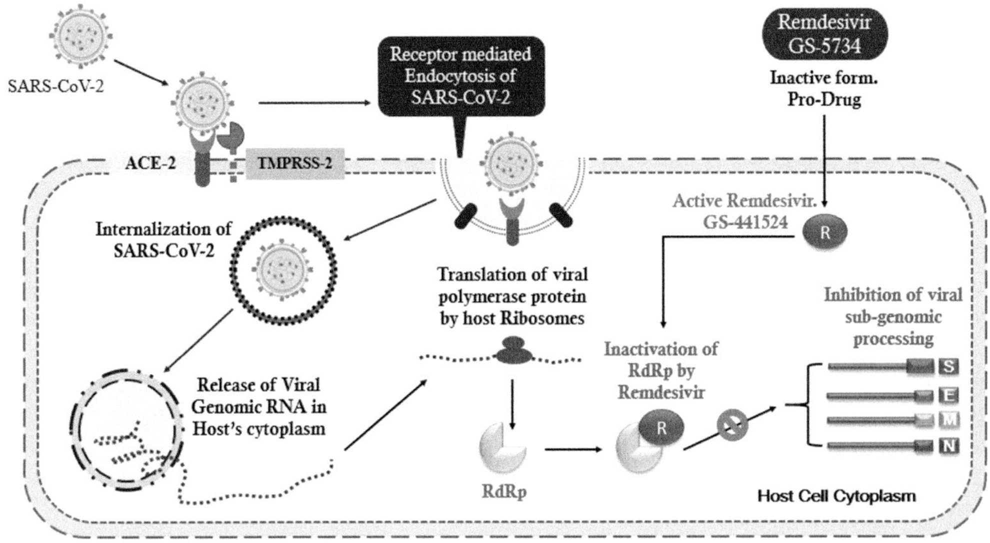

Figure 9.3 Simple representation of the mechanism of action of remdesivir (GS-5734).

is 3'-5' exoribonuclease (proofreading) activity. It is a viral protein produced from the original viral RNA template. This protein possesses the ability to detect and fix abnormalities in the viral RNA strand. If RdRp is making viral RNA with artificial adenosine, it detects the anomaly and corrects it. The adverse reactions caused by remdesivir include severe headaches, tachycardia or bradycardia, wheezing and shortness of breath, acute respiratory failure, facial swelling, nausea and vomiting, fever with chills and shivering, dizziness, increase in aminotransferase level, liver complications, and renal complications. On November 20, 2020, the World Health Organization issued a report recommending against the use of remdesivir in hospitalized patients regardless of disease severity as there is currently no evidence that remdesivir improves survival and other outcomes in these patients, but there is ample evidence showing adverse drug reactions and iatrogenic complications associated with its use (Dey et al., 2020; Wang et al., 2020; Lo et al., 2019; WHO, 2020b).

Antiviral Agent: Ribavirin (Guanine Analog – RdRp Inhibitor)

The experimental antiviral drug ribavirin (tribavirin), currently undergoing clinical trials for its effectivity against COVID-19, is a guanine analog capable of inhibiting viral RdRp activity. Currently under emergency use authorization, this drug was originally developed to deal with complications arising from RSV infection, hepatitis C, bunyavirus infection, herpesvirus infection, poxvirus infection, and hemorrhagic fevers. The beneficial effect of this drug in the treatment of COVID-19 has been inconclusive but adverse reactions like drug-induced hemolytic anemia, acute cardiac failure, increase in bilirubin level, arthralgia, hypocalcemia, hypomagnesemia, and increased toxicity levels of associated medications. The research community does not recommend the use of this drug in the treatment of COVID-19 patients because of dose-dependent adverse reactions (Knowles et al., 2003; Crotty et al., 2002; Khalili et al., 2020).

Antiviral Agent: Favipiravir (RNA-dependent RNA Polymerase Inhibitor)

Developed by Toyama Chemical in 2014 (Japan), favipiravir, the experimental antiviral drug is an RdRp inhibitor. It acts as a molecular mimic by structurally resembling guanine. It was originally developed to deal with diseases like influenza A, influenza B, Ebola, and norovirus infection. Favipiravir (the guanine analog) is known to disrupt viral RNA synthesis by competitively binding in the place of natural guanine, thus disrupting the structure and rendering RdRp ineffective (see Figure 9.4). Clinical trials revealed that the positive effect of favipiravir on critically ill COVID-19 patients was not significant but a range of adverse reactions like gastrointestinal complications (diarrhea, nausea, vomiting, abdominal pain, duodenal ulcer, hematochezia, gastritis), hyperuricemia, increased level of transaminases, decrease in neutrophil count, teratogenic effect and embryotoxicity, hypersensitivity reactions (rashes, eczema, pruritus), hepatic complications (increased AST, increased ALT, increased γ-GTP, hyperbilirubinemia), respiratory complications (asthma, inflammatory condition of upper respiratory tract), metabolic complications (hypokalemia, increased blood triglyceride levels), and disturbed neurological coordination have been documented in relation to the treatment of COVID-19 patients. Favipiravir is still under clinical trial (Lam et al., 2020; Furuta, 2017; McKee et al., 2020).

DRUGS INHIBITING VIRAL PROTEIN SYNTHESIS

Antiviral Agent: Lopinavir-Ritonavir (3CL Protease Inhibitor)

Lopinavir-ritonavir is a combination of two antiviral agents that act as a 3CL protease inhibitor, used in the management of patients suffering from HIV infection. This combination is known to inhibit viral assembly by disrupting the protease activity required for the process. Ritonavir increases and prolongs the activity and bioavailability of lopinavir in patients. In clinical trials, no positive effect was reported in relation to COVID-19 patients but few adverse reactions were

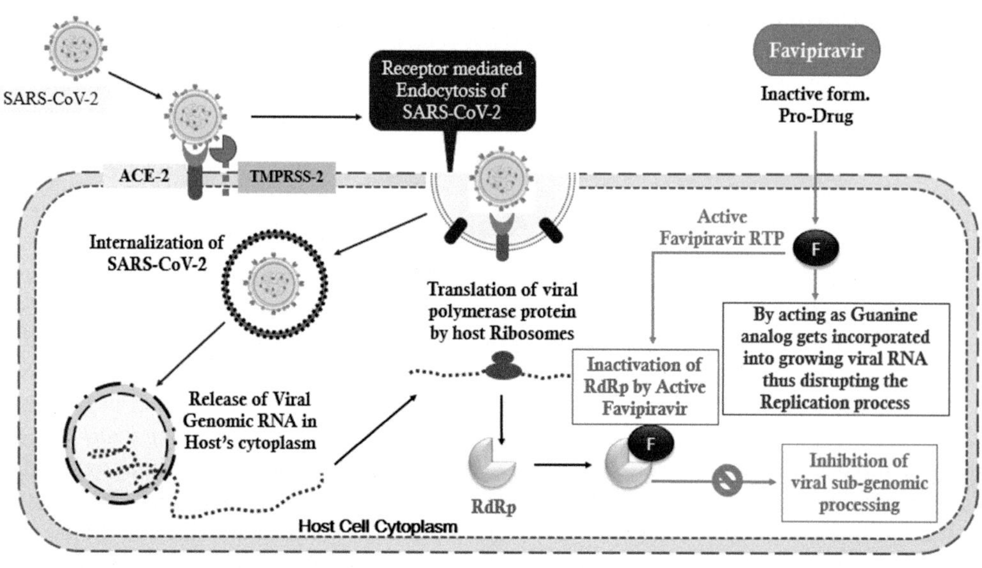

Figure 9.4 Simple representation of the mechanism of action of favipiravir.

documented, which included gastrointestinal complications, increased transaminase level, increased bleeding, hyperlipidemia, hyperglycemia, resistance to insulin, prolonged QT, renal dysfunction, yellowing of skin or eyes, and skin rashes (Chen et al., 2020; Anand, 2003; WHO, 2020a).

Antiviral Agent: Oseltamivir (Neuraminidase Inhibitor)

Oseltamivir, a neuraminidase inhibitor, is an antiviral agent originally implemented for the management of influenza A and influenza B. This antiviral agent under clinical trials failed to show promising results in relation to the treatment of COVID-19 cases with adverse reactions like gastrointestinal complications, arrhythmia, hepatic complications, and anaphylaxis. The research community does not recommend its use for COVID-19 patients as extensive studies are required (Tan et al., 2020; US National Library of Medicine, 2020b).

IMMUNOMODULATORY AND ANTI-INFLAMMATORY AGENTS

Tocilizumab (Interleukin-6 Inhibitor)

Tocilizumab is a humanized monoclonal antibody targeted toward the interleukin-6 receptor (IL-6R) intended to inhibit interleukin-6 activity. It is an immunosuppressive drug approved for addressing conditions like cytokine release syndrome (CRS). The data obtained from ongoing clinical trials are not sufficient enough to make any conclusion about the effectiveness of tocilizumab in the management of COVID-19 cases. The documented adverse reactions include infusion reactions, perforations in the gastrointestinal tract, increased neutrophil levels, decreased platelet count, neutropenia, urinary tract infections, liver complications, painful blistering and rashes on the skin, inflammation of the upper respiratory tract, and stools with blood. Clinical trials for the safety and effectiveness of tocilizumab for COVID-19 are in progress. Figure 9.5 represents the concise mechanism of action of Tocilizumab (Office of the Commissioner, 2021b; Actemra® (Tocilizumab) EUA | Patient, n.d.; Ramiro, 2020; AIFA, 2020).

Interferons (Interferon-α or Interferon-β)

Interferons are immunomodulatory chemicals (cytokines) that may be used as a non-specific antiviral agent. Interferon-α and interferon-β are major pharmacological candidates among others that have shown significant response in the management of COVID-19 patients and are still under clinical trials. The binding of interferon-α and interferon-β to their specific receptors (INF-αR and INF-βR, respectively) leads to the phosphorylation of several transcription factors including STAT-1. The phosphorylated STAT-1 gets translocated into the nucleus where it associates with interferon-stimulated genes (ISGs). This association leads to immunomodulatory and antiviral effects and thus interferes with the viral replication process. Due to a lack of convincing data, the use of interferons for the treatment of COVID-19 patients is not recommended at present (Zhou, 2020; Interferons, 2020; Alavi Darazam et al., 2021).

Plasma Therapy

Plasma containing antibodies specific for SARS-CoV-2 collected from eligible donors who have recovered from COVID-19. Although it has shown some degree of momentary benefit, its inability

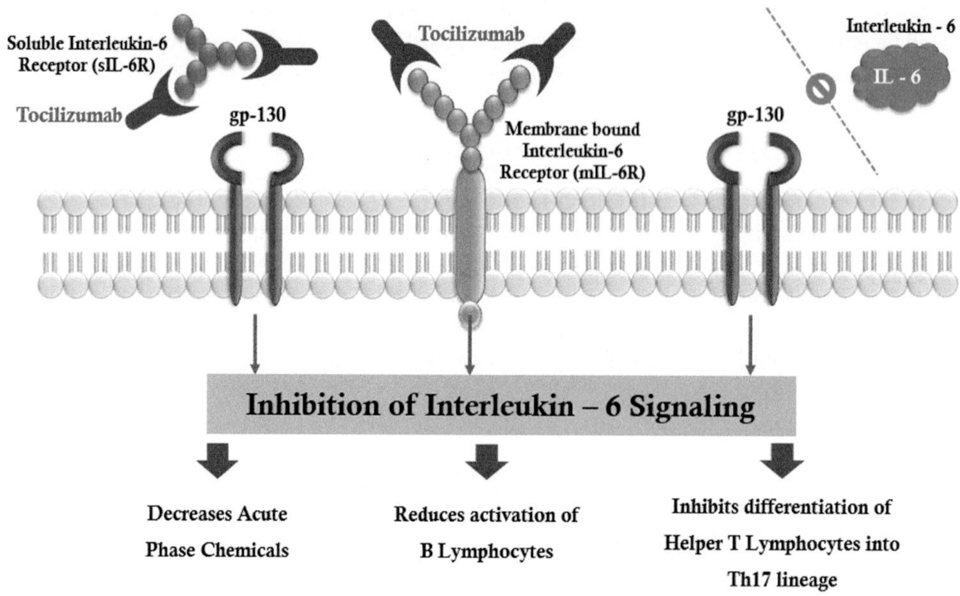

Figure 9.5 Simple representation of the mechanism of action of tocilizumab.

to provide long-term benefits along with the adverse reactions it possesses means that the FDA has not approved its use. The FDA recommended a thorough investigation for the determination of safety and efficacy through regulated clinical trials before declaring it a therapy for COVID-19 (Tang et al., 2020; Coppola, 2020; Office of the Commissioner, 2021a).

NON-ANTIVIRAL/ADJUNCTIVE AGENTS

Azithromycin (Antibacterial Substance)

The antibiotic azithromycin is conventionally used to treat respiratory infections caused by intracellular gram-positive bacteria. This antibiotic was used with other antiviral drugs for synergistic antiviral effects. Under FDA emergency use authorization, azithromycin in combination with hydroxychloroquine was being administered to COVID-19 patients as a primary treatment. This combination showed no significant effects, instead, it was found that the risks of cardiovascular failure and death were increased. Other adverse reactions included gastrointestinal disturbances and hepatotoxicity. The use of azithromycin in combination or standalone is not recommended for COVID-19 patients (Patel et al., 2021; Butler et al., 2021).

Corticosteroids (Cytokine Gene Expression Inhibitors)

Under emergency use authorization, corticosteroids, such as methylprednisolone, were implemented in the management of COVID-19 cases based on the idea that it acts within the lungs, reducing the host inflammatory response, thus providing protection from acute lung injury and ARDS. Corticosteroids are known to suppress cytokine gene expression and are used in the management of pneumonia and severe systemic inflammation. Treatment with corticosteroids leads to iatrogenic immunosuppression, rendering the patient vulnerable to life-threatening secondary infections like mucormycosis. The adverse reactions caused by corticosteroids include weight gain, mood swings, muscle weakness, blurred vision, easy bruising, suppressed immunity, lower resistance to infection, worsening of diabetes, worsening of hypertension, gastrointestinal disturbances, adrenal suppression, and nervous system dysfunction. Minimized doses of corticosteroids may be useful in patients with severe COVID-19 and other clinical indications, such as ARDS, sepsis, or septic shock, but due to a lack of direct evidence, corticosteroids should be implemented with extra caution for managing COVID-19 patients (Russel et al., 2020; Mishra & Mulani, 2021).

Oxygen Therapy

So far, according to experience and knowledge gathered from two waves of the COVID-19 outbreak, oxygen proved the most effective and perhaps only effective drug used. So, the use of oxygen is a must in COVID-19 and the basics of oxygen therapy are given as follows.

Oxygen cascade: Atmosphere (158–150 mmHg) → Alveoli (104 mmHg) → Arterial blood (95–100 mmHg) → Tissue extraction → Venous blood (40 mmHg)

Three terminologies are important in relation to oxygen therapy: anoxia (no oxygen availability in tissue), hypoxia (lack of oxygen availability in tissues), and hypoxemia (lack of oxygen in the blood). Hypoxia is of two types, first, acute hypoxia which includes restlessness, disorientation, confusion, impaired judgment, and second, chronic hypoxia which includes fatigue, drowsiness, decreased work capacity, inattentiveness, apathy, and delayed reaction time. Common effects of both acute and chronic hypoxia include hyperventilation, air hunger, and circulatory changes. To maintain adequate tissue oxygenation while minimizing cardiopulmonary work is the main goal of managing COVID-19 cases with hypoxia/hypoxemia. Indications for oxygen therapy include acute hypoxia ($PaO_2 < 60$ mmHg or $SpO_2 < 92\%$), arrest (cardiac or respiratory), idiopathic hypotension, low cardiac output with metabolic acidosis, and respiratory distress with $SpO_2 < 92\%$. The low flow variable performance devices include nasal cannulas, nasal catheters, and trans-tracheal catheters. Reservoir systems include reservoir cannulas, simple face masks, partial rebreathing masks, non-rebreathing masks, and tracheostomy masks. The high-flow fixed performance devices include ventimask (HAFOE), aerosol masks, and T-piece with nebulizers. The toxicity of normobaric oxygen may lead to pulmonary complications (like atelectasis and alveolar collapse), cardiac complications (depressed contractility and decreased cardiac output), vasoconstriction, V/Q changes, a reduced buffering capacity of blood, CO_2 narcosis, retrolental fibroplasia, and suppressed hemopoiesis. Toxicity of normobaric oxygen occurs if there is 100% oxygen given for more than 12 hours, 80% oxygen given for more than 24 hours, or 60% oxygen given for more than 36 hours. It is to be understood that oxygen is a drug. When appropriately used, it is extremely beneficial but when misused or abused, it is potentially harmful (Oxygenation and Ventilation, 2021; Daher et al., 2021).

CHALLENGES IN DRUG DEVELOPMENT FOR COVID-19

In conventional systems of medicine, studying the effects of experimental drugs on animal models is essential to understand the mechanisms of action and safety and efficacy issues. At present, cell culture methods are used for pharmacological studies but they are not as significant as actual animal models. Since present research of COVID-19 experimental drugs is being performed on Vero cells, their outcome in actual clinical settings (when applied to patients) varies greatly. Also, all the drugs mentioned in the previous sections are not proven for effectivity on COVID-19 and are currently under clinical trials. All the experimental drugs were implemented under emergency use authorization. To date, no drug has been available with international recommendations. Besides, due to their documented adverse reactions on patients, these drugs cannot be used directly against COVID-19. Furthermore, physiological changes must be considered, which arise because of drug action. Cytotoxicity is one of the major assays performed in cases of drug development as it determines the viability of cells against the developed drug. Being popular drugs used to treat COVID-19, both chloroquine and hydroxychloroquine are reported to cause ventricular dysrhythmias, hyperkalemia, and systemic lupus erythematosus (SLE) in cases of abnormal dosages. In addition to this, many of the drugs have not cleared QT analysis, which is essential for the normal functioning of ECG, including hydroxychloroquine. Considering these factors, the need to identify a potential drug has been the need of the hour. Alongside the dosage aspects, treating COVID-19 patients with non-COVID-19 diseases/disorders becomes hectic due to the drug–drug reactions between COVID-19 and non-COVID-19 therapeutic agents. As a result, patients who can be successfully tested for drug use against COVID-19 cannot be tested for other drugs because of the effect of other non-COVID-19 therapeutic agents. Therefore, it becomes difficult to accurately analyze the pharmacological effect of a COVID-19 drug in the presence of a non-COVID-19 drug. As of December 2021, no drug is available in conventional medicine that helps prevent, treat, and manage COVID-19 patients (Clinical Management Protocol: Covid-19, 2020; Li et al., 2020; Shi et al., 2020).

REFERENCES

Actemra® (tocilizumab) EUA | Patient. (n.d.). *Actemra*. Retrieved November 24, 2021, from https://www.actemra.com/covid-19.html

AIFA Covid 19: studio randomizzato italiano, nessun beneficio dal tocilizumab 18 giugno 2020. Available from: https://www.aifa.gov. it/-/covid-19-studio-randomizzato-italiano-nessun-beneficio-dal-tocilizumab. Accessed December 14, 2020.

Alavi Darazam, I., Shokouhi, S., Pourhoseingholi, M.A., Naghibi Irvani, S.S., Mokhtari, M., Shabani, M., Amirdosara, M., Torabinavid, P., Golmohammadi, M., Hashemi, S., Azimi, A., Jafarazadeh Maivan, M.H., Rezaei, O., Zali, A., Hajiesmaeili, M., Shabanpour Dehbsneh, H., Hoseyni Kusha, A., Taleb Shoushtari, M., Khalili, N., … Khoshkar, A.. Role of interferon therapy in severe COVID-19: the COVIFERON randomized controlled trial. *Sci. Rep.* 2021;11(1). https://doi.org/10.1038/s41598-021-86859-y

Al-Tawfiq, J.A., Al-Homoud, A.H., & Memish, Z.A.. Remdesivir as a possible therapeutic option for the COVID-19. *Travel. Med. Infect. Dis.* 2020;34:101615. https://doi.org/10.1016/j.tmaid.2020.101615

Anand, K., Ziebuhr, J., Wadhwani, P., Mesters, J.R., & Hilgenfeld, R. Coronavirus main proteinase (3CLpro) structure: basis for design of anti-SARS drugs. *Science.* 2003;300(5626):1763–1767. doi:https://doi.org/10.1126/science.1085658

Available from: https://emergency.cdc.gov/coca/ppt/2020/V4_Combined_Critically-Ill-Adults-COCA-4.2.2020.pdf. Accessed December 14, 2020.

Booth, C.M., Matukas, L.M., Tomlinson, G.A., et al. Clinical features and short-term outcomes of 144 patients with SARS in the greater Toronto area. *JAMA* 2003;289(21):2801–2809.

Browning, D.J. (2014) Pharmacology of chloroquine and hydroxychloroquine. In: *Hydroxychloroquine and Chloroquine Retinopathy.* Springer, New York. https://doi.org/10.1007/978-1-4939-0597-3_2

Butler, C.C., Dorward, J., Yu, L.M., Gbinigie, O., Hayward, G., Saville, B.R., van Hecke, O., Berry, N., Detry, M., Saunders, C., Fitzgerald, M., Harris, V., Patel, M.G., de Lusignan, S., Ogburn, E., Evans, P.H.,

Thomas, N.P., & Hobbs, F.R. Azithromycin for community treatment of suspected COVID-19 in people at increased risk of an adverse clinical course in the UK (PRINCIPLE): a randomised, controlled, open-label, adaptive platform trial. *Lancet* 2021;397(10279):1063–1074. https://doi.org/10.1016/s0140-6736(21)00461-x

Cai, Q., Yang, M., Liu, D., Chen, J., Shu, D., Xia, J., Liao, X., Gu, Y., Cai, Q., Yang, Y., Shen, C., Li, X., Peng, L., Huang, D., Zhang, J., Zhang, S., Wang, F., Liu, J., Chen, L., Chen, S., … Liu, L. Experimental treatment with favipiravir for COVID-19: An open-label control study. *Engineering (Beijing, China).* 2020;6(10):1192–1198. https://doi.org/10.1016/j.eng.2020.03.007

Calabrese, F., Pezzuto, F., Fortarezza, F., et al. Pulmonary pathology and COVID-19: lessons from autopsy. The experience of European Pulmonary Pathologists. *Virchows Arch.* 2020;477(3):359–372.

Chan, J.F., Yuan, S., Kok, K.H., et al. A familial cluster of pneumonia associated with the 2019 novel coronavirus indicating person-to-person transmission: a study of a family cluster. *Lancet.* 2020;395(10223):514–23.

Chen, Y.W., Yiu, C.B., & Wong, K.Y. Prediction of the SARS-CoV-2 (2019-nCoV) 3C-like protease (3CL (pro)) structure: virtual screening reveals velpatasvir, ledipasvir, and other drug repurposing candidates. *F1000Res.* 2020;9:129.

Clinical Management Protocol: Covid-19; Government of India; Ministry of Health and Family Welfare Directorate General of Health Services (EMR Division) Version 3; 13.06.20.

Coppola, A., Lombardi, M., Tassoni, M.I., et al. COVID-19, thromboembolic risk and thromboprophylaxis: learning lessons from the bedside, awaiting evidence. *Blood Transfus.* 2020;18(3):226–229. doi:10.2450/2020.0113-20

Crotty, S., Cameron, C., & Andino, R. Ribavirin's antiviral mechanism of action: lethal mutagenesis? *J. Mol. Med.* 2002; 80(2):86–95.

Daher, A., Balfanz, P., Aetou, M., Hartmann, B., Müller-Wieland, D., Müller, T., Marx, N., Dreher, M., & Cornelissen, C.G.. Clinical course of COVID-19 patients needing supplemental oxygen outside the intensive care unit. *Sci. Rep.* 2021;11(1). https://doi.org/10.1038/s41598-021-81444-9

Dey, S., Saini, M., Dhembla, C., et al. Suramin, penciclovir and anidulafungin bind Nsp12, which governs the RNA-dependent- RNA polymerase activity of Sars-cov-2, with similar interaction energy as remdesivir-triphosphate, indicating potential in the treatment of COVID-19 infection. OSF. 2020. doi:10.31219/osf.io/ urxwh

Dutta, J., Goswami, S., & Mitra, A. *COVID-19 and Emerging Environmental Trends: A Way Forward* (1st ed.). CRC Press. 2020. https://doi.org/10.1201/9781003108887

EMA. COVID-19: reminder of risk serious side effects with chloroquine and hydroxychloroquine. (2020, June 19). European Medicines Agency. Retrieved November 3, 2021, from https://www.ema.europa.eu/en/news/covid-19-reminder-risk-serious-side-effects-chloroquine-hydroxychloroquine

Furuta, Y., Komeno, T., & Nakamura, T. Favipiravir (T-705), a broad spectrum inhibitor of viral RNA polymerase. *Proc. Japan. Acad. Ser. B.* 2017;93(7):449–463.

Huang, D., Yu, H., Wang, T., Yang, H., Yao, R., & Liang, Z. Efficacy and safety of umifenovir for coronavirus disease 2019 (COVID-19): a systematic review and meta-analysis. *J. Med. Virol.* 2021;93(1):481–490. https://doi.org/10.1002/jmv.26256

Interferons. (2020, August 27). *COVID-19 Treatment Guidelines.* Retrieved November 24, 2021, from https://www.covid19treatmentguidelines.nih.gov/therapies/immunomodulators/interferons/

Khalili, J.S., Zhu, H., Mak, N.S.A., Yan, Y., & Zhu, Y.. Novel coronavirus treatment with ribavirin: groundwork for an evaluation concerning COVID-19. *J. Med. Virol.* 2020;92(7):740–746. https://doi.org/10.1002/jmv.25798

Knowles, S.R., Phillips, E.J., Dresser, L., & Matukas, L. Common adverse events associated with the use of ribavirin for severe acute respiratory syndrome in Canada. *Clin. Infect. Dis.* 2003;37(8):1139–1142.

Lam, S., Lombardi, A., & Ouanounou, A.. COVID-19: a review of the proposed pharmacological treatments. *Eur. J. Pharmacol.* 2020;886:173451. https://doi.org/10.1016/j.ejphar.2020.173451

Li, H., Liu, S.M., Yu, X.H., Tang, S.L., & Tang, K. Coronavirus disease 2019 (COVID-19): current status and future perspectives. *Int. J. Antimicrobial. Agents.* 2020; 55 (5):105951.

Lo, M.K., Feldmann, F., Gary, J.M., et al. Remdesivir (GS-5734) protects African green monkeys from Nipah virus challenge. *Sci. Transl. Med.* 2019;11(494):eaau9242.

McKee, D.L., Sternberg, A., Stange, U., Laufer, S., & Naujokat, C.. Candidate drugs against SARS-CoV-2 and COVID-19. *Pharmacol. Res.* 2020;157:104859. https://doi.org/10.1016/j.phrs.2020.104859

Mishra, G.P., & Mulani, J. Corticosteroids for COVID-19: the search for an optimum duration of therapy. *Lancet Resp. Med.* 2021;9(1):e8. https://doi.org/10.1016/s2213-2600(20)30530-0

Nojomi, M., Yassin, Z., Keyvani, H. et al. Effect of Arbidol (Umifenovir) on COVID-19: a randomized controlled trial. *BMC Infect Dis* 2020;20:954. https://doi.org/10.1186/s12879-020-05698-w

Office of the Commissioner. (2020, June 15). Coronavirus (COVID-19) update: FDA revokes emergency use authorization for chloroquine and hydroxychloroquine. US Food and Drug Administration. Retrieved November 3, 2021, from https://www.fda.gov/news-events/press-announcements/coronavirus-covid-19-update-fda-revokes-emergency-use-authorization-chloroquine-and

Office of the Commissioner. (2021a, February 4). *FDA In Brief: FDA Updates Emergency Use Authorization for COVID-19 Convalescent Plasma to Reflect New Data*. US Food and Drug Administration. Retrieved November 23, 2021, from https://www.fda.gov/news-events/fda-brief/fda-brief-fda-updates-emergency-use-authorization-covid-19-convalescent-plasma-reflect-new-data

Office of the Commissioner. (2021b, June 24). *Coronavirus (COVID-19) Update: FDA Authorizes Drug for Treatment of COVID-19*. US Food and Drug Administration. Retrieved November 24, 2021, from https://www.fda.gov/news-events/press-announcements/coronavirus-covid-19-update-fda-authorizes-drug-treatment-covid-19

Oxygenation and Ventilation. (2021, October 19). *COVID-19 Treatment Guidelines*. Retrieved November 23, 2021, from https://www.covid19treatmentguidelines.nih.gov/management/critical-care/oxygenation-and-ventilation/

Patel, J., Berezowski, I., Abdelmonem, A., Taylor, D., & Pourmand, A. Azithromycin for mild-to-moderate COVID-19. *Lancet Resp. Med.* 2021;9(10):e99. https://doi.org/10.1016/s2213-2600(21)00379-9

Qingxian. A trial of lopinavir–titonavir in Covid-1. *N. Engl. J. Med.* 2020; 382(21):e68. https://doi.org/10.1056/nejmc2008043

Ramiro, S., Mostard, R.L.M., Magro-Checa, C., et al. Historically controlled comparison of glucocorticoids with or without tocilizumab versus supportive care only in patients with COVID-19-associated cytokine storm syndrome: results of the CHIC study. *Ann Rheum Dis.* 2020;79(9):1143–1151.107.

Russell, C.D., Millar, J.E., & Baillie, J.K. Clinical evidence does not support corticosteroid treatment for 2019-nCoV lung injury. *Lancet.* 2020;395(10223):473–475.

Shereen, M.A., Khan, S., Kazmi, A., et al. COVID-19 infection: origin, transmission, and characteristics of human coronaviruses. *J. Adv. Res.* 2020;24:91–98.

Shi, J., Xiao, Y., Zhang, Y., Geng, D., Cong, D., Shi, K.X., & Knapp, R.J. Challenges of drug development during the COVID-19 pandemic: key considerations for clinical trial designs. *Br. J. Clin. Pharmacol.*, 2020;87(5):2170–2185. https://doi.org/10.1111/bcp.14629

Tan, Q., Duan, L., Ma, Y., Wu, F., Huang, Q., Mao, K., Xiao, W., Xia, H., Zhang, S., Zhou, E., Ma, P., Song, S., Li, Y., Zhao, Z., Sun, Y., Li, Z., Geng, W., Yin, Z., & Jin, Y. Is oseltamivir suitable for fighting against COVID-19: in silico assessment, in vitro and retrospective study. *Bioorg. Chem.* 2020;104:104257. https://doi.org/10.1016/j.bioorg.2020.104257

Tang, N., Bai, H., Chen, X., et al. Anticoagulant treatment is associated with decreased mortality in severe coronavirus disease 2019 patients with coagulopathy. *J. Thromb Haemost.* 2020;18(5):1094–1099.

US National Library of Medicine. Umifenovir in Hospitalized COVID-19 Patients – Full Text View – ClinicalTrials.gov. (2020a, April 20). US National Library of Medicine. Retrieved November 22, 2021, from https://clinicaltrials.gov/ct2/show/NCT04350684

US National Library of Medicine. *Hydroxychloroquine, Oseltamivir and Azithromycin for the Treatment of COVID-19 Infection: An RCT – Full Text View – ClinicalTrials.gov.* (2020b, July 15). US National Library of Medicine. Retrieved November 24, 2021, from https://clinicaltrials.gov/ct2/show/NCT04338698

Wang, W., Xu, Y., Gao, R., et al. Detection of SARS-CoV-2 in different types of clinical specimens. *JAMA.* 2020;323(18):1843–1844. https://doi.org/10.1001/jama.2020.3786

WHO. *WHO discontinues hydroxychloroquine and lopinavir/ritonavir treatment arms for COVID-19.* (2020a, July 4). World Health Organization. Retrieved November 24, 2021, from https://www.who.int/news/item/04-07-2020-who-discontinues-hydroxychloroquine-and-lopinavir-ritonavir-treatment-arms-for-covid-19

WHO. (2020b, November 20). *WHO recommends against the use of remdesivir in COVID-19 patients*. World Health Organization. Retrieved November 24, 2021, from https://www.who.int/news-room/feature-stories/detail/who-recommends-against-the-use-of-remdesivir-in-covid-19-patients

Wrapp, D., Wang, N., Corbett, K.S., et al. Cryo-EM structure of the 2019-nCoV spike in the prefusion conformation. *Science* (80). 2020;67(6483):1260–1263.

Wu, C., Chen, X., Cai, Y., et al. Risk factors associated with acute respiratory distress syndrome and death in patients with coronavirus disease 2019 pneumonia in Wuhan, China. *JAMA Intern Med.* 2020;180(7):1–11.

Yang, P., & Wang, X. COVID-19: a new challenge for human beings. *Cell. Mol. Immunol.* 2020;17(5):555–557.

Zhou, Q., Chen, V., Shannon, C.P., et al. Interferon-α2b treatment for COVID-19. *Front Immunol.* 2020;11:1061.

Chapter 10

Research and Development for COVID-19 Vaccines

Srijan Goswami* and Ushmita Gupta Bakshi

CONTENTS

INTRODUCTION

The COVID–19 pandemic has caused fear and concern regarding global health safety. Scientists and policymakers around the world are currently working in collaboration to find out evidence-based treatments and ways of implementing them in order to treat patients with COVID–19. Globally, institutions, pharmaceutical companies, universities, non-government organizations, and several groups of independent researchers are involved in the research and development of vaccines, new antiviral agents, medical devices, and so on (Naqvi et al., 2020).

Since the beginning of the COVID–19 pandemic, scientists all around the world have been working tirelessly with the sole aim of developing a permanent treatment for COVID–19. Several kinds of approaches are being implemented and have been put to trial for the development of a vaccine for COVID–19. Even if the scientific community is progressing with speed, the process

DOI: 10.1201/9781003178514-12

of vaccine development takes time. It is the responsibility of vaccine regulatory authorities to make sure the vaccine is safe for humans before it is approved for therapeutic use. All vaccines go through a rigorous process to make sure they are safe and effective. Vaccine effectivity and safety are assessed through clinical trials having multiple phases. Currently, the vaccines developed by Pfizer-BioNTech, Moderna, and AstraZeneca-Oxford are authorized for emergency use in the prevention of COVID-19 by the Food and Drug Administration (FDA), United States (Office of the Commissioner, 2021).

The world has witnessed a concerning and unprecedented rat race for the development of COVID-19 vaccines, fueled by a sense of global competition to become the "first COVID-19 vaccine developer" or to claim the title of "number one" at any cost. This tight race against time for the development of COVID-19 vaccines is not a healthy scientific practice and opens up avenues for scientific studies to be guided by a sense of greed, economic profit, and global monopoly. The sheer volume of expected sales for such a vaccine at the moment is breathtaking. It is a big-money game running into billions of dollars. Hence, it is not a surprise that many companies want to win this jackpot. But these aspects must not distract the scientific community from the path of honesty and integrity. Dr. Sreejith Rajasekharan, virologist at the Laboratory of Molecular Virology, International Center for Genetic Engineering and Biotechnology, Italy, mentioned in an interview that due to the severity of the circumstances, companies are requesting the FDA for an early deployment of vaccines even before the clinical trials end. The scientific data provided by these companies thus far show that their respective vaccines are indeed effective. However, the current clinical trials being carried out are not double-blind, and therefore there is an ethical responsibility to let the volunteers know whether they are in the placebo group or not once the study becomes unblind. Dr. Rajasekharan also clarified that nobody can be directly blamed in this context because the demand and pressure are unprecedented from various interest groups. As soon as the vaccine will be made available, these volunteers have the right to take the vaccine, and therefore can no longer be included in the control group. If too many volunteers cross over, the study might not have sufficiently large control groups to obtain statistically significant results for certain long-term goals (Deccan Chronicle, 2021).

This race for the vaccine has several challenges and ethical issues such as compressed timelines, generation and proper management of resources and finances, risks to the participating volunteers due to the curtailed research trial processes, geopolitical contentions, misinformation through social media, and a parallel race with drugs. The scientific community feel that the fundamental principles of ethics – autonomy, beneficence, non-maleficence, and justice – should not be violated in this hastened vaccine development process (Kamble & Dubhashi, 2020). The standard vaccine development cycle, including research and development (phase I to IV of clinical trials), manufacturing, approvals, licensing, distribution, and deployment take several years. But the COVID-19 pandemic storm has compressed the timelines of coronavirus vaccine development to a few months. The major threat to the compressed timeline is curtailment and compromise in different steps of research and development. Many manufacturing companies have started mass production of vaccines, accepting the risk of failure of vaccines during trials. Others are working with regulators in multiple countries simultaneously, looking for the quickest path to market (Kamble & Dubhashi, 2020; Thanh Le et al., 2020; Deccan Chronicle., 2021).

This chapter covers the research and development of potential vaccines and their merits and demerits in relation to COVID–19. It is to be understood that research and development are progressing at a rapid pace and new data are becoming available every day, thus the information presented here about vaccine research may change over time.

VACCINES FOR COVID-19: THE PHASES OF DEVELOPMENT

We all talk about vaccines but rarely do we realize the steps that a candidate vaccine goes through to receive FDA approval (in this case emergency use authorization [EUA]). Although there are several intricate stages of vaccine development, two of them are particularly important (in relation to EUA) and will be discussed in this section (CDC, 2014; COVID-19 Vaccination, 2020; Juda, 2021).

- **Safety** is the first goal of vaccine development and is of utmost priority. This stage is implemented to make sure any side effects are monitored. Any serious or deadly side effects related to the vaccine are observed and documented (CDC, 2014; COVID-19 Vaccination, 2020; Juda, 2021).
- **Efficacy** is the second and equally important goal of vaccine development. Efficacy can be thought of in two ways, efficacy of the vaccines to prevent infection and efficacy of the vaccines to prevent disease. COVID-19, the disease caused by SARS-CoV-2, either may present with symptoms ranging from mild to moderate to critical, where hospitalization and emergency care are required, or they could be completely asymptomatic and not develop mild, moderate, or severe cases. Ensuring the effectiveness of vaccines in preventing disease severity or preventing asymptomatic infections is very important. The primary focus of COVID-19 vaccine development is on the efficacy of the vaccine for protection from the disease (CDC, 2014; COVID-19 Vaccination, 2020; Juda, 2021).

The following are the fundamental stages of vaccine development in reference to the assessment of safety and efficacy (CDC, 2014; COVID-19 Vaccination, 2020; Juda, 2021):

1. **Exploratory stage**. This is the first and research-intensive stage in the development of any kind of vaccine. The objective of this stage is to identify antigens or chemical molecules that might help prevent or treat a disease condition.
2. **Pre-clinical stage.** This is primarily a phase where the testing on cell-culture systems, tissue-culture systems, and laboratory animals is performed. If animal testing is found to be safe and effective, the study is moved to the human trial.
3. **Clinical stage**. A human trial is performed in the clinical stage. The organization performing the study registers a detailed proposal for an investigational new drug (IND) to the FDA that includes the findings to date and an explanation of how the candidate vaccine will be created and tested. The approval process is performed by the expert review group of the FDA and may take around 30 days. Once the proposal has been approved, the candidate vaccine must qualify through three phases.
   a. **Phase 1**. A human trial is performed on a small population size. The primary aim of this stage determines whether the candidate vaccine is safe for humans, and also document the spectrum of responses it generates on the test subjects. If it is found to be effective and safe, the study is taken to phase 2.
   b. **Phase 2**. A human trial is performed on a larger sample size as compared with phase 1. If still safe and effective, the study is taken to phase 3.
   c. **Phase 3**. Contains a larger human population compared with phase 2.
4. **Approval stage**. Finally, if it has met all the safety and effectiveness goals it had planned for safety and efficacy, it is sent for FDA approval. In this case, because of the COVID-19 pandemic, we are looking for EUA. This will be followed by follow-up studies.
5. **Manufacturing and distribution.** The governing and regulatory authorities have ensured the timely manufacturing and distribution of vaccines that have received FDA approval or EUA.

6. **Tracking safety using vaccine monitoring systems.** As vaccines are distributed outside clinical trials under EUA, several systems and protocols for tracking the safety of vaccines in real-time have been implemented. Regulatory authorities like the CDC and the FDA are closely monitoring safety issues through centralized reporting systems like the Vaccine Adverse Event Reporting System (VAERS), the Vaccine Safety Datalink (VSD), and V-safe. This step is implemented to ensure vaccine safety and efficacy as they are being given to the global population in real-world settings (Figure 10.1).

PRE-CLINICAL STAGE

In the pre-clinical stage, the candidate vaccines are tested on cell-culture, tissue-culture systems, and laboratory animals. It consists of the following important events.

1. Administration of candidate vaccines to laboratory animals.
2. Monitoring of adverse drug reactions.
3. Monitoring of efficacy.
4. Intentional introduction of virus (SARS-CoV-2) into test animals.
5. Final observation (ensuring whether the candidate vaccine is able to prevent disease development in test animals) (Figure 10.2).

The candidate vaccines are administered to laboratory animals (like mice or primates) and observed for any kind of adverse effects (like skin irritation, fatigue, fever, or death). Alongside the safety studies, the efficacy of the candidate vaccine is also monitored in the laboratory animals, as are any positive reactions like the development of desired antibodies and their effectiveness in combating the disease (COVID-19). After the laboratory animals are injected with the candidate vaccines, they are intentionally infected with the virus against which the vaccine effectiveness is being monitored. The test animals are monitored to ensure whether the candidate vaccine can prevent the disease. If the outcome of the assessment in this pre-clinical stage is positive, the candidate vaccine is taken to the next stage of vaccine development (CDC, 2014; COVID-19 Vaccination, 2020; Juda, 2021) (Figures 10.3 and 10.4).

CLINICAL STAGE

The clinical stage is performed on humans (volunteers enrolled for clinical trials) and contains three phases:

- **Phase I.** In phase I of a clinical trial, the candidate vaccines are tested on humans. The sample size is very small in this phase and may consist of generally less than 100 participants. The participants must be healthy and not have any comorbidities or underlying illnesses because the aim is to ensure that it is the candidate vaccine that causes any kind of adverse reaction leading to vaccine-induced disease conditions. Alongside the vaccine-induced adverse drug reactions, the optimum and effective dosage (the upper limit and lower limit) are also monitored. If the outcome of phase I is found to be fruitful, the study is taken to phase II (CDC, 2014; COVID-19 Vaccination, 2020; Juda, 2021).

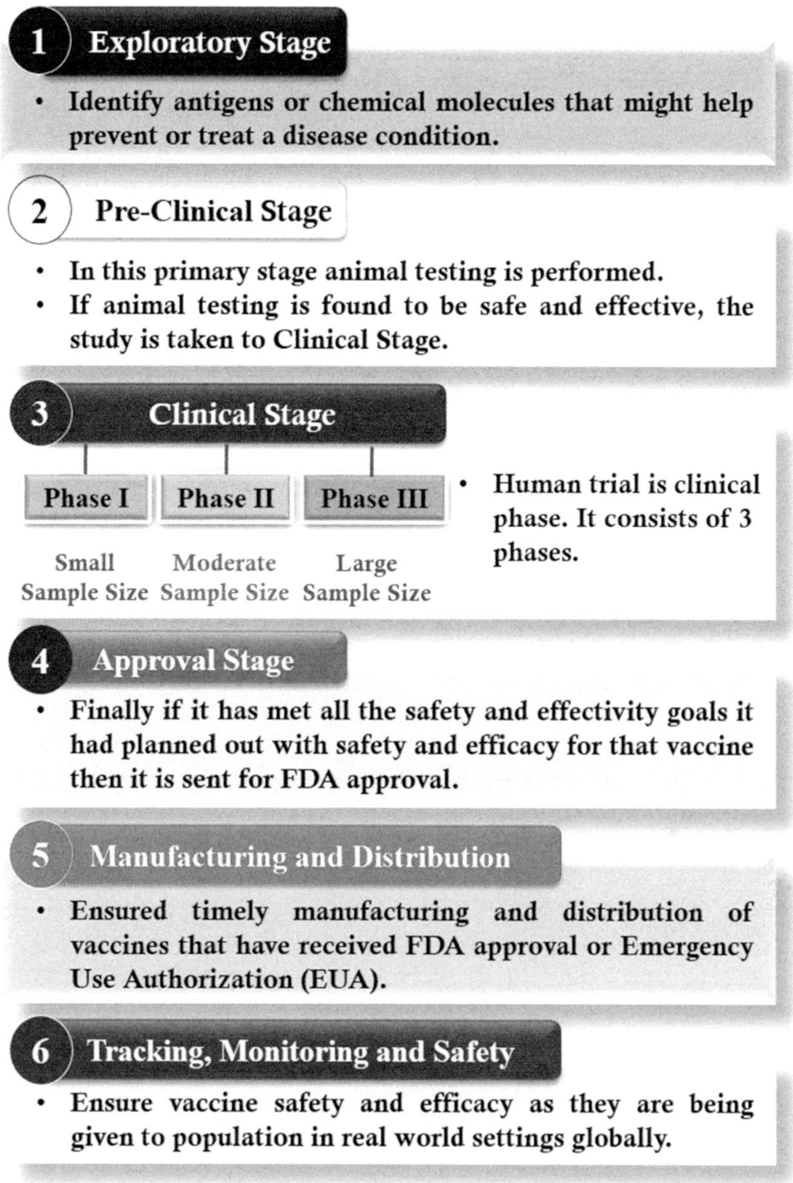

Figure 10.1 Major phases of vaccine development.

- **Phase II**. Phase II is a human trial but with a moderate sample (~100 to 1000 patients) size as compared with phase I. The volunteers are recruited to match the demographics like age, race, gender, and underlying comorbidities. In this phase, healthy individuals are not considered as volunteers, instead, the candidate vaccines are administered to individuals with health conditions or underlying comorbidities. These kinds of

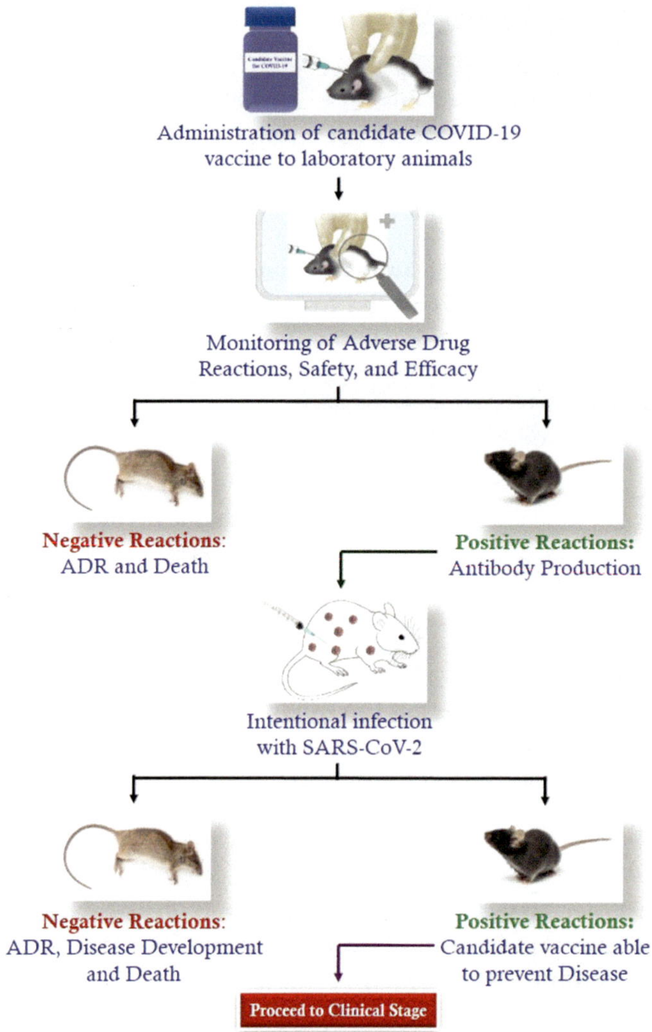

Figure 10.2 The pre-clinical stage of vaccine development.

demographic analyses provide a better statistical representation of the possible outcome. In phase II, the first aim is to monitor and document the adverse vaccine reactions (if any) and ensure the effectiveness and efficacy of dosage limits recorded in phase I. If the outcome of phase II is found to be fruitful, the study is taken to phase III (CDC, 2014; COVID-19 Vaccination, 2020; Juda, 2021).

- **Phase III.** Phase III is a human trial but with a large sample (~1000 to 10,000 patients) size as compared with phases I and II. This phase is critical for receiving approval from the Food and Drug Administration (FDA) for EUA. The major criteria for selection at this phase are that the demographics of the recruited volunteers should match with the demography of the people receiving the vaccine after the approval. Individuals with

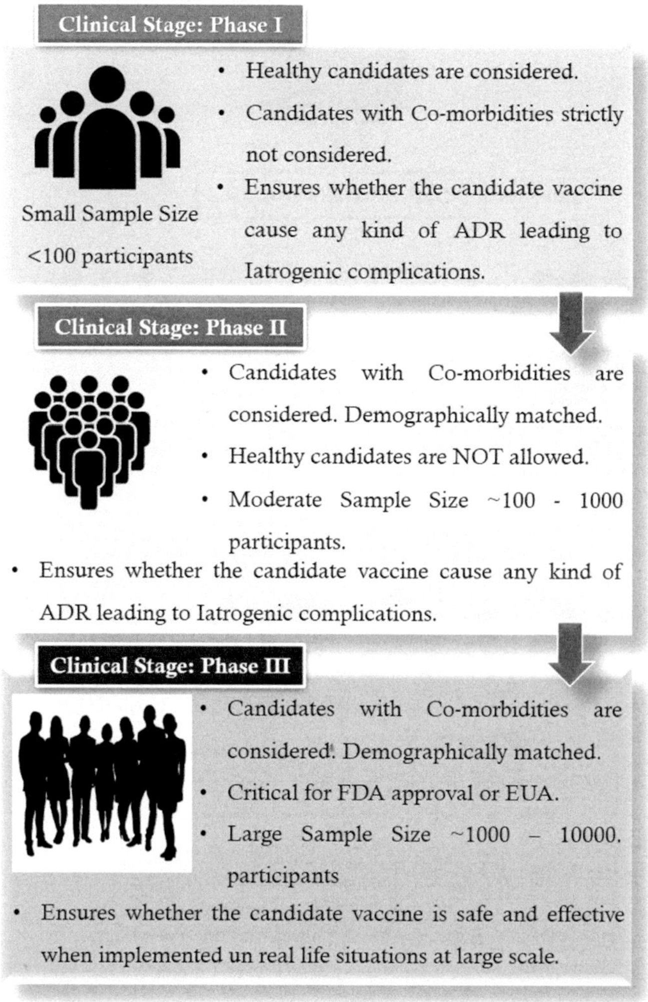

Figure 10.3 Phases of the clinical stage of vaccine development.

health conditions or underlying comorbidities are recruited. This kind of demographic analysis provides a better statistical representation of the possible outcomes than obtained through phase II. The goal is to record the safety and efficacy of the candidate vaccines in real-life situations.

The candidate vaccines are administered to volunteers, following that, they are allowed to go out and perform all their normal daily activities. During this time span, the volunteers are monitored by the organization(s) performing the trials for symptoms and deviations from health, followed by RT-PCR testing to confirm the diagnosis. The objective of these real-life monitoring situations is to ensure some of the volunteers went out in the real world doing normal daily activities and contracted the disease. Alongside the vaccinated volunteer group, another group called the placebo group or

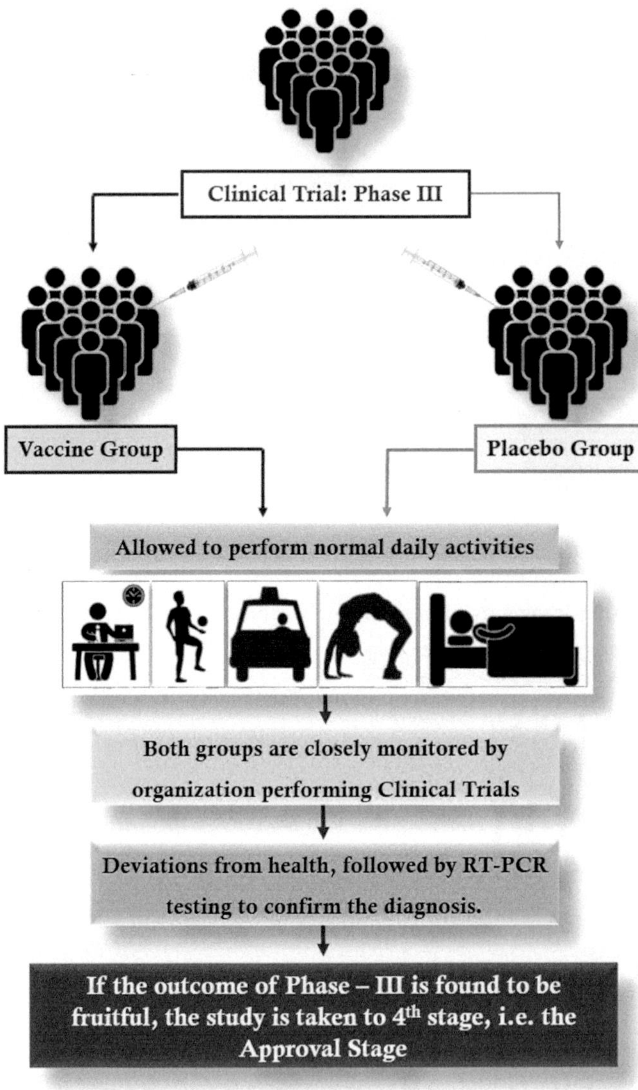

Figure 10.4 General representation of various steps involved in vaccine clinical trials.

the control group is also taken into consideration. Instead of active candidate vaccines, non-medicinal substances or saline are administered to individuals in the placebo/control group, following that, they are allowed to go out and perform all their normal daily activities (like individuals of the vaccine group). During this time span, the individuals of the placebo/control group are monitored by the organization(s) performing the trials for any kind of symptoms and deviations from health, followed by RT-PCR testing to confirm the diagnosis. If the outcome of phase III is found to be fruitful, the study is taken to the fourth stage, i.e., the approval stage (CDC, 2014; COVID-19 Vaccination, 2020; Juda, 2021).

APPROVAL STAGE

Once the candidate vaccine has gone through all these stages and the safety and efficacy are confirmed (in an evidence-based manner), then it is considered for FDA approval or EUA. Following formal approval and authorization by the concerned authorities, the vaccine can be administered to the general population (CDC, 2014; COVID-19 Vaccination, 2020; Juda, 2021).

COVID-19 VACCINES: MECHANISM OF ACTION

As of August 2021, the vaccines developed by Moderna, Pfizer-BioNTech, and AstraZeneca-Oxford are approved for use under EUA. In this section, we will discuss how these vaccines produce an immune response inside the recipient. Moderna and Pfizer-BioNTech implement mRNA technology for developing vaccines but AstraZeneca-Oxford uses viral vector (genetically modified virus) as the basic ingredient of their vaccines.

Moderna and Pfizer-BioNTech Vaccines

Moderna and Pfizer-BioNTech use mRNA technology for preparing their vaccines. For developing COVID-19 vaccines, the therapeutic mRNA is wrapped around a lipid nanoparticle (a phospholipid bilayer). The phospholipid nanoparticle acts as a vehicle or transport mechanism for therapeutic mRNA into the recipient cells. The therapeutic mRNA is obtained from the SARS-CoV-2 spike protein gene, as this particular surface protein is involved with infection and pathogenicity. The reverse genetic technology has been implemented to trace the corresponding mRNA sequence from the SARS-CoV-2 spike protein itself. Then the SARS-CoV-2 spike protein mRNA is incorporated inside a phospholipid nanoparticle and used as the functional component of their COVID-19 vaccines.

After injection, the phospholipid nanoparticle containing the therapeutic mRNA infects the recipient's cell by fusing with the recipient's cell membrane. Following the fusion of phospholipid nanoparticles from vaccines with the recipient's cell membrane, the therapeutic mRNA (for the spike protein) is released into the cytoplasm. The researchers reported that the therapeutic mRNA from the vaccine does not get incorporated inside the recipient's DNA. Instead, the mRNA (from the vaccine) interacts with the recipient cell's ribosomes (on rough endoplasmic reticulum) for synthesizing viral proteins (in this case, the spike protein of SARS-CoV-2) through the process of translation. The newly synthesized viral protein particles are expressed on the membrane of the recipient's cells through the process of antigen presentation. The newly synthesized viral protein (the antigen) is presented through two types of cell surface receptors: major histocompatibility complex class-I (MHC-I) and major histocompatibility complex class-II (MHC-II). In human beings, the MHC-II surface molecules are present on the antigen-presenting cells (APCs) such as the dendritic cells, macrophages, and B lymphocytes, while the MHC-I surface molecules are found in all nucleated cells. When the newly synthesized viral protein (the antigen) is presented by the receptors on the recipient cells, the other cells and molecules of the immune system are activated and attracted toward the site. A type of lymphocyte called the helper T lymphocyte (T_H cells) binds to the newly synthesized viral protein (presented by MHC-II) using a structure called T-cell receptor (TCR) present on its surface. The helper T lymphocytes have another cell surface protein called cluster of differentiation 4 (CD4+) that interacts directly with the MHC-II protein presenting the antigen. The synchronized interaction between antigen-TCR and MHC-II-CD4+ strengthens the interaction and activates the helper T lymphocytes. When activated, the helper T lymphocytes start producing and releasing a range of cytokines, mainly interleukin-2, interleukin-4, interleukin-5, interleukin-10, transforming growth factor-β, tumor necrosis factor, and interferon-γ, which performs several critical roles in mediating the immune response. One such function is the activation, proliferation, and differentiation of B lymphocytes. The activation, proliferation, and differentiation of B lymphocytes by specific cytokines lead to the production of antibody-secreting plasma cells. These antibodies are specific for the spike protein of SARS-CoV-2 and thus possess the ability to neutralize the virus or enhance the destruction of the virus. The cytokines secreted as a result of helper T lymphocyte activation not only lead to the proliferation of B lymphocytes to make plasma cells and memory B lymphocytes but also stimulate helper T lymphocytes to proliferate and produce effector and memory T lymphocytes. These sequences of events are important for mounting a proper immune response. There is another type of T lymphocyte called the cytotoxic T lymphocyte (T_C Cells), which binds to the newly synthesized viral protein (presented by MHC-I) using TCR (of T_C cells) present on its surface. The cytotoxic T lymphocytes have another cell surface protein called cluster of differentiation 8 (CD8+) that interacts directly with the MHC-I protein presenting the antigen. The synchronized interaction between antigen-TCR (of T_C cells) and MHC-I-CD8+ strengthens the interaction and activates the cytotoxic T lymphocytes. This interaction leads to the production of cytokines like interleukin-4, interleukin-12, interleukin-22, transforming growth factor-α, transforming growth factor-β, and tumor necrosis factor-α that have specific abilities to recognize and destroy recipient cells that are infected with SARS-CoV-2 in the future, and not the recipient cells processing the vaccines at that time. This is the basic mechanism of action of Moderna and Pfizer-BioNTech vaccines in generating an immune response against SARS-CoV-2 and may provide protection against COVID-19. But the real-time safety and effectiveness is uncertain and may change drastically in relation to the data available at this point in time (US Department of Health and Human Services, 2021; ModernaTX, Inc., 2021; Pfizer-BioNTech, 2021; Abbas et al., 2016).

AstraZeneca-Oxford University COVID-19 Vaccine

The AstraZeneca-Oxford University vaccine does not implement mRNA technology, instead, it has therapeutic DNA incorporated inside an adenovirus vector. In this case, the therapeutic DNA is inserted inside an adenovirus that acts as a vehicle or transport mechanism for therapeutic DNA into the recipient cells. As a spike protein is involved with infection and pathogenicity, the therapeutic DNA, capable of producing the spike protein, is obtained from SARS-CoV-2 using reverse genetics technology. Then the SARS-CoV-2 DNA (encoding only the spike protein) is incorporated inside the adenoviral vector and is used as the functional component of the COVID-19 vaccine. Like phospholipid nanoparticles, the adenovirus (from the vaccine) fuses with the plasma membrane of the recipient's cell and thus releases the therapeutic DNA (having the ability to encode spike proteins) into the cytoplasm. Following release, the therapeutic DNA (from the vaccine) enters the recipient cell's nucleus. The researchers reported that the therapeutic DNA (from the vaccine) does not get integrated with the recipient's DNA and instead uses the enzymes present in the nucleus and the machinery (like ribosomes on the endoplasmic reticulum) for its transcription and translation. The viral protein thus produced will be expressed on the recipient's cell membrane (plasma membrane). Following injection, the adenoviral vector containing the therapeutic DNA then infects the recipient's cell by fusing with the recipient's plasma membrane. Following fusion of the cell membrane of the adenoviral vector from the vaccine with the recipient's cell membrane, the therapeutic DNA (capable of producing spike proteins) is released into the cytoplasm and subsequently migrates inside the nucleus. The researchers reported that the therapeutic DNA from the vaccine does not get incorporated inside the recipient's DNA (US Department of Health and Human Services, 2021; AstraZeneca, 2021; Abbas et al., 2016) (Figure 10.5).

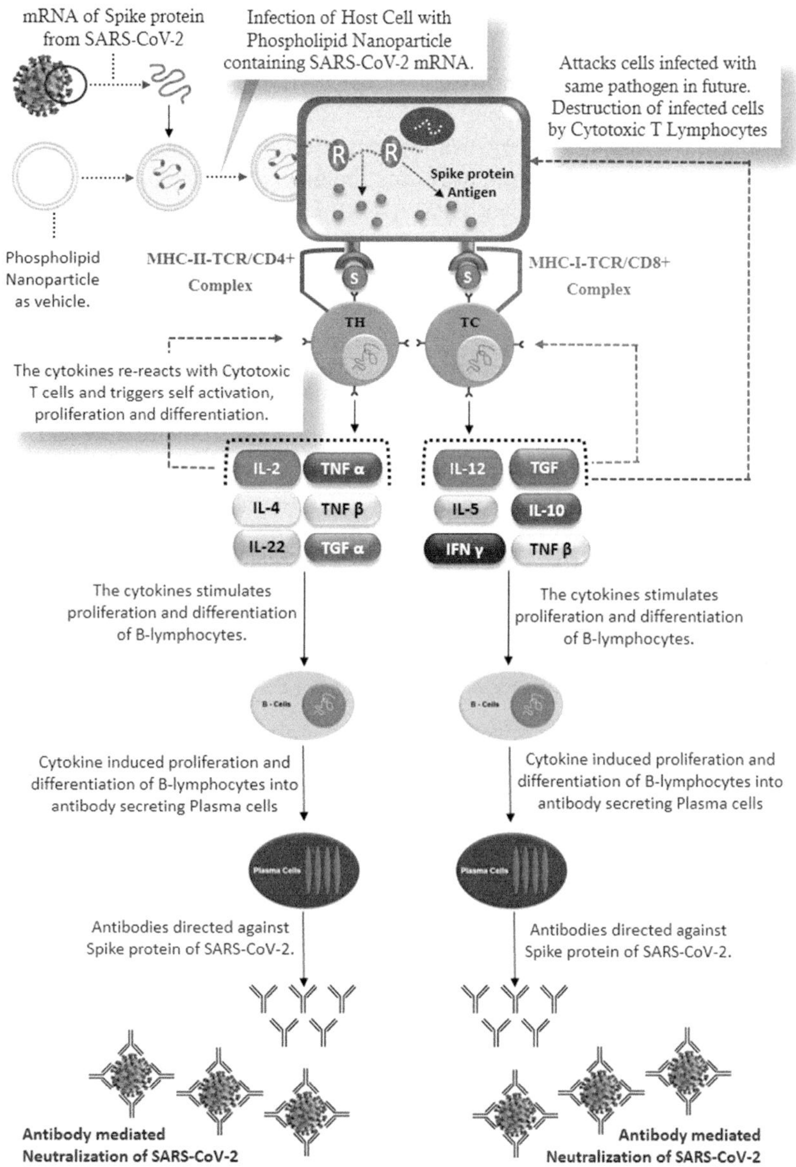

Figure 10.5 Generalized mechanism of action of Moderna and Pfizer-BioNTech COVID-19 vaccines.

Instead, the DNA (from the vaccine) interacts with the recipient cell's nuclear enzymes and cytoplasmic components to facilitate its transcription and translation in order to synthesize viral proteins (in this case, the spike protein of SARS-CoV-2). The newly synthesized viral protein then gets expressed on the membrane of the recipient's cells through the process of antigen presentation. The newly synthesized viral protein (the antigen) is presented through two types of cell surface receptors: MHC-I and MHC-II. In human beings, the MHC-II surface molecules are present on the APCs such as the dendritic cells, macrophages, and B lymphocytes, while the MHC-I surface molecules are found in all nucleated cells. When the newly synthesized viral protein (the antigen) is presented by the receptors on recipient cells, the other cells and molecules of the immune system are activated and attracted toward the site. T_H cells bind to the newly synthesized viral protein (presented by MHC-II) using TCR present on its surface. The helper T lymphocytes have another cell surface protein, CD4+, which interacts directly with the MHC-II protein presenting the antigen. The synchronized interaction between antigen-TCR and MHC-II-CD4+ strengthens the interaction and activates the helper T lymphocytes. When activated, the helper T lymphocytes start producing and releasing a range of cytokines mainly interleukin-2, interleukin-4, interleukin-5, interleukin-10, transforming growth factor-β, tumor necrosis factor, and interferon-γ, which perform several critical roles in mediating the immune response. One such function is the activation, proliferation, and differentiation of B lymphocytes. The activation, proliferation, and differentiation of B lymphocytes by specific cytokines lead to the production of antibody-secreting plasma cells. These antibodies are specific for the spike protein of SARS-CoV-2 and thus possess the ability to neutralize the virus or enhance the destruction of the virus. The cytokines secreted as a result of helper T lymphocyte activation not only lead to the proliferation of B lymphocytes to make plasma cells and memory B lymphocytes but also stimulate helper T lymphocytes to proliferate and produce effector and memory T lymphocytes. These sequences of events are important for mounting a proper immune response (US Department of Health and Human Services, 2021; AstraZeneca, 2021). T_C Cells bind to the newly synthesized viral protein (presented by MHC-I) using TCR (of T_C Cells) present on its surface. CD8+ interacts directly with the MHC-I protein presenting the antigen. The synchronized interaction between antigen-TCR (of T_C Cells) and MHC-I-CD8+ strengthens the interaction and activates cytotoxic T lymphocytes. This interaction leads to the production of cytokines like interleukin-4, interleukin-12, interleukin-22, transforming growth factor-α, transforming growth factor-β, and tumor necrosis factor-α that have specific abilities to recognize and destroy recipient cells that are infected with SARS-CoV-2 in the future, and not the recipient cells processing the vaccines at that time. This is the basic mechanism of action of the AstraZeneca-Oxford University vaccine. The vaccine aids in generating an immune response against SARS-CoV-2 and may provide protection against COVID-19. But the real-time safety and effectiveness is uncertain and may change drastically in relation to the data available at this point in time (US Department of Health and Human Services, 2021; AstraZeneca, 2021; Abbas et al., 2016).

COVID-19 VACCINES: INGREDIENTS AND COMPONENTS

Moderna, Pfizer-BioNTech, and AstraZeneca Vaccines

- **Moderna vaccines.** The basic ingredients include both active and inactive ingredients. Active ingredients consist of nucleoside modified mRNA encoding the viral spike(S) glycoprotein of SARS-CoV-2. The inactive agents are PEG2000-DMG:

1,2-dimyristoyl-rac-glycerol, methoxypolyethylene glycol, 1,2-distearoyl-sn-glycero -3-phosphocholine, cholesterol, SM-102: heptadecan-9-yl 8-((2-hydroxyethyl) (6-oxo-6-(undecyloxy) hexyl) amino) octanoate, tromethamine, tromethamine hydrochloride, acetic acid, sodium acetate, and sucrose (ModernaTX, Inc., 2021); Oxford Vaccine Group 2020, 2021) (Figure 10.6).

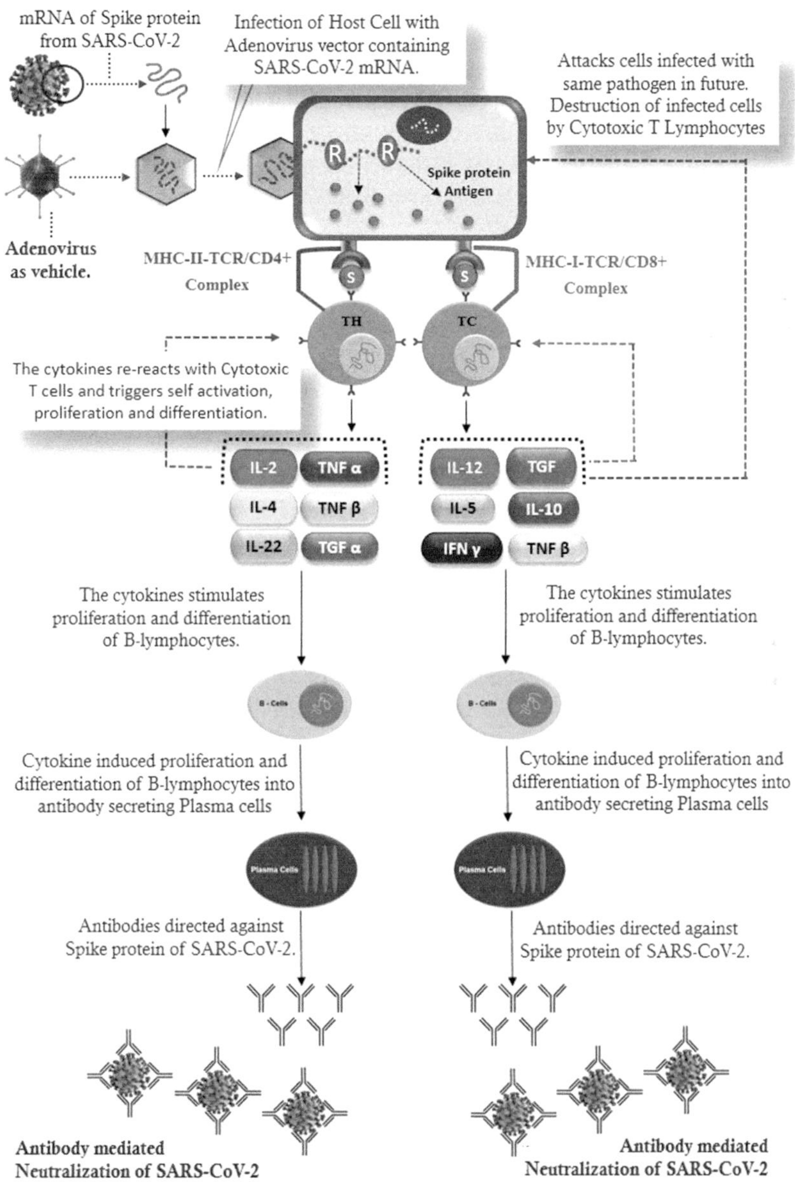

Figure 10.6 Generalized mechanism of action of the AstraZeneca COVID-19 vaccine.

- **Pfizer-BioNTech**. The basic ingredients include both active and inactive ingredients. Active ingredient consists of nucleoside modified mRNA encoding the viral spike(S) glycoprotein of SARS-CoV-2. The inactive agents are 2[(polyethylene glycol (PEG))-2000]-N,N-ditetradecylacetamide, 1,2-distearoyl-sn-glycero-3-phosphocholine, cholesterol, (4-hydroxybutyl)azanediyl)bis(hexane-6,1-diyl)bis(2-hexyldecanoate), sodium chloride, monobasic potassium phosphate, potassium chloride, dibasic sodium phosphate dehydrate, and sucrose (Pfizer-BioNTech, 2021; Oxford Vaccine Group 2020, 2021).
- **AstraZeneca-Oxford University**. The manufacturing process for the AstraZeneca-Oxford University vaccine involves the production of a virus, the adenovirus, which carries the genetic material to the cells inside the body. To produce this virus in the laboratory, a "host" cell line is needed. For some vaccines, chicken cells are used for this process, and for others, human cell lines are used to produce the virus. The Oxford-AstraZeneca vaccine uses a cell line called HEK-293 cells. HEK-293 is the name given to a specific line of cells used in various scientific applications. The original cells were taken from the kidney of a legally aborted fetus in 1973. HEK-293 cells used nowadays are clones of those original cells but are not themselves the cells of the aborted fetus. Each dose of the vaccine (0.5 ml) is known to contain the COVID-19 vaccine (ChAdOx1-S recombinant) 5×1010 viral particles (vp), and recombinant, replication-deficient chimpanzee adenovirus vector encoding the SARS-CoV-2 spike (S) glycoprotein (AstraZeneca, 2021; Oxford Vaccine Group 2020, 2021).

COVID-19 VACCINES: ADMINISTRATION, SAFETY CONCERNS, AND POSSIBLE ADVERSE REACTIONS

Moderna Vaccines

The COVID-19 vaccine developed by Moderna is administered intramuscularly in two separate doses at one-month intervals. As per the revised report of August 27, 2021, this is an unapproved vaccine authorized under EUA by the FDA to be administered to individuals 18 years and older. Individuals having conditions such as allergy or autoimmune conditions, inflammatory cardiovascular disorders, tendency of fever, bleeding disorders, using blood thinning medications, compromised immune system, using immunosuppressive treatments, are pregnant or planning to conceive, are breastfeeding, have received a different COVID-19 vaccine, or other underlying conditions should consult their physician before taking the vaccine. The vaccine is not recommended for individuals who had severe allergic reactions after the first dose of the vaccine and/or are allergic to any ingredients of the vaccine. After receiving the first dose, it is recommended that the second dose must be completed within the given time period. A third dose of the vaccine may be administered to immunocompromised individuals. During ongoing clinical trials, ~15,400 candidates of 18 years of age and above received at least one dose of the COVID-19 vaccine developed by Moderna. The mentioned vaccine was reported to be able to prevent COVID-19 during clinical trials. But the researchers do not guarantee full protection, and the duration of protection provided by the vaccine cannot be determined. It is recommended that physical hygiene precautions for preventing COVID-19 be maintained. There may be a possibility of adverse reactions in individuals receiving the vaccine, which include severe allergic reactions such as difficulty breathing, swelling of the face and throat, tachycardia, skin rashes, dizziness, severe weakness, myocarditis, and pericarditis as recorded during clinical trials. General common side effects include injection site reactions, fatigue, headache, muscle pain, joint pain, chills, nausea, vomiting, and fever. According to the FDA, the possible range of adverse vaccine reactions is still not completely known and there is a possibility of unknown unexpected adverse reactions. In case any individual experiences unknown unexpected adverse reactions after receiving the vaccine, they should seek emergency medical attention at the nearest emergency healthcare facility. There are no prominent data to confirm or deny the impact of the Moderna COVID-19 vaccine on pregnant or breastfeeding mothers (US Department of Health and Human Services, 2021; ModernaTX, Inc., 2021).

Pfizer-BioNTech Vaccines

The FDA authorized Pfizer-BioNTech vaccine for COVID-19 (also known as COMIRNATY: COVID-19 mRNA vaccine) has been implemented under EUA. COMIRNATY is the brand name for the COVID-19 vaccine developed by Pfizer-BioNTech with no change in formulation or mechanism of action (CDC, 2021). The Pfizer-BioNTech vaccine for COVID-19 has been authorized to be administered in individuals of 16 years of age and older in two separate doses, and for individuals from 12 years to 15 years of age in two separate doses. The booster dose of the same vaccine may be applicable for individuals above 65 years of age or having a high risk of susceptibility to COVID-19. It is not recommended for individuals who had severe allergic reactions after the first dose of the vaccine and/or are allergic to any ingredients of the vaccine. After receiving the first dose, it is recommended that the second dose must be completed within the given time period. Individuals with conditions such as allergy or autoimmune conditions, inflammatory cardiovascular disorders, tendency of fever, bleeding disorders, using blood thinning medications, compromised immune system, using immunosuppressive treatments, are pregnant or planning to conceive, are breastfeeding, or have received a different COVID-19 vaccine, or other underlying conditions should consult their physician before taking the vaccines. During ongoing clinical trials, ~23,000 candidates of 12 years of age and above received at least one dose of the COVID-19 vaccine developed by Pfizer-BioNTech. The mentioned vaccine was reported to be able to prevent COVID-19 during clinical trials. But the researchers do not guarantee full protection, and the duration of protection provided by the vaccine is yet to be determined. According to the FDA, the possible range of adverse vaccine reactions is still not completely known and there is a possibility of unknown unexpected adverse reactions. The adverse vaccine reactions documented during clinical trials included severe allergic reactions such as difficulty breathing, swelling of the face and throat, tachycardia, skin rashes, dizziness, severe weakness, myocarditis, and pericarditis as recorded during clinical trials. Also, some common side effects include injection site reactions, fatigue, headache, muscle pain, joint pain, chills, lymphadenopathy, nausea, vomiting, loss of appetite, diarrhea, and fever. In case any individual experiences unknown unexpected adverse reactions after receiving the vaccine, they should seek emergency medical attention at the nearest emergency healthcare facility. There are no prominent data to confirm or deny the impact of the Pfizer-BioNTech COVID-19 vaccine on pregnant or breastfeeding mothers (Pfizer-BioNTech, 2021; US Department of Health and Human Services, 2021).

AstraZeneca-Oxford University Vaccines

The COVID-19 vaccine developed by AstraZeneca-Oxford University known as AZD1222 (ChAdOx1 [Recombinant]) is authorized by the FDA to be used under EUA. According to the reports published by the World Health Organization, the AZD1222 vaccine against COVID-19 has an efficacy of 63.09% against symptomatic SARS-CoV-2 infection. The AZD1222 vaccine for COVID-19 has been authorized to be administered in individuals of 18 years of age and older in two separate doses of 0.5 ml each with an interval of about 12 weeks. During ongoing clinical trials, ~23,745 candidates of 18 years of age and above received at least one dose of the COVID-19 vaccine developed by AstraZeneca. The mentioned vaccine was reported to be able to prevent COVID-19 during clinical trials. It is recommended that pregnant, breastfeeding women, or women willing to conceive should avoid taking this vaccine as a precautionary measure because no safety studies are available and there are anticipated risks that should not be excluded. It is not known whether this vaccine impacts the reproductive capability of people receiving it because developmental and reproductive toxicology studies are not complete and genotoxicity and carcinogenicity studies have not been conducted. According to the FDA, the possible range of adverse vaccine reactions is still not completely known and there is a possibility of unknown or unexpected adverse reactions. Recent research shows association of this vaccine with vaccine-induced thrombosis with thrombocytopenia (TTS), which includes neurological symptoms, severe persistent headache, blurred vision, shortness of breath, chest pain, persistent gastrointestinal disturbance, and peripheral edema and blood spots under the skin. Common side effects include injection site reactions, fatigue, headache, muscle pain, joint pain, chills, lymphadenopathy, nausea, vomiting, loss of appetite, diarrhea, and fever. As per the revised reports released by AstraZeneca (January 2021), the duration of protection given by this vaccine is not known and the vaccination may not protect all recipients from the disease. It is not recommended for individuals who had severe allergic reactions after the first dose of the vaccine and/or are allergic to any ingredients of the vaccine. Individuals having conditions such as allergy or autoimmune conditions, inflammatory cardiovascular disorders, tendency of fever, bleeding disorders, using blood thinning medications, compromised immune system, using immunosuppressive treatments, are pregnant or planning to conceive, are breastfeeding, or have received different COVID-19 vaccine, or other underlying conditions should consult their physician before taking the vaccine (Queensland, 2021; AstraZeneca, 2021; US Department of Health and Human Services, 2021).

COVID-19 VACCINES: EMERGENCY USE AUTHORIZATION, NORMAL APPROVAL, AND FUTURE CONSIDERATIONS

During this ongoing pandemic, we have witnessed the implementation of many experimental drugs and vaccines under EUA in order to deal with the COVID-19 situation. It is to be understood that EUA approval and regular FDA approval are not the same thing. Supported by the Secretary of Health and Human Services (HHS), the EUA is implemented to justify the emergency use of experimental unapproved drugs, vaccines, or biological products during the COVID-19 situation. None of the approved drugs or vaccines have undergone the same type of scrutiny as to receive regular FDA approval or as FDA cleared products.

REFERENCES

Abbas, A., Lichtman, A., & Pillai, S. (2016). *Cellular and Molecular Immunology* (9th ed.). Elsevier.

AstraZeneca. (2021, January). *PI-for-COVID-19-Vaccine-AstraZeneca*. Doc ID-004379265 v. 2.0.

CDC. (2014, May 1). Vaccine Testing and Approval Process. Centers for Disease Control and Prevention. https://www.cdc.gov/vaccines/basics/test-approve.html

CDC. (2021, October 28). Information about the Pfizer-BioNTech COVID-19 Vaccine. Centers for Disease Control and Prevention. Retrieved November 10, 2021, from https://www.cdc.gov/coronavirus/2019-ncov/vaccines/different-vaccines/Pfizer-BioNTech.html

COVID-19 Vaccination. (2020, February 11). Centers for Disease Control and Prevention. https://www.cdc.gov/coronavirus/2019-ncov/vaccines/safety/safety-of-vaccines.html

DECCAN CHRONICLE. (2021, January 10). The rat race for COVID vaccine. *DECCAN CHRONICLE*. https://www.deccanchronicle.com/lifestyle/health-and-wellbeing/071220/the-rat-race-for-covid-vaccine.html

Juda, E. (2021, July 19). *Producing Prevention: How Vaccines Are Developed | Online Public Health*. GW-UMT. https://onlinepublichealth.gwu.edu/resources/producing-prevention-the-complex-development-of-vaccines/

Kamble, P. H., & Dubhashi, S. P. (2020). Expedited COVID-19 vaccine trials: A rat-race with challenges and ethical issues. *Pan African Medical Journal, 36*, 206. https://doi.org/10.11604/pamj.2020.36.206.23977

ModernaTX, Inc. (2021, August). *Emergency Use Authorization (EUA) of the Moderna COVID-19 Vaccine to Prevent Coronavirus Disease 2019 (COVID-19) in Individuals 18 Years of Age and Older*. Moderna.

Naqvi, A. A. T., Fatima, K., Mohammad, T., Fatima, U., Singh, I. K., Singh, A., Atif, S. M., Hariprasad, G., Hasan, G. M., & Hassan, M. I. (2020). Insights into SARS-CoV-2 genome, structure, evolution, pathogenesis and therapies: Structural genomics approach. *Biochimica et Biophysica Acta (BBA): Molecular Basis of Disease, 1866*(10), 165878. https://doi.org/10.1016/j.bbadis.2020.165878

Office of the Commissioner. (2021, October 5). *COVID-19 Vaccines*. U.S. Food and Drug Administration. https://www.fda.gov/emergency-preparedness-and-response/coronavirus-disease-2019-covid-19/covid-19-vaccines

Oxford Vaccine Group 2020. (2021, October 15). COVID-19 Vaccines | Vaccine Knowledge. Retrieved October 16, 2021, from https://vk.ovg.ox.ac.uk/vk/covid-19-vaccines

Pfizer-BioNTech. (2021, October). *Vaccine Information Fact Sheet for Recipients and Caregivers about Comirnaty (COVID-19 Vaccine, mRNA) and Pfizer-BioNTech COVID-19 Vaccine to Prevent Coronavirus Disease 2019 (COVID-19)*. Pfizer-BioNTech.

Queensland; C. O. S. O. (2021, November 2). *Side Effects*. Health and Wellbeing | Queensland Government. Retrieved November 10, 2021, from https://www.qld.gov.au/health/conditions/health-alerts/coronavirus-covid-19/protect-yourself-others/covid-19-vaccine/about/side-effects

Thanh Le, T., Andreadakis, Z., Kumar, A., Gómez Román, R., Tollefsen, S., Saville, M., & Mayhew, S. (2020). The COVID-19 vaccine development landscape. *Nature Reviews Drug Discovery, 19*(5), 305–306. https://doi.org/10.1038/d41573-020-00073-5

US Department of Health and Human Services. (2021, May). *Emergency Use Authorization for Vaccines to Prevent COVID-19: Guidance for Industry*. U.S. Department of Health and Human Services. Food and Drug Administration. Center for Biologics Evaluation and Research.

Chapter 11

Mucormycosis

Post-COVID-19 Complications in Patients with Diabetes and the State of Immunosuppression

Soumyajit Dutta* and Srijan Goswami

CONTENTS

INTRODUCTION TO THE PRESENT SITUATION

The world has been suffering from the COVID-19 pandemic since December 2019. One wave after the other has made the situation worse. Conventional treatment protocols and experimental pharmacological interventions have condemned the individuals recovering from active SARS-CoV-2 infection to an iatrogenic immunosuppressive state. These iatrogenic immunosuppressive states have the potential to increase the chances of developing secondary opportunistic diseases. In the midst of this ongoing crisis, another threat has emerged as a challenge in the form of COVID-associated mucormycosis or wrongly termed as "The Black Fungus Disease". Opportunistic fungal infections have been reported in patients with severe COVID-19 or those recovering from the disease and have been associated with severe illness and death. According to the World Health Organization (*WHO)*, the prevention of COVID-associated mucormycosis needs to focus on aiming for better glycemic control in COVID-19 patients and monitoring the use of systemic corticosteroids in treating severe cases. The incidence rate of mucormycosis globally varies from 0.005 to 1.7 per million population. In India, the prevalence of mucormycosis is estimated as 140 per million population, which is about 80 times higher than the prevalence in developed countries. Following the surge of COVID-19 associated mucormycosis and the Government of India directive, several states in India made mucormycosis a notifiable disease in May 2021. This will provide better insights into the disease burden, population characteristics,

DOI: 10.1201/9781003178514-13

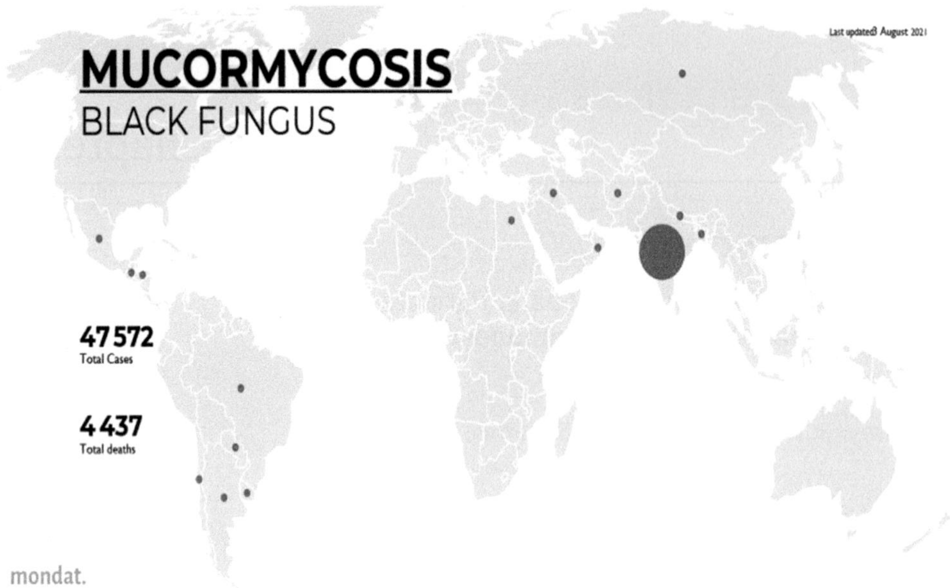

Figure 11.1 World situation report of mucormycosis cases.

risk factors, clinical spectrum, and outcomes of these patients. Current trends indicate that the surge is higher in those with pre-existing diabetes and those on systemic corticosteroids. It is being observed in both people with COVID-19, and those recovering from the disease (Singh et al., 2021). Much is not known to the scientific community about the connection between COVID-19 infection and mucormycosis. Through this chapter, the authors intend to present the available information regarding COVID-associated-mucormycosis in a simple, elaborate, and easily understandable sequence. We have to understand that research and development are progressing at an exponential rate and treatment protocols may change from time to time, but the fundamental concepts will remain the same (Figures 11.1 and 11.2).

COVID-ASSOCIATED MUCORMYCOSIS: THE DISEASE PRESENTATION

Mucormycosis is an angioinvasive, non-contagious but serious life-threatening disease known to be caused by a group of fungi called mucormycetes. The word "mucormycosis" is derived from two Latin words *Mucor* and *mycosis*. The word *Mucor* (Latin) refers to mold and *mycosis* (Latin) refers to "the presence of fungi as parasites in the body". The mucormycetes group of fungi can be found everywhere in the environment especially on surfaces with dead and decaying organic matter. Encounters with these fungi groups are completely unavoidable but they are not harmful to the majority of the human population. However, in individuals with immunosuppressive conditions, inhalation of the spores from the fungi may cause pulmonary infection and inflammation of nasal sinuses or may even spread to different locations of the body, thus causing a serious pathological state (WHO, 2021; CDC, 2021). Mucormycosis may be caused by several types of fungi belonging to the order Mucorales. According to the Centers for Disease Control and Prevention (CDC), *Rhizopus* and *Mucor* are the two most common species of fungus that are known to cause

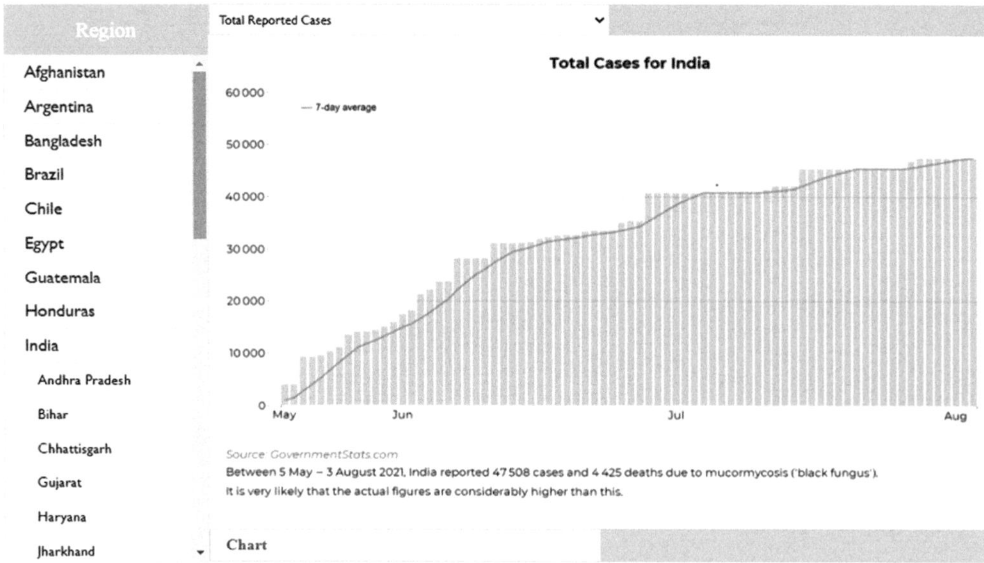

Figure 11.2 Indian situation report of mucormycosis cases.

mucormycosis, the other possible names include *Rhizomucor* species, *Cunninghamella bertholletiae*, *Apophysomyces*, *Lichtheimia*, and *Saksenaea* (WHO, 2021; CDC, 2021).

The group of fungi responsible for mucormycosis tends to enter the body through the respiratory tract, and then depending on the condition, progresses to the other organs of the body. The symptoms and clinical presentation of mucormycosis depend on the regions of the body that are involved. The general signs and symptoms may include facial pain, painful sinuses, teeth, and gums, decreased sensation over half of the face (paresthesia), blackish discoloration of the skin over the alae nasi, blackish nasal discharge, periorbital swelling, blurred vision, loosening of teeth and discoloration of the palate, degeneration of respiratory functions, and so on (DGHS India, 2021).

According to reports published by the WHO and CDC, mucormycosis may be classified into five categories, namely rhino-cerebral mucormycosis (involving nasal sinuses and brain), pulmonary mucormycosis (involving the lungs), cutaneous mucormycosis (involving the skin), gastrointestinal mucormycosis (involving the digestive tract), and disseminated mucormycosis. Table 11.1 points out the clinical signs and symptoms depending on the type of mucormycosis.

COVID-associated mucormycosis does not spread from one person to another. The fungus may enter the body through inhalation or the ingestion of spores that are present in the surrounding environment. These fungal spores only survive in an environment containing dead and decaying organic matter. So, an individual having diseased and decaying organic matter in their system has increased chances of developing complications of mucormycosis. The fungal spores may also enter the body through injuries or breaks on skin surfaces like abscesses, burns, lacerated wounds, cuts, or any type of injuries caused on the skin. Also, many non-sterile medical devices and objects like hospital linen, wound dressing bandages, tongue depressors, negative pressure rooms, and buildings may contain the spores. The infection is commonly visible in the rhino-cerebral context as the spore enters the system through the upper respiratory tract. Individuals suffering or recovering from severe COVID-19 or other life-threatening illnesses like

TABLE 11.1 THE TYPES AND SYMPTOMS OF MUCORMYCOSIS ACCORDING TO INFORMATION PROVIDED BY THE WHO AND CDC (CDC, 2021)

S. No	Mucormycosis Type	Clinical Signs and Symptoms
1.	Rhino-cerebral	Nasal or sinus congestion
		One-sided facial swelling
		Severe headache and fever
		Black lesions on the nasal bridge or the roof of the mouth that progressively become more severe
		Lethargy, seizures, slurred speech, partial paralysis
2.	Pulmonary	Cough and fever
		Chest pain and shortness of breath
		Hemoptysis
3.	Cutaneous	Ulcer or blister-like skin lesion
		The affected area progressively turns black
		Pain, warmth, redness, or swelling (inflammation) around the wound
4.	Gastrointestinal	Abdominal pain
		Nausea and vomiting
		Bleeding from the gastrointestinal tract
5.	Disseminated	Occurs in individuals with co-morbid conditions
		Differentiation of symptoms specific to mucormycosis is very difficult

acquired immunodeficiency syndrome (HIV-AIDS), diabetes, immunosuppressive treatments, cancers, and respiratory complications are at higher risk of contracting opportunistic fungal infections like mucormycosis (Cornely et al., 2019; Shakir et al., 2021; Chauhan et al., 2021; CDC, 2021; ICMR, 2021; Pongas et al., 2009; Lewis et al., 2011; Trifilio et al., 2007; AIIMS, 2021) (Figure 11.3).

COVID-ASSOCIATED MUCORMYCOSIS: IMMUNOSUPPRESSION

Individuals with suppressed immune systems are more susceptible to opportunistic infections. The complications associated with COVID-19 occur due to the cytokine storm happening inside the patient's body. The cytokine storm comprising of interleukin-1, interleukin-6, interleukin-8, tumor necrosis factor-α, and various chemokines damage vital organs like the liver, heart, lungs, and kidneys, thus leading to a state of multisystem organ failure. In order to protect the patient from multisystem organ failure, immunosuppressive treatments are provided. These immunosuppressive treatments include steroids and associated immunosuppressive drugs, the dosage and duration of which far exceeded the safety recommendations of the World Health Organization. This treatment not only induces an immunosuppressive state but also leads to an increase in blood sugar levels, thus rendering the patient a higher susceptibility to COVID-associated mucormycosis. Also, individuals under conventional treatment for malignancies,

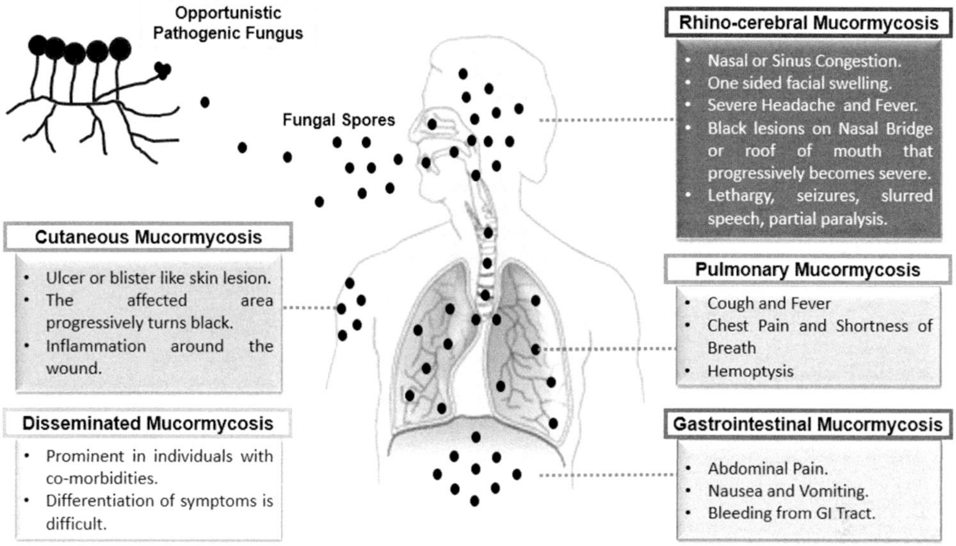

Figure 11.3 Various types of mucormycosis based on the location they infect.

burns, or traumatic injuries, or who have undergone organ or bone marrow transplantation, suffer from a drug-induced immunosuppressive state. These drugs maintain a systemic immunosuppressive state and thus make an individual more susceptible to opportunistic infections (CDC, 2021; ICMR, 2021; Pongas et al., 2009) (Figure 11.4).

COVID-ASSOCIATED MUCORMYCOSIS: DIABETES OR HYPERGLYCEMIA

In general, patients having hyperglycemia or abnormally high amounts of glucose in the blood, commonly known as diabetes mellitus, are vulnerable to various kinds of life-threatening opportunistic infections. The Directorate General of Health Services (DGHS-India) reported a significant increase in cases of mucormycosis in COVID-19 patients having pre-existing uncontrolled hyperglycemia (DGHS India, 2021). From May 5, 2021, to June 12, 2021, 41,512 cases and 3554 deaths were documented to be associated with COVID-associated mucormycosis. Based on the reports of May 10, 2021, COVID-associated mucormycosis was declared an epidemic by the Central Government of India (Singh et al., 2021; ASM, 2021; Mucormycosis, n.d.).

It is important to understand why hyperglycemia increases the risk of being affected by mucormycosis. It is known to the scientific community that fungus thrives on carbohydrates like glucose, fructose, mannose, maltose, and so on. When more than the required amount of glucose starts accumulating in the blood, the pH changes to an acidic side. The blood with acidic pH causes damage to the cells of the body, thus leading to a cascade of systemic inflammation and metabolic disruption. Studies have shown that an increase in blood glucose levels creates a significant decrease in the immune function and regulation of the body, confirming that hyperglycemia causes immunosuppression. Thus, the acidic pH of the blood and the continuous immunosuppressive state of the body leads to progressive degradation of the cellular components, thus developing a suitable environment for

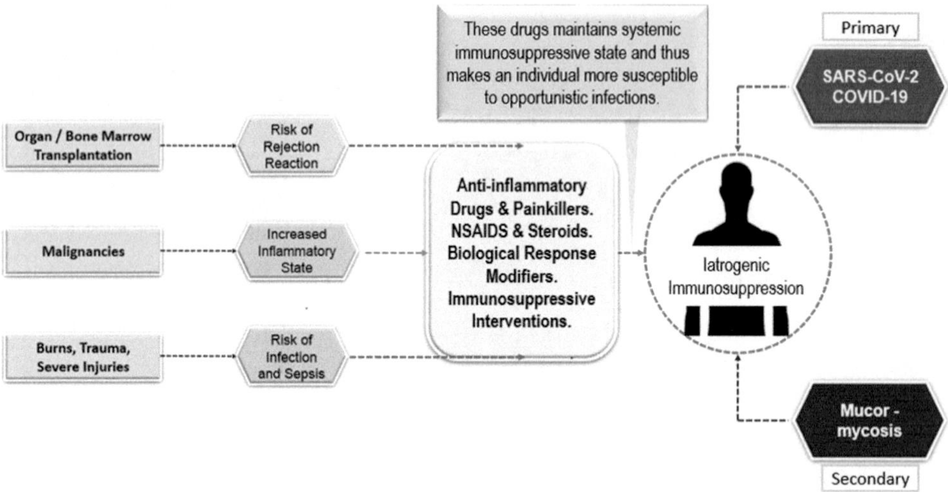

Figure 11.4 Conventional treatment-induced immunosuppression and vulnerability to opportunistic life-threatening secondary infectious diseases like mucormycosis.

the opportunistic group of fungi to thrive. The fungus gets all the required nutrients from the decaying organic compounds present in the circulation of the patient and aggressively spreads to different parts in the absence of a functional host immune response. So, as a preventive measure, it is very important to lower the consumption of refined sugar as much as possible. When the consumption of glucose decreases, the concentration of glucose in the blood also decreases, as a result, the pH of the blood returns to its normal state. When the homeostasis of circulating blood is restored, the opportunistic fungus finds the environment unsuitable for their survival and thus may lead to lowering of the pathological impact. Individuals having unchecked hyperglycemia may need to follow a treatment regimen that helps manage hyperglycemia, so that these life-threatening secondary diseases can be prevented (Singh et al., 2021; ASM, 2021; Mucormycosis, n.d.).

COVID-ASSOCIATED MUCORMYCOSIS: HOST–MICROBE INTERACTION

The human body is made up of approximately 10^{-14} human cells and 10^{-14} million microorganisms (called human microbiome comprising of ~9 million germ genes). These human microbiomes have a symbiotic relationship with the human being and are equally important as any vital organ of the body. Disturbance in the balance between the human microbiome and human cells leads to life-threatening complications. So the "germs" are not our enemy, but friends, essential for survival. But overuse and misuse of antimicrobial agents in our daily life create a state of dysbiosis and resistance. On top of that, the intensive immunosuppressive treatment protocols with evidence of having iatrogenic consequences further create a physical environment that is habitable for opportunistic pathogens to survive and proliferate. The destruction of the host's natural microbiome makes the immune response non-functional. In the absence of a host microbiome, opportunistic pathogens cause life-threatening diseases (Cornely et al., 2019; Shakir et al., 2021; Chauhan et al., 2021; 13CDC, 2021; ICMR, 2021; Pongas et al., 2009; Lewis et al., 2011; Trifilio et al., 2007;

AIIMS, 2021). The lack of proper composition and population of the host microbiome makes the host's immune system non-functional or less powerful, this condition leads to the increased impact of the SARS-CoV-2 virus. When SARS-CoV-2 enters the upper respiratory tract and gradually progresses toward the lower respiratory tract, it keeps on damaging the epithelial cell linings of respiratory mucosa. The destruction of respiratory mucosal cells triggers the release of pro-inflammatory cytokines that in turn cause unwanted damage to the organ(s). The abnormal and poor regulation of the host's immune response leads to pathological changes. These progressive degenerative pathological changes, along with iatrogenic immunosuppression, force the body's healing mechanisms to shut down. The damaged and dying tissues generate chemicals that are suitable for the survival of the opportunistic fungus group and thus mucormycosis is seen to be associated with recovering severe COVID-19 cases (Cornely et al., 2019; Shakir et al., 2021; Chauhan et al., 2021; 13CDC, 2021; ICMR, 2021; Pongas et al., 2009; Lewis et al., 2011; Trifilio et al., 2007; AIIMS, 2021).

COVID-ASSOCIATED ORAL MANIFESTATIONS: RHINO-MAXILLARY MUCORMYCOSIS

COVID-19 and associated treatment procedures lead to a state of immunosuppression and damage to the nasopharyngeal and oropharyngeal route. The tongue contains multiple follicles that help in taste sensation. Loss of taste is one of the primary and most common oral symptoms of COVID-19 and is caused by the destruction of the follicles. Oral manifestations associated with COVID-19 were grouped based on their etiology, including iatrogenic lesions caused by intubation and opportunistic infections. Post-COVID-mucormycosis is one of the severe oral complications requiring surgical intervention. The common manifestation of rhino-cerebral mucormycosis is seen in oral, nasal, orbital, and cerebral regions. The common signs and symptoms include halitosis, gingivitis, and discharge of pus from the gum, loosening of teeth in the upper jaw, ulceration, discoloration and ischemic necrosis of the palate, soft tissue growth of the palate, one-sided facial swelling, and headache. Necrosis of the palate occurs due to thrombosis of turbinate because of injuries caused to the sphenopalatine and greater palatine arteries. The fungal infection begins at the nasal mucosal surface, the palate, followed by paranasal sinuses, cribriform palate, and the brain. After coming in contact with circulating blood, the fungus creates damage to the endothelial lining of the arterial wall, thus causing intravascular thrombosis, infarction, and tissue necrosis. Rhino-maxillary mucormycosis is less critical as compared with rhino-cerebral mucormycosis, which is both progressively invasive and lethal. Since mucormycosis is a progressive and fatal disease, early detection is the key to minimizing complications. Since the signs and symptoms of rhino-maxillary mucormycosis overlap with the symptoms of diseases like osteomyelitis, squamous cell carcinoma, syphilis, or chronic suppurative periodontitis, proper differential diagnosis of the disease is very important. The radiographic methods used for diagnosis include PNS CBCT, CT, and MRI. CBCT findings may be opacification of nasopharyngeal sinuses, filled with a thick layer of mucus and pus, and degeneration of bones around the jaw. Tissue culture and biopsy may also be performed with H and E, PAS, and GMS staining while culture is performed on Sabouraud Dextrose Agar (Cornely et al., 2019; Shakir et al., 2021; Chauhan et al., 2021; 13CDC, 2021; ICMR, 2021; Pongas et al., 2009; Lewis et al., 2011; Trifilio et al., 2007; AIIMS, 2021). Some clinical images are presented that sequentially indicate instances from the surgical management of rhino-maxillary mucormycosis (Figures 11.5–11.9).

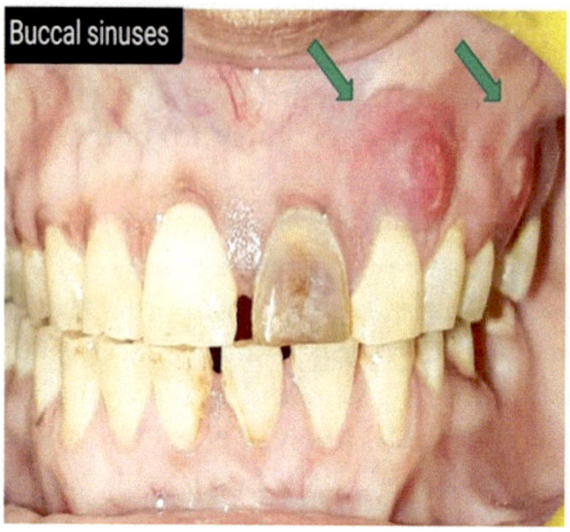

Plate 01: Pre operative image, buccal aspect.

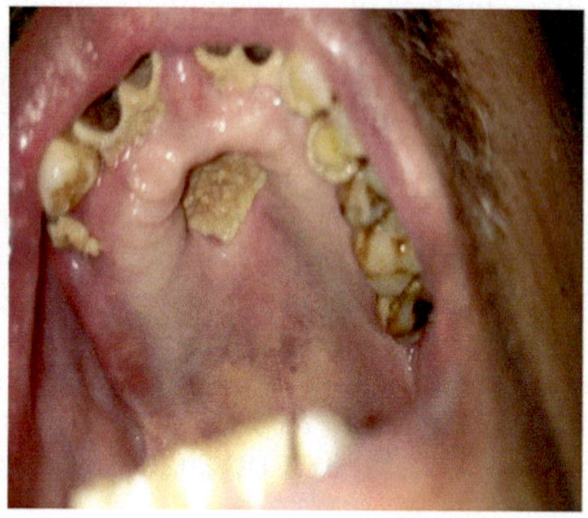

Plate 02: pre operative intra oral clinical image.

Figure 11.5 Plate 1: Pre-operative image, buccal aspect. Plate 2: Pre-operative intraoral clinical image. Picture courtesy of Dr. Sankalp Mittal (Oral and Maxillofacial Surgeon and Implantologist. BDS. MDS. MOMSRCPS. Diplomate of International Congress of Oral Implantologist, USA) and Dr. Amit Harsh (BDS. Rajasthan University of Health Sciences).

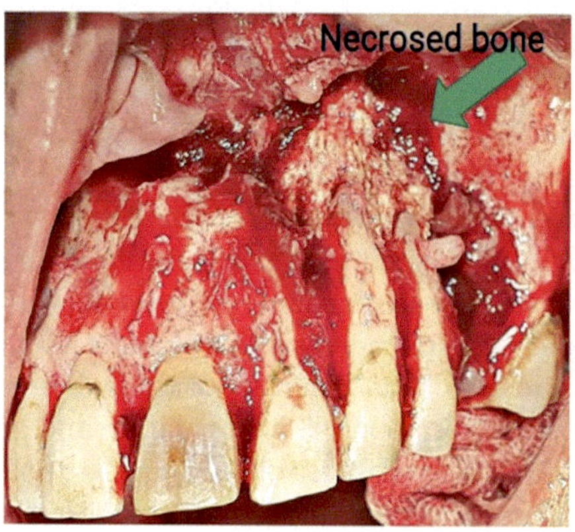

Plate 03: reflection of buccal muco periosteal flap with exposure of the necrotic bone.

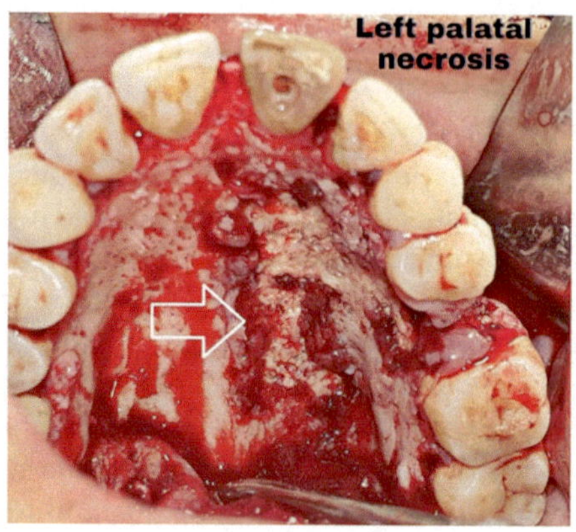

Plate 04: Reflection of the palatal flap shows necrosis of the palatal bone.

Figure 11.6 Plate 3: Reflection of buccal muco periosteal flap with exposure of the necrotic bone. Plate 4: Reflection of the palatal flap shows necrosis of the palatal bone. Picture courtesy of Dr. Sankalp Mittal (Oral and Maxillofacial Surgeon and Implantologist. BDS. MDS. MOMSRCPS. Diplomate of International Congress of Oral Implantologist, USA) and Dr. Amit Harsh (BDS. Rajasthan University of Health Sciences).

DIAGNOSIS OF COVID-ASSOCIATED MUCORMYCOSIS

According to the CDC, the National Center for Emerging and Zoonotic Infectious Diseases (NCEZID), and the Division of Foodborne, Waterborne, and Environmental Diseases (DFWED), like any other infectious disease, the diagnosis of COVID-associated mucormycosis involves consideration of medical history, signs and symptoms, physical examination, and laboratory-based investigations (Singh et al., 2021; ASM, 2021).

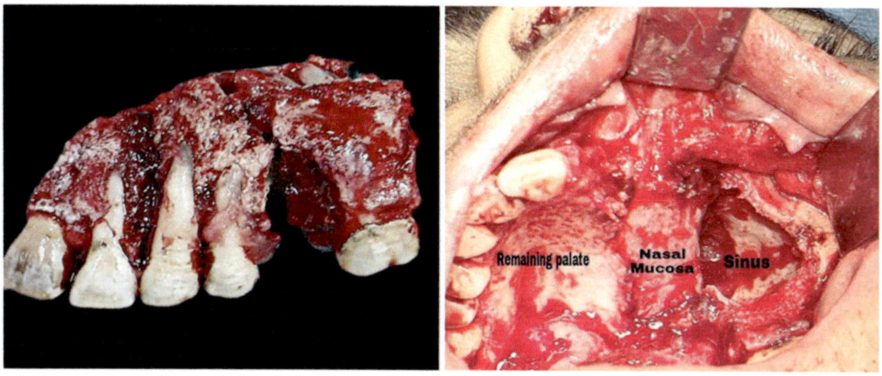

Plate 05: resection of the necrosed bone.

Plate 06: Remaining palatal bone, nasal mucosa, maxillary sinus , all on healthy bone margin.

Figure 11.7 Plate 5: Resection of necrosed bone. Plate 6: Remaining palatal bone, nasal mucosa, maxillary sinus, all on healthy bone margin. Picture courtesy of Dr. Sankalp Mittal (Oral and Maxillofacial Surgeon and Implantologist. BDS. MDS. MOMSRCPS. Diplomate of International Congress of Oral Implantologist, USA) and Dr. Amit Harsh (BDS. Rajasthan University of Health Sciences).

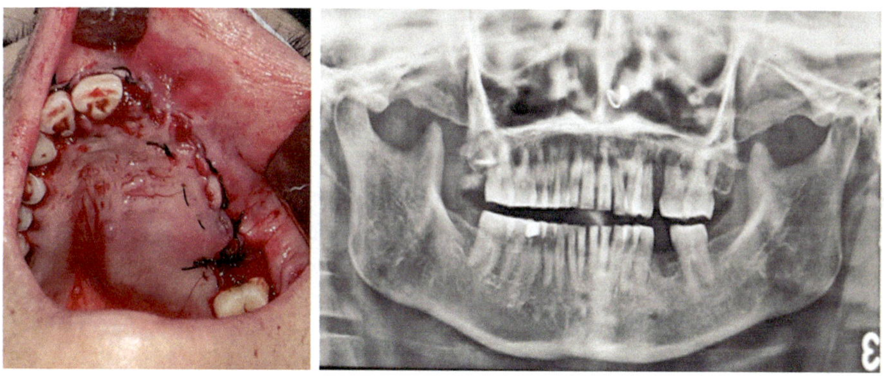

Plate 07: Final suturing of the patient

Plate 08: Orthopantomograph

Figure 11.8 Plate 7: Final suturing of the patient. Plate 8: Orthopantomograph. Picture courtesy of Dr. Sankalp Mittal (Oral and Maxillofacial Surgeon and Implantologist. BDS. MDS. MOMSRCPS. Diplomate of International Congress of Oral Implantologist, USA) and Dr. Amit Harsh (BDS. Rajasthan University of Health Sciences).

If rhino-cerebral or pulmonary complications are suspected then a fluid specimen from nasal sinuses or the respiratory tract is collected for analysis, also a tissue biopsy may be collected for histopathological studies as well as fungal culture for microscopic examination at cellular level. Advanced imaging techniques like CT may also be performed for scanning lungs, sinuses, or other parts of the body depending on the indication. Investigative and diagnostic processes that may be implemented include the following (Cornely et al., 2019; Shakir et al., 2021; Chauhan et

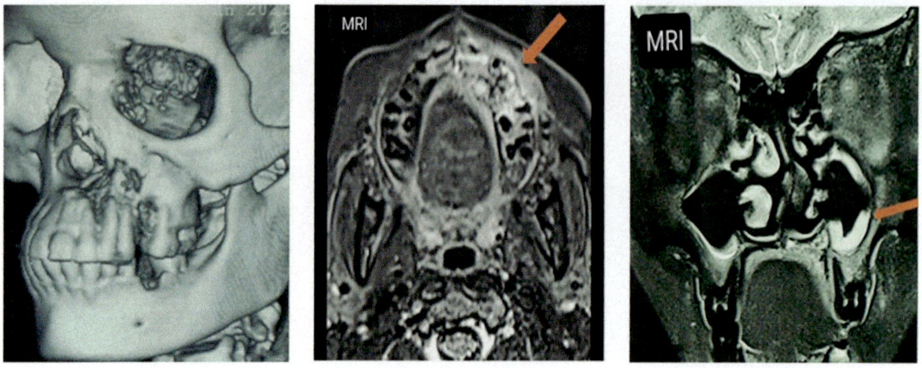

Plate 09: Preoperative 3D reconstructive image showing extensive erosion of the maxillary bone

Plate 10: MRI showing extensive damage of the maxillary bone by the necrosed tissue.

Plate 11 : MRI showing extensive damage of the maxillary bone by the necrosed tissue.

Figure 11.9 Plate 9: Pre-operative 3D reconstructive image showing extensive erosion of the maxillary bone. Plate 10: MRI showing extensive damage of the maxillary bone by the necrosed tissue. Plate 11: MRI showing extensive damage of the maxillary bone by the necrosed tissue. Picture courtesy of Dr. Sankalp Mittal (Oral and Maxillofacial Surgeon and Implantologist. BDS. MDS. MOMSRCPS. Diplomate of International Congress of Oral Implantologist, USA) and Dr. Amit Harsh (BDS. Rajasthan University of Health Sciences).

al., 2021; CDC, 2021; ICMR, 2021; Pongas et al., 2009; Lewis et al., 2011; Trifilio et al., 2007; AIIMS, 2021);

- NCCT-PNS: Non-contrast computed tomography (NCCT) of paranasal sinuses (PNS) is advised in suspected cases having an inflammation of the sinuses.
- HRCT chest: High resolution computed tomography of the thorax may be advised to suspected patients. Multiple nodules ($\geq$10 nodules), pleural effusion, and reverse halo sign are some of the key features.
- MRI-brain may be performed as per indication.
- K-OH staining for microscopic analysis may be performed for general fungal identification.
- Fungal cell culture and biopsy for histopathological analysis.
- MALDI-TOF: Matrix-assisted laser desorption/ionization (MALDI)-time of flight (TOF) is a mass spectrometric (MS) technique and is one of the accurate methodologies for identifying fungal specimens, and is widely used in microbiological analysis.

PREVENTION AND CLINICAL MANAGEMENT OF COVID-19-ASSOCIATED MUCORMYCOSIS

Prevention of COVID-associated mucormycosis is focused on managing the underlying health conditions like glycemic index control, judicial use of corticosteroids, and monitoring and preventing the unnecessary use of antibiotics, antifungal drugs, and other immunomodulators

(Shakir et al., 2021; Chauhan et al., 2021; CDC, 2021; ICMR, 2021; Pongas et al., 2009; Lewis et al., 2011; Trifilio et al., 2007; AIIMS, 2021). For preventing the spread of the pathogen, IPC guidelines are to be implemented thoroughly that include the following:

- Sterilization and disinfection of equipment used by multiple patients (tracheal tubes, ventilators) and ventilation systems (if there is poor ventilation in the hospital that can contribute to dampness and dust).
- Proper wound management (bandage, tape, and adhesives including tapes to secure medical devices such as endotracheal tubes; ostomy devices must be sterilized and changed regularly)
- Proper line management in health facilities. One should have a high index of suspicion of invasive fungal infections such as mucormycosis in the presence of predisposing conditions as mentioned previously. Timely initiation of treatment reduces mortality. A multidisciplinary team approach is required. Treatment of mucormycosis involves a combination of surgical debridement and antifungal therapy.
- Liposomal amphotericin B in an initial dose of 5 mg/kg body weight (10 mg/kg body weight in case of CNS involvement) is the treatment of choice. Each vial contains 50 mg. It should be diluted in 5% or 10% dextrose. It is incompatible with normal saline/Ringer lactate. It has to be continued until a favorable response is achieved and the disease is stabilized, which may take several weeks, following which, step down to oral posaconazole (300 mg delayed-release tablets twice a day for one day followed by 300 mg daily) or isavuconazole (200 mg, one tablet three times daily for two days followed by 200 mg daily) can be done.
- The therapy has to be continued until the clinical resolution of signs and symptoms of infection, as well as the resolution of the radiological signs of active disease and the elimination of predisposing risk factors such as hyperglycemia, immunosuppression, and so on. It may have to be given for an extended period of time.
- Conventional amphotericin B (deoxycholate) with a dose of 1–1.5 mg/kg may be used if the liposomal form is not available and renal functions and serum electrolytes are within normal limits.

REFERENCES

AIIMS. (2021). Mucormycosis in COVID 19. *AIIMS Guidance*. https://covid.aiims.edu/mucormycosis-in-covid-19 accessed 26 May 2021.

ASM. (2021, July). COVID-19-Associated Mucormycosis: Triple Threat of the Pandemic. ASM.Org. Retrieved November 28, 2021, from https://asm.org/Articles/2021/July/COVID-19-Associated-Mucormycosis-Triple-Threat-of

CDC. (2021). Where Mucormycosis Comes From | Mucormycosis | CDC. Centers for Disease Control and Prevention (CDC). Retrieved September 26, 2021, from https://www.cdc.gov/fungal/diseases/mucormycosis/causes.html

Chauhan, K., Soni, D., Sarkar, D., Karuna, T., Sharma, B., Singh, S., & Karkhur, S. (2021). Mucormycosis after COVID-19 in a patient with diabetes. *The Lancet*, *398*(10301), e10. https://doi.org/10.1016/s0140-6736(21)01641-x

Cornely, O. A., Alastruey-Izquierdo, A., Arenz, D., Chen, S., Dannaoui, E., Hochhegger, B., Hoenigl, M., Jensen, H. E., Lagrou, K., Lewis, R. E., Mellinghoff, S. C., Mer, M., Pana, Z. D., Seidel, D., Sheppard, D. C., Wahba, R., Akova, M., Alanio, A., Al-Hatmi, A., Arikan-Akdagli, S., … Mucormycosis ECMM MSG Global Guideline Writing Group (2019). Global guideline for the diagnosis and management of mucormycosis: an initiative of the European Confederation of Medical Mycology in cooperation with the Mycoses Study Group Education and Research Consortium. *The Lancet. Infectious Diseases*, *19*(12), e405–e421. https://doi.org/10.1016/S1473-3099(19)30312-3

DGHS India. (2021). Guideline for management of Mucormycosis in Covid-19 patients. https://dghs.gov.in/WriteReadData/News/202105171119301555988MucormycosismanagementinCovid-19.pdf

ICMR. (2021). Evidence based advisory in the times of COVID-19. https://www.icmr.gov.in/pdf/covid/techdoc/Mucormycosis_ADVISORY_FROM_ICMR_In_COVID19_time.pdf accessed 26 May 2021

Lewis, R. E., Liao, G., Wang, W., Prince, R. A., & Kontoyiannis, D. P. (2011). Voriconazole pre-exposure selects for breakthrough mucormycosis in a mixed model of Aspergillus fumigatus-Rhizopus oryzaepulmonary infection. *Virulence*, *2*(4), 348–355. https://doi.org/10.4161/viru.2.4.17074

Pongas, G., Lewis, R., Samonis, G., & Kontoyiannis, D. (2009). Voriconazole-associated zygomycosis: A significant consequence of evolving antifungal prophylaxis and immunosuppression practices? *Clinical Microbiology and Infection*, *15*(Supplement 5), 93–97. https://doi.org/10.1111/j.1469-0691.2009.02988.x

Shakir, M., Maan, M. H. A., & Waheed, S. (2021). Mucormycosis in a patient with COVID-19 with uncontrolled diabetes. *BMJ Case Reports*, *14*(7), e245343. https://doi.org/10.1136/bcr-2021-245343

Singh, A. K., Singh, R., Joshi, S. R., & Misra, A. (2021). Mucormycosis in COVID-19: A systematic review of cases reported worldwide and in India. *Diabetes & Metabolic Syndrome*, *15*(4), 102146. https://doi.org/10.1016/j.dsx.2021.05.019

Trifilio, S. M., Bennett, C. L., Yarnold, P. R., McKoy, J. M., Parada, J., Mehta, J., Chamilos, G., Palella, F., Kennedy, L., Mullane, K., Tallman, M. S., Evens, A., Scheetz, M. H., Blum, W., & Kontoyiannis, D. P. (2007). Breakthrough zygomycosis after voriconazole administration among patients with hematologic malignancies who receive hematopoietic stem-cell transplants or intensive chemotherapy. *Bone Marrow Transplantation*, *39*(7), 425–429. https://doi.org/10.1038/sj.bmt.1705614

WHO. (2021). Mucormycosis. World Health Organization. Retrieved November 28, 2021, from https://www.who.int/india/emergencies/coronavirus-disease-(covid-19)/mucormycosis

Chapter 12

Impact of COVID–19 on Reproductive, Maternal and Child Health

Sonali Sain* and Chiranjeeb Dey

CONTENTS

COVID-19 AND REPRODUCTIVE HEALTH: INTRODUCTION

The world has lived with the COVID-19 pandemic since December 2019 and it is still ongoing. It was recognised to have begun in Wuhan, China. SARS-COV-2 is the new variant of human coronavirus that has caused the COVID pandemic. The spectrum of disease ranges from asymptomatic patients to severe complicated cases with full-blown clinical features of a cytokine storm (Coronavirus, 2020). SARS-CoV-2 infects the human body by binding with the angiotensin-converting enzyme-2 (ACE-2) receptor, which is in various human tissues like the lung, intestine, kidney, testis, ovary, uterus and vagina. Although the virus is found in semen and vaginal secretion, its potential for sexual transmission and resulting subfertility has not been established until now (Morelli et al., 2021). As the ACE-2 receptor is commonly found in Leydig cells and seminiferous tubules of the testis, SARS-CoV-2 can easily affect those areas. It may lead to orchitis but a full evaluation of reproductive function following SARS-CoV-2 infection is under research (Fan et al., 2021; Wang & Xu, 2020). Female reproductive processes necessitate the renin-angiotensin-aldosterone system. It helps in folliculogenesis, steroid genesis, oocyte maturation and ovulation (Li et al., 2020). Although no definite evidence of involvement in the female reproductive tract has been established, it has been postulated that the SARS-CoV-2 virus might affect ovarian tissue, including granulosa cells, leading to subfertility and miscarriage. ACE receptors are expressed in the endometrium, thus it might affect the endometrium and the implantation of the embryo.

The natural history of Covid-19 infection is under research. The possibility of sexual transmission of the disease has not yet been established. Both male and female subfertility along with miscarriage may occur following Covid-19 infection (Li et al., 2020).

DOI: 10.1201/9781003178514-14

CONTRACEPTION AND FAMILY PLANNING DURING THE COVID-19 PANDEMIC

The routine care delivery in the health system was severely compromised during the current pandemic. But the right to sexual and reproductive health care should be respected. Any modern method of contraception can be used to prevent undesirable pregnancy, which is acceptable and safe to them. These methods can include condoms, the pill or mini-pill, emergency contraception pills and DMPA-SC and can be used as a self-care method. A correctly used condom is the only method to prevent sexually transmitted infections, including HIV, along with the prevention of unintended pregnancy. Emergency contraceptive pills can be used safely during the pandemic, and they can prevent conception in up to 95% of cases if used correctly. Regular hand washing, keeping a physical distance of one meter with other people, avoiding touching the face, avoiding large gatherings, self-isolation if unwell and vaccination can prevent SARS-CoV-2 infection. Prevention of COVID-19 can curb all the COVID-19 related reproductive system complications (Headquarters, 2021). The majority of COVID-19 infected mothers present as asymptomatic patients. They were only diagnosed during routine screening. Those who were symptomatic had mild to moderate symptoms. There is very little evidence of mother to child transmission of Covid-19. Even if there is vertical transmission of Covid-19, it is very uncommon. However, a more severe form of infection is found in pregnancy, especially in the later phase. Intensive care admission is more common in Covid-19 affected pregnant women compared with non-pregnant women (Chen et al., 2020). Covid-19 infection in early pregnancy may lead to miscarriage because of the effect on the endometrium. It might lead to preterm birth but most preterm birth is due to iatrogenic causes following symptomatic maternal infection. Vertical transmission of Covid-19 occurs during the antenatal and intranatal period. This transmission is not affected by mode of delivery, delayed cord clamping, skin-to-skin contact and rooming-in (Chen et al., 2020). Apart from preterm birth, there is almost no adverse effect on the foetus. There is no reported increased incidence of congenital anomaly, stillbirth or neonatal death among newborns (Chen et al., 2020). Pregnant mothers should be advised to carry on with routine antenatal care, if possible via teleconsultation. NICE recommended screening for gestational diabetes in all pregnant women during the pandemic to assess the risk of Covid-19 infection following exposure to a suspected case (NICE, 2021).

BREASTFEEDING AND COVID-19

Breast milk is the best source of nutrition for newborn infants, even if mothers have confirmed or suspected COVID-19 infection. Until now, COVID-19 has not been detected in breast milk. Breast milk contains secretory antibodies and other immunological factors that help in the growth and development of a baby and also protects against several infections including respiratory and intestinal infections. It also prevents obesity and non-communicable diseases later in life. Mothers should exclusively breastfeed their babies for the first six months of life and thereafter continue until the child is two years of age. If the mother is very sick then expressed breast milk, relactation (the process of resuming breastfeeding after a period of no breastfeeding or very little breastfeeding) and donor human milk from certified milk banks can be used (World Health Organization, 2021b). Thus, an infected mother should breastfeed her child while taking proper personal protection.

IMPACT OF COVID-19 ON NEWBORN HEALTH

Clinical features of Covid-19 infection in children are similar to that of adult infection. Prevalent symptoms are of the respiratory system (Coronavirus Disease 2019 (COVID-19), 2020b). Infants and children with certain conditions like obesity, asthma or respiratory disease, cardiac disease, diabetes, sickle cell disease and immunocompromised conditions are more prone to a severe form of Covid-19 infection. A newborn baby to a Covid-19 infected mother very rarely presents symptoms. They might be infected from an adult but are mostly asymptomatic (Chawla et al., 2020). Perinatal transmission of infection is very rare and prevention of maternal infection can prevent neonatal infection. Various methods can be adopted to curb maternal infection. The infected neonate can be treated in isolation with proper hygiene controls. Rooming-in and direct breastfeeding can be safely adopted. Breastfeeding should be continued. Recommended national guidelines include fluid therapy, oxygen therapy, antibiotics, management of shock and respiratory support for hypoxemic respiratory failure (Chawla et al., 2020; Wastnedge et al., 2021).

IMPACT OF COVID-19 ON CHILDREN AND ADOLESCENTS

Since the inception of Covid-19 in December 2019, children were found to be less affected by the SARS-CoV-2 virus compared with the adult population. Even if they were affected, they showed a milder form of the disease and mortality was significantly less (Esposito et al., 2021). SARS-CoV-2 spreads directly from person to person, indirectly through contaminated objects or surfaces and/or through close contact with asymptomatic and predominantly symptomatic patients. Infected people spread the infection through oral and/or nasal secretions. Pathophysiology could be explained by the different expression levels of the ACE-2 receptor, the functional receptor for SARS-CoV-2, in children compared with adults. ACE-2 is highly prevalent in organs such as the lungs, heart, gut, kidney and bladder. The following reasons were postulated for different expressions (Adeyinka et al., 2021):

- ACE-2 expression is low children
- Children have different responses to coronavirus qualitatively as a result of thymic involution, continuous antigenic stimulation and so on
- Competition of the SARS-CoV-2 virus with other viruses for respiratory epithelial lining attachment

Children and adolescents were mostly asymptomatic or mild to moderate (96%) with minimum fatalities (0.08%) (Ludvigsson, 2020). Worsening of conditions among the paediatric age group was usually associated with factors like disease severity, associated comorbidity, immune-compromised conditions such as organ transplant, steroid therapy and so on and family compliance. Moderate to severe bronchial asthma increased morbidity and mortality from Covid-19 infection (Abrams & Szefler, 2020). But children with haemato-oncological diseases were not more susceptible to Covid-19 infection compared with the general population (Balduzzi et al., 2020). SARS-CoV-2 resulted in a hypercoagulation state following a cytokine storm in severe types of disease. There was evidence of immune dysregulation, endotheliitis, a hypercoagulation state which led to widespread microvascular thrombosis in the lung parenchyma, causing severe respiratory morbidity. As a result of this hypercoagulable state, there was disseminated intravascular coagulation (Loi et al., 2020; Bhattacharyya et al., 2020). Multisystemic inflammatory syndrome (MIS-C) is a hyperinflammatory syndrome following exposure to the SARS-CoV-2 virus in children and adolescents. It usually occurs two to six weeks after infection. Patients commonly present with persistent fever (>38°C), a systemic inflammatory state with the elevation of inflammation markers, neutrophilic leukocytosis, lymphopenia and organ dysfunction. It has to be substantiated by laboratory or epidemiological evidence of SARS-CoV-2 infection and the exclusion of other microbiological causes. It has clinical-laboratory similarities to Kawasaki's disease, toxic shock syndrome and macrophage activation syndrome. The Royal College of Paediatrics and Child Health coined this condition as paediatric inflammatory multisystem syndrome. It was temporarily associated with the SARS-CoV-2 virus. It defined clinical case definition as persistent fever and the evidence of single or multiorgan dysfunction (shock, cardiac, respiratory, renal, gastrointestinal or neurological disorder) with additional features of full or partial criteria for Kawasaki disease (RCPCH, n.d.). Kawasaki disease (KD) is a medium vessel vasculitis of undetermined aetiology. It usually affects children below five years of age. It was hypothesised as an unidentified respiratory infectious agent, commonly a virus with tropism to vascular tissue. This coronavirus resulted in persistent infection in the bronchial epithelium and macrophages with intracytoplasmic inclusions (Kabeerdoss et al., 2020).

Several studies showed that children, regardless of age and sex, suffered from neuropsychiatric disorders with long-term effects. Commonly found disorders were anxiety and depression. These were due to stressful factors such as lack of school attendance, lack of social contact, quarantine and stressful situations at home. The closure of schools plays an important factor in social, behavioural and psychological consequences (Imai et al., 2020; Viner et al., 2020). Maintenance of all school activities following proper Covid-19 protocols may help to curb the psychological impact of changing lifestyles because of school closures, especially in older children and adolescents (Esposito et al., 2021).

Different preventive measures can be adopted against SARS-CoV-2 in children and adolescents. Children are mainly infected within households, while transmission within educational services is rare. Younger children (preschool and primary) transmit SARS-CoV-2 less often than adolescents while transmissions by adolescents occur with the same frequency as adults in the family and community. Physical distancing (interpersonal distance of at least one meter), use of face masks (nose and mouth cover) in crowded or poorly ventilated environments, proper and regular handwashing with soap and water or an alcoholic product and the frequent cleaning of surfaces all play an important role in breaking the chain of transmission. In addition, there should be the isolation of patients, tracking of close contacts (from 48 h before symptoms appear), control of the source of infection, quarantining the close contacts of infected persons and active surveillance. Protection of the susceptible population can be ensured by proper vaccination along with routine immunisation (Esposito et al., 2021). Hydroxychloroquine has little or no effect on the severity or fatality of the disease in Covid-19 infected patients. It has no effect on the risk of death and the progression to mechanical ventilation (Singh et al., 2020).

COVID-19 VACCINATION AND RELATED CONCERNS FOR PREGNANT WOMEN AND CHILDREN

Although pregnancy is an immune-suppressing condition, it does not increase the risk of SARS-CoV-2 infection. But if a pregnant mother is infected with SARS-CoV-2, then there is an increased risk of adverse pregnancy outcomes like preterm birth. There is also a higher chance of neonatal morbidity (Wei et al., 2021). Most COVID-19 infected mothers remain asymptomatic, but those who become symptomatic and with comorbidities show signs and symptoms of complications. These mothers often require hospitalisation. Pregnant mothers infected with a complicated Covid-19 infection are at an increased risk of iatrogenic preterm birth and neonatal hospitalisation, leading to neonatal death (Chawla et al., 2020). Thus, it is necessary to protect mothers by vaccinating against COVID-19. The World Health Organization recommends vaccinating against COVID-19 in pregnant and lactating mothers as the benefits of vaccination to the pregnant woman outweigh the potential risks. Pregnant women with comorbidities are at high-risk for severe COVID-19 disease. Thus, mothers with comorbidities such as diabetes, organ transplant recipients, chronic respiratory conditions like COPD, asthma, cystic fibrosis, homozygous sickle cell disease, receiving immunosuppression therapies, on dialysis or advanced chronic kidney disease, congenital or acquired heart disease are the priority groups for vaccination against COVID-19 infection. If the pregnant woman has already been infected with COVID-19 during the current pregnancy, then she should be vaccinated after the delivery of the baby. Pregnant women should avoid vaccination if they have had a history of an anaphylactic or allergic reaction to the previous dose of the COVID-19 vaccine or an allergic reaction to vaccines or injectable medicines, especially the penicillin group of drugs. If COVID-19 infection occurs, then vaccination is to be deferred for 12 weeks from infection or four to eight weeks from recovery or if treated with anti-COVID-19 monoclonal antibodies or convalescent plasma. The World Health Organization does not recommend prior pregnancy testing for vaccination. The International Federation of Gynecology and Obstetrics (FIGO) and the Royal College of Obstetricians and Gynaecologists (RCOG) also advised not to discriminate against pregnant women regarding vaccination. The American College of Obstetricians and Gynecologists (ACOG) also recommends that the vaccine should be administered to pregnant women and those who are considering pregnancy in the near future. Countries like Australia, Canada, Israel, Singapore, the UK and the US are vaccinating pregnant women with COVID-19 vaccines (Royal College of Obstetricians and Gynaecologists, 2021; American College of Obstetricians and Gynecologists, 2020). Most children are protected from the severity of Covid-19 infection. They usually recover with basic medication and hydration. Although some children suffer from multisystemic inflammatory syndrome (MIS-C), Kawasaki's disease and so on, the vaccine is still essential to prevent infection. The CDC recommends the Covid-19 vaccination for everyone 12 years and above. Children between two and 12 years should follow Covid-19 appropriate behaviour (CDC, 2021).

As per the revised reports released by AstraZeneca (January 2021), the duration of protection given by this vaccine is not known and the vaccination may not protect all recipients from the disease. It is not recommended for individuals who had severe allergic reactions after the first dose of the vaccine and/or are allergic to any ingredients of the concerned vaccine. Individuals having conditions such as allergies or autoimmune conditions, inflammatory cardiovascular disorders, tendency of fever, bleeding disorders, under blood-thinning medications, a compromised immune system, under immunosuppressive treatments, are pregnant or planning to conceive, are breastfeeding, having received different COVID-19 vaccines or other underlying conditions should consult their physician before taking the vaccines (Queensland; 2021; AstraZeneca, 2021; US Department of Health and Human Services, 2021).

According to the FDA, the possible range of adverse vaccine reactions of the Pfizer vaccines are still not completely known and there is a possibility of unknown or unexpected adverse reactions. The adverse vaccine reactions documented during clinical trials include severe allergic reactions such as difficulty breathing, swelling of the face and throat, tachycardia, skin rashes, dizziness, severe weakness, myocarditis and pericarditis. Also, some common side effects include injection site reactions, fatigue, headache, muscle pain, joint pain, chills, lymphadenopathy, nausea, vomiting, loss of appetite, diarrhoea and fever. In cases of an individual experiencing unknown or unexpected adverse reactions after receiving the vaccine, they should seek emergency medical attention at the nearest emergency healthcare facility. There are no prominent data to confirm or deny the impact of the Pfizer-BioNTech COVID-19 vaccine on pregnant or breastfeeding mothers (Pfizer-BioNTech, 2021; US Department of Health and Human Services, 2021).

There may be the possibility of adverse reactions in individuals receiving the Moderna vaccine, which include severe allergic reactions such as difficulty breathing, swelling of the face and throat, tachycardia, skin rashes, dizziness, severe weakness, myocarditis and pericarditis as recorded during clinical trials. General common side effects include injection site reactions, fatigue, headache, muscle pain, joint pain, chills, nausea, vomiting and fever. According to the FDA, the possible range of adverse vaccine reactions are still not completely known and there is a possibility of unknown or unexpected adverse reactions. Where any individual experiences unknown or unexpected adverse reactions after receiving the vaccine, they should seek emergency medical attention at the nearest emergency healthcare facility. There are no prominent data to confirm or deny the impact of the Moderna COVID-19 vaccine on pregnant or breastfeeding mothers (US Department of Health and Human Services, 2021; ModernaTX, Inc., 2021).

REFERENCES

Abrams, E. M., & Szefler, S. J. (2020). Managing asthma during coronavirus disease-2019: An example for other chronic conditions in children and adolescents. *The Journal of Pediatrics, 222*, 221–226. https://doi.org/10.1016/j.jpeds.2020.04.049

Accessed from https://www.acog.org/clinical/clinical-guidance/practice-advisory/articles/2020/12/covid-19-vaccination-considerations-for-obstetric-gynecologic-care Accessed on 8 October 2021

Accessed from https://www.cdc.gov/coronavirus/2019-ncov/vaccines/recommendations/adolescents Accessed on 8 October 2021.

Accessed from https://www.icmr.gov.in Accessed on 8 October 2021.

Accessed from https://www.rcog.org.uk/en/guidelines-research-services/coronavirus-covid-19-pregnancy-and-womens-health/covid-19-vaccines-and-pregnancy/covid-19-vaccines-pregnancy-and-breastfeeding Accessed on 8 October 2021.

Accessed from https://www.unicef.org/india/coronavirus/covid-19/faq Accessed on 8 October 2021.

Accessed from https://www.who.int/immunization/sage/Guidelines_development_recommendations.pdf Accessed on 8 October 2021.

Accessed from Royal College of Obstetricians and Gynaecologists (RCOG). COVID-19 vaccines, pregnancy and breastfeeding. https://www.rcog.org.uk/en/guidelines-research-services/coronavirus-covid-19-pregnancy-and-womens-health/covid-19-vaccines-and-pregnancy/covid-19-vaccines-pregnancy-and-breastfeeding/ Accessed on 25 February 2022.

Adeyinka, A., Bailey, K., Pierre, L., & Kondamudi, N. (2021). COVID 19 infection: Pediatric perspectives. *Journal of the American College of Emergency Physicians Open, 2*(1). https://doi.org/10.1002/emp2.12375

American College of Obstetricians and Gynecologists. (2020). *COVID-19 Vaccination Considerations for Obstetric–Gynecologic Care*. Retrieved March 8, 2022, from https://www.acog.org/clinical/clinical-guidance/practice-advisory/articles/2020/12/covid-19-vaccination-considerations-for-obstetric-gynecologic-care

AstraZeneca. (2021, January). *PI-for-COVID-19-Vaccine-AstraZeneca*. Doc ID-004379265 v. 2.0.

Balduzzi, A., Brivio, E., Rovelli, A., Rizzari, C., Gasperini, S., Melzi, M. L., Conter, V., & Biondi, A. (2020). *Lessons After the Early Management of the COVID-19 Outbreak in a Pediatric Transplant and Hemato-Oncology Center Embedded within a COVID-19*. Dedicated Hospital in Lombardia, Italy. *Estote Parati*. (Be Ready.). SSRN *Electronic Journal*. Published. https://doi.org/10.2139/ssrn.3559560

Bhattacharyya, R., Iyer, P., Phua, G. C., & Lee, J. H. (2020). The interplay between coagulation and inflammation pathways in COVID-19-associated respiratory failure: A narrative review. *Pulmonary Therapy, 6*(2), 215–231. https://doi.org/10.1007/s41030-020-00126-5

Chawla, D., Chirla, D., Dalwai, S., Deorari, A. K., Ganatra, A., Gandhi, A., Kabra, N. S., Kumar, P., Mittal, P., Parekh, B. J., Sankar, M. J., Singhal, T., Sivanandan, S., & Tank, P. (2020). Perinatal-neonatal management of COVID-19 infection: Guidelines of the Federation of Obstetric and Gynaecological Societies of India (FOGSI), National Neonatology Forum of India (NNF), and Indian Academy of Pediatrics (IAP). *Indian Pediatrics, 57*(6), 536–548. https://doi.org/10.1007/s13312-020-1852-4

Chen, H., Guo, J., Wang, C., Luo, F., Yu, X., Zhang, W., Li, J., Zhao, D., Xu, D., Gong, Q., Liao, J., Yang, H., Hou, W., & Zhang, Y. (2020). Clinical characteristics and intrauterine vertical transmission potential of COVID-19 infection in nine pregnant women: A retrospective review of medical records. *The Lancet, 395*(10226), 809–815. https://doi.org/10.1016/s0140-6736(20)30360-3

Coronavirus. (2020, January 10). World Health Organization. Retrieved 24 August 2021, from https://www.who.int/health-topics/coronavirus#tab=tab_1

Coronavirus Disease 2019 (COVID-19). (2020b, February 11). Centers for Disease Control and Prevention. Retrieved 27 August 2021, from https://www.cdc.gov/coronavirus/2019-ncov/groups/families-children.html

Esposito, S., Giannitto, N., Squarcia, A., Neglia, C., Argentiero, A., Minichetti, P., Cotugno, N., & Principi, N. (2021a). Development of psychological problems among adolescents during school closures because of the COVID-19 lockdown phase in Italy: A cross-sectional survey. *Frontiers in Pediatrics, 8*. https://doi.org/10.3389/fped.2020.628072

Esposito, S., Marchetti, F., Lanari, M., Caramelli, F., de Fanti, A., Vergine, G., Iughetti, L., Fornaro, M., Suppiej, A., Zona, S., Pession, A., & Biasucci, G. (2021b). COVID-19 management in the pediatric age: Consensus document of the COVID-19 working group in paediatrics of the Emilia-Romagna region (RE-CO-Ped), Italy. *International Journal of Environmental Research and Public Health, 18*(8), 3919. https://doi.org/10.3390/ijerph18083919

Fan, C., Lu, W., Li, K., Ding, Y., & Wang, J. (2021). ACE2 expression in kidney and testis may cause kidney and testis infection in COVID-19 patients. *Frontiers in Medicine, 7*. https://doi.org/10.3389/fmed.2020.563893

Headquarters, W. H. O. (2021, January 25). *COVID-19 Clinical management: Living guidance.* World Health Organization. Retrieved 20 October 2021, from https://www.who.int/publications/i/item/WHO-2019-nCoV-clinical-2021-1

Imai, N., Gaythorpe, K. A., Abbott, S., Bhatia, S., van Elsland, S., Prem, K., Liu, Y., & Ferguson, N. M. (2020). Adoption and impact of non-pharmaceutical interventions for COVID-19. *Wellcome Open Research, 5*, 59. https://doi.org/10.12688/wellcomeopenres.15808.1

Kabeerdoss, J., Pilania, R. K., Karkhele, R., Kumar, T. S., Danda, D., & Singh, S. (2020). Severe COVID-19, multisystem inflammatory syndrome in children, and Kawasaki disease: Immunological mechanisms, clinical manifestations and management. *Rheumatology International, 41*(1), 19–32. https://doi.org/10.1007/s00296-020-04749-4

Li, R., Yin, T., Fang, F., Li, Q., Chen, J., Wang, Y., Hao, Y., Wu, G., Duan, P., Wang, Y., Cheng, D., Zhou, Q., Zafar, M. I., Xiong, C., Li, H., Yang, J., & Qiao, J. (2020). Potential risks of SARS-CoV-2 infection on reproductive health. *Reproductive BioMedicine Online, 41*(1), 89–95. https://doi.org/10.1016/j.rbmo.2020.04.018

Loi, M., Branchford, B., Kim, J., Self, C., & Nuss, R. (2020). COVID-19 anticoagulation recommendations in children. *Pediatric Blood & Cancer, 67*(9). https://doi.org/10.1002/pbc.28485

Ludvigsson, J. F. (2020). Systematic review of COVID-19 in children shows milder cases and a better prognosis than adults. *Acta Paediatrica, 109*(6), 1088–1095. https://doi.org/10.1111/apa.15270

ModernaTX, Inc. (2021, August). *Emergency Use Authorization (EUA) of the Moderna COVID-19 Vaccine to Prevent Coronavirus Disease 2019 (COVID-19) in Individuals 18 Years of Age and Older.* Moderna.

Morelli, F., Meirelles, L. E. D. F., de Souza, M. V. F., Mari, N. L., Mesquita, C. S. S., Dartibale, C. B., Damke, G. M. Z. F., Damke, E., da Silva, V. R. S., Souza, R. P., & Consolaro, M. E. L. (2021). COVID-19 infection in the human reproductive tract of men and nonpregnant women. *The American Journal of Tropical Medicine and Hygiene.* https://doi.org/10.4269/ajtmh.20-1098

NICE. (2021, May 27). National Institute for Health and Care Excellence (NICE). Retrieved 27 August 2021, from https://www.nice.org.uk/guidance/conditions-and-diseases/respiratory-conditions/covid19

Pfizer-BioNTech. (2021, October). *Vaccine Information Fact Sheet for Recipients and Caregivers About Comirnaty (COVID-19 Vaccine, mRNA) and Pfizer-BioNTech COVID-19 Vaccine to Prevent Coronavirus Disease 2019 (COVID-19).*

RCPCH. (n.d.) *Paediatric Multisystem Inflammatory Syndrome Temporally Associated with COVID-19 (PIMS): Guidance for Clinicians.* RCPCH. Retrieved 27 August 2021, from https://www.rcpch.ac.uk/resources/paediatric-multisystem-inflammatory-syndrome-temporally-associated-covid-19-pims-guidance

Royal College of Obstetricians & Gynaecologists. (2021, August 25). *Coronavirus (COVID-19) Infection and Pregnancy.* Retrieved 27 August 2021, from https://www.rcog.org.uk/coronavirus-pregnancy

Queensland, COSO. (2021, November 2). *Side Effects*. Health and Wellbeing | Queensland Government. Retrieved 10 November 2021, from https://www.qld.gov.au/health/conditions/health-alerts/coronavirus-covid-19/protect-yourself-others/covid-19-vaccine/about/side-effects

Singh, B., Ryan, H., Kredo, T., Chaplin, M., & Fletcher, T. (2020). Chloroquine or hydroxychloroquine for prevention and treatment of COVID-19. *Cochrane Database of Systematic Reviews*. Published. https://doi.org/10.1002/14651858.cd013587

US Department of Health and Human Services. (2021, May). *Emergency Use Authorization for Vaccines to Prevent COVID-19: Guidance for Industry*. US Department of Health and Human Services. Food and Drug Administration. Center for Biologics Evaluation and Research.

Viner, R., Russell, S., Croker, H., Packer, J., Ward, J., Stansfield, C., Mytton, O., & Booy, R. (2020). School closure and management practices during coronavirus outbreaks including COVID-19: A rapid narrative systematic review. *SSRN Electronic Journal*. Published. https://doi.org/10.2139/ssrn.3556648

Wang, Z., & Xu, X. (2020). scRNA-seq Profiling of human testes reveals the presence of the ACE2 receptor, a target for SARS-CoV-2 infection in spermatogonia, leydig and sertoli cells. *Cells*, *9*(4), 920. https://doi.org/10.3390/cells9040920

Wastnedge, E. A. N., Reynolds, R. M., van Boeckel, S. R., Stock, S. J., Denison, F. C., Maybin, J. A., & Critchley, H. O. D. (2021). Pregnancy and COVID-19. *Physiological Reviews*, *101*(1), 303–318. https://doi.org/10.1152/physrev.00024.2020

Wei, S. Q., Bilodeau-Bertrand, M., Liu, S., & Auger, N. (2021). The impact of COVID-19 on pregnancy outcomes: A systematic review and meta-analysis. *Canadian Medical Association Journal*, *193*(16), E540–E548. https://doi.org/10.1503/cmaj.202604

World Health Organization. (2021b, August 4). *WHO Recommends Continuing Breastfeeding during COVID-19 Infection and after Vaccination*. World Health Organization, Regional Office for Europe. Retrieved 27 August 2021, from https://www.euro.who.int/en/media-centre/sections/press-releases/2021/who-recommends-continuing-breastfeeding-during-covid-19-infection-and-after-vaccination

Part III

COVID-19 and Supportive, Complementary, and Alternative Treatment Strategies

Chapter 13

Ayurveda and COVID-19

C. R. Desai*

CONTENTS

DOI: 10.1201/9781003178514-16

INTRODUCTION

In the past few decades, healthcare has evolved from local family doctors who took care of all ailments for the whole family, to specialists trained in specific skills, and, finally, to capital-intensive mammoth hospitals with state-of-art diagnostic equipment and the latest gadgetry for advanced surgical procedures. To date, the approach to healthcare has been a reaction to disease in the form of prevention, vaccination, eradication programs, early detection, and early intervention drives. Advanced techniques in diagnostics, newer molecules for the treatment of various diseases, lasers, advanced surgical equipment, and robotic surgery have taken healthcare to the next level. However, we are doing more and more for a fewer number of patients and diseases. Ninety per cent of healthcare is concentrating on less than 10% of diseases and patients. The focus is more on treating a few treatable diseases with expensive, sophisticated procedures. Raising the health status of not-yet-ill people does not receive enough attention. In fact, health *per se* has no identity.

Only 5% of humanity needs medical attention and that too mostly in the first and last year of life; in the first year to avoid death and in the last year to postpone it. The rest of the population, called the not-yet-ill, are left to their own means with a psychological blanket of medical insurance that they believe will compensate them if they fall ill. Healthcare needs to ensure health, not just insure it. The Covid-19 pandemic of 2020 has thrown the spotlight on the elephant in the room. *Healthcare* is a misnomer; it should be called 'disease care'. Life insurance is a misnomer and should be called death insurance; like fire insurance and riot insurance, you get compensation only if there is a fire, a riot, or if you die. Your health is given attention if you fall ill or are an insurance risk. At a huge cost in the form of human life, the pandemic showed us that while we were busy looking after a few diseases, the health of the population has steadily declined, leaving people vulnerable to a virus like Covid-19. The pandemic has clearly shown us this. The first and last line of defence is robust health and a strong immune system.

We are standing at the edge of a precipice; it is time we shifted our attention from disease care to health care. We need a disruptive, innovative approach to healthcare; more of the same will not work. Digging the same hole deeper is not the answer; we need to dig a new hole. But then do we know where to begin? The pandemic has also given us the clue to where we can begin. A large percentage of the people who died or suffered most in the pandemic had co-morbidities like diabetes, hypertension, cardiac, or pulmonary diseases, or in some way had a compromised immune system. These co-morbidities are known as non-communicable diseases (NCD). Today, there are millions suffering from NCDs. In fact, 70% of deaths are due to NCDs. Paying attention to NCDs will be a good point at which to begin.

We are not sure about the aetiology of NCDs; we call them lifestyle diseases or stress-induced disorders. There are multiple factors contributing to the development of NCDs. Our current strategy of 'one cause-one disease-one standardized cure' will not work. It is clear that we need a comprehensive solution that includes diet, lifestyle, exercise, and many other aspects of health. In addition, the solution that we seek has to address health at the physical, physiological, psychological, and social levels; the healthcare solution has to be multidimensional.

Another cause of rising concern is morbidity due to the adverse effects of medicines prescribed to treat NCDs. The situation begs us to reconsider our approach to the 'one size fits all' standardized approach to healthcare. The fact is, considering the differences in the genetic profiles, gender, age, upbringing, geo-climatic conditions, current health status, diet, and lifestyle, each individual is unique. Obviously, the advice given cannot be standardized; it has to be personalized to all these aspects of the individual. Hence, the solution that we seek should be personalized. We need a comprehensive, multidimensional, and personalized healthcare solution in order to ensure robust health. Luckily for us, we need not reinvent the wheel. Ayurveda, the ancient Indian system of medicine, is precisely the solution that we are looking for. It is multidimensional, comprehensive, and personalized. Ayurveda is not only a medical system; it is the science of life. *Ayuh* means life and *Veda* means science. According to Ayurveda, balance is health. For a *vaidya* (Ayurveda doctor), the most important thing is to maintain the balance of the individual at the physical, physiological, mental, and spiritual levels. Thus, the approach is **multidimensional**.

Ayurveda has identified ten major factors influencing the health of an individual. These include *Ahar* (diet), *Vihar* (vocation), *Achar* (habits, addictions, and hobbies), *Vichar* (values, principles, and attitude), *Nidra* (sleep pattern), *Maithun* (sex life), *Dinacharya* (lifestyle), *Rutucharya* (changes in lifestyle with seasons), *Desh* (infrastructure, facilities, and amenities), and *Kaal* (geopolitical conditions and religious practices).

There is a branch in Ayurveda called Swasthavrutta, dealing with a healthy regime. Swasthavrutta is an in-depth study of the effects of influencing factors on the health of the individual. It is designed to make subtle changes in the ten factors that influence the health of the individual to maintain balance. This makes Ayurveda a **comprehensive** solution.

The third requirement is the ability to personalize the multidimensional and comprehensive advice. This is where we see the sheer brilliance of the sages who designed Ayurveda. The whole Ayurvedic system is based on the Science of Classification or the Tridosha System of Classification (*Tri* means three and *dosha* means tendency). The natural tendency of any phenomenon or entity (animate and inanimate) is known as its dosha; it can be read as its default setting. All flora, fauna, and phenomena, including the human being, are classified under the Tridosha System of Classification. The constitution of the individual is known as his Prakruti. The resultant of an interaction between an individual and any dietary item, lifestyle practice, climate, change of season, and even habit can be predicted through the Science of Classification. It becomes possible to derive the algorithm, based on which the advice given can be personalized to the Prakruti, age, gender, diet, and lifestyle of every individual. We thus have a system that can also give us **personalized** health advice.

To sum up, *Ayurveda offers us a multidimensional, comprehensive, and personalized healthcare system.*

The one factor that separates human beings from other life forms is their free will or freedom to choose. It is common knowledge that the wrong use of free will in choosing junk food, addictions, and negative emotions and actions harm the individual. As we delve deeper into Ayurveda and Indian philosophy, we realize that the same free will can be used to enhance health. Patanjali Yogasutra is the technology of enhancing the health of the individual by empowering the individual to enhance his health at the physical, physiological, mental, intellectual, and spiritual levels. We can choose health over disease by harnessing our free will. With its advanced techniques of yogasanas, Pranayama, and meditation, Patanjali Yogasutra offers a **proactive** healthcare solution. We thus have a healthcare system that empowers the individual to proactively participate in enhancing health. There is, however, another aspect of health that merits serious consideration, namely, mental health. Whenever we think of mental health, we think about stress, depression, and psychological and psychiatric disorders. By default, we think of mental diseases instead of mental health. Eastern philosophy has never separated the mind from the body, and has, hence, thought about mental health as a continuum of physical health and life itself. The aim is to harness the mind and intellect of the individual to raise him to the next stage of evolution, *from where he is to where he can yet be.*

Karl Marx, in his book on humanity, says that when we are born, we are born as animals; when we fulfil our physiological needs and start thinking about our psychological needs, our birth as a human being begins. He finishes by saying that it is unfortunate that most people die before being born. Having good health is ensuring that we have a well-sharpened tool; it is the first step towards healthy living. Knowing what to do with this tool is the first step towards happy living.

Maslow has identified the hierarchy of needs of the human being: survival, security, belonging, appreciation, and self-actualization. As each of these needs is fulfilled, the individual evolves to the next stage of evolution. Recognizing that our physical and physiological needs are fulfilled is the first step towards living a meaningful life. The key, however, is to become aware of the fact that the previous need is fulfilled; the key to evolving lies in satiation at the physical level, contentment at the mental level, and satisfaction at the level of existence. As Karl Marx said, this is when our birth as a human being begins.

Currently, the world is in the grip of a simple philosophy—more is better. The feeling is that if a thing gives me happiness, more of it will give me more happiness. Eastern philosophy teaches us that happiness is like salt in cooking. More is not better; more is more and better is better. They suggest the Madhya Marg—the path of the golden mean. Balance at the physical, physiological, mental, and intellectual levels is health but this is the first step of living. Real living is in going beyond balance. But what is beyond balance?

It is common knowledge and proven by quantum physics that everything in the universe is constantly changing according to the laws of physics, chemistry, and biology. In fact, change is the only constant. However, there is one power in this universe that has the capacity to participate in and give direction to change. That power is the free will of the human being. We are the power in the universe that can participate in change and direct it with our free will. The buildings, roads, dams, civilization, scientific invention, and art that one sees all around could not have been the products of mindless laws of physics; they are the work of the creativity of the human being.

This is the finger pointing to the moon, towards what lies beyond balance.

Dr Paul Maclean, in his Theory of the Triune Brain, describes the three stages of evolution of the brain, namely, reptilian, mammalian, and neocortex. The reptilian and mammalian brains are designed to take care of the physical and physiological needs. The neocortex is responsible for creativity, innovation, love, compassion, altruism, and all the human qualities that give meaning to human life. Indian and Chinese philosophies have studied the human mind in-depth. There is a lot that one can learn from these ancient cultures. Recent research in genetics and endocrinology has unearthed the brilliant design of nature that helps the individual to discover himself and give meaning to life. The main motivators of human life are pleasure, happiness, and joy. Understanding these will provide the key to happy living. This will help us shift our focus from mental illness to mental wellness, and, further, to the joy of living.

However, there is one last problem that we need to deal with. We will have to find a way to make this solution available and accessible to each individual. This is where information technology (IT), machine learning (ML), and artificial intelligence (AI) come into the picture. With the help of the latest technology, wisdom can be brought within the reach of every individual. This chapter is an integration of ancient wisdom, modern science, and state-of-art technology that will trace the path of the journey of an individual from illness to wellness, and further towards excellence, making it possible for every individual to lead a productive, happy, and meaningful life. This is the solution that we are going to develop, a confluence of ancient wisdom, modern science, and state-of-art technology. This is the Science of Living.

THE SCIENCE OF LIVING

Step-by-step, we will develop the Science of Living.

1. Imbalance to balance
2. Maintaining balance
3. Balance to excellence
4. Going beyond balance—being human

Imbalance to Balance

> No man is an island entire of itself; every man is a piece of the continent a part of the main…
>
> Any man's death diminishes me, because I am involved in mankind;
>
> And therefore never send to know for whom the bells toll; it always tolls for thee.
>
> John Donne

Humanity was rudely woken up to the gravity of the words of John Donne by the Covid-19 pandemic. The pandemic broke down all barriers of caste, creed, influence, affluence, nation, and continent. It showed us that the fate of each individual is tied together with that of the rest of humanity; no man is an island. Going a step further, the pandemic has made us aware of the Butterfly Effect. The flap of the wings of a bat in Wuhan can start a pandemic and disrupt the very fabric of the world. We have learnt that the human being is just a part of the intricately interwoven fabric of the biosphere of the earth that includes the entire gamut of flora, fauna, and microbes. The human body itself is teaming with a wide range of commensal bacteria and viruses. For instance, the vitamins thiamine, riboflavin, pantothenic acid, and a large part of vitamin K in the body are generated by friendly bacteria living in the gut. We have a symbiotic relationship with them and contribute to each other's growth and survival.

Some scientists believe that the earth is one living throbbing, breathing organism. Organic matter continuously interacts with inorganic matter to form a synergistic, self-regulatory system that makes it possible for life to survive on the planet earth. This hypothesis was put forth by James Lovelock. It is known as the Gaia Hypothesis. Gaia is the Greek goddess who is supposed to have drawn life out of the chaos in the universe. Oxygen, nitrogen, and carbon dioxide from the atmosphere, steam, water vapour, and water from the hydrosphere, and calcium, iron, and other chemicals from the lithosphere are constantly interacting with plants and animals. Plants convert carbon dioxide to oxygen and nitrates to nutrition with the help of chlorophyll and sunlight. Animals breathe in oxygen and give out carbon dioxide. There is seamless continuity at the subtle and gross levels between the biosphere, atmosphere, hydrosphere, and lithosphere. Together they help to maintain the temperature, composition of gases, and water on earth, within the range that supports life. It is a system that sustains, regenerates, and maintains itself at an equilibrium away from the equilibrium of the rest of the universe.

It is clear that we have to learn to live as a part of and not apart from the rest of the world.

The foundation of Indian philosophy is the concept of *Advaita* (*A* means not, *dvaita* means dualism), non-dualism or not twoness. The Bible of Yoga is Patanjali Yogasutra. According to Sage Patanjali, the author of Patanjali Yogasutra, the final stage of evolution that an individual can reach is known as *Kaivalya* (only-ness or oneness). Chinese philosophy believes that Tao is where Yin merges with Yang; where there is no dualism. There is a lot to learn from these philosophies.

We depend on the world around us for our very existence, survival, sustenance, and growth. Everything that happens in the world affects us and our health. We cannot live *without* the world, so we need to live *within* it. We just cannot isolate ourselves from the rest of the world.

At the same time, it will be a folly to think that the human being is an insignificant speck of sand on the shore of the world. The free will of the human being is the only power that can wilfully make or break the world and humanity. The collective action of humanity and the choices made by each individual, culture, community, and nation has an effect on the rest of the world. When the United States dropped nuclear bombs on Hiroshima and Nagasaki, humanity almost destroyed all life on planet earth. Global warming, nuclear waste, plastic, and other non-degradable wastes that are choking the soil, the animals, and even the fish in the ocean are proof enough of the destructive power of humanity. On the other hand, the progress in architecture, science, art, philosophy, and evolution of the human being as a species is proof of the constructive power of humanity. It is time we realized the power that we as a species have been vested with. We have to understand that our well-being and happiness are directly linked to the well-being of the rest of the world. We have to learn that judicious use of our free will as an individual, community, nation, and species is the only way to live happily.

Awareness of the sanctity of our birth as a human being and respect for the tremendous power vested in us by nature are the first signs of health. Along with the freedom to choose comes the responsibility of choosing judiciously. To do so, our focus has to shift from imbalance or disease to balance or health. Balance at the physical level ensures that our body is fit. Balance at the mental level ensures that we make intelligent and judicious choices of action each moment of our life. Balance at the spiritual level helps us strike a balance between actions motivated by self (*swartha*) and those motivated by non-self (*paramartha*). That is the way to live a productive, happy, and meaningful life and to justify our birth as a human being. This is the Science of Living.

Maintaining Balance

The law of nature is that everything that is born lives for a stipulated time and eventually dies. Everyone knows it and yet there is a multitude of literature on trying not to die. There is no need to add more to it. What one dies of is a matter of statistics; what matters, however, is how one lives. Life is nothing but time between birth and death. The only difference between other animals and human beings is that the human being has the power to choose. The choices we make during this time decide how good or bad our life will be. The choices we make will be right for us only when we know the areas in which we have a choice, the options that we have, and the logic behind making the right choice. Equally important is to be in a state of balance at the physical, mental, social, and spiritual levels in order to be able to make unbiased and correct choices. It is important to understand the grand design of nature and all that it has to offer the individual.

We have seen in the Gaia hypothesis *(Wikipedia)* that nature is constantly fine-tuning the gaseous composition of the atmosphere, the temperature of the planet, the regularity of the seasons, and the proportion of growth of plants, microbes, and animals in order to maintain the balance on earth. It is only because of this that life has sustained on earth for millions and millions of years. Nature, however, has not been merely a repetitive cycle, there is a definite direction in which the changes are going. Life is evolving towards higher and higher complexity. What we learn from this is that we, as human beings, are not an accident of nature. We are part of an unbroken chain that is definitely leading towards higher evolved life forms.

We are part of a relay and cannot afford to drop the baton or disrupt the game. At the same time, being part of an unbroken chain gives us a sense of belonging and makes us start thinking that maybe there really is a purpose to life. Nobody is sure whether there is life anywhere else in the universe and if there is what form it will be in, or at what stage of evolution; but the journey started billions of years ago. It has been going on since and, in all probability, will go on for billions of years. Evolution can be perceived as a mammoth software development program. According to the latest scientific theory, it began with the Big Bang about 14 billion years ago. At first, there was just a matter-energy soup. Within a very short time (ten raised to the power of minus 35 seconds), the algorithm of gravity manifested itself, followed by electromagnetism, the strong force, and the weak force. It took nature almost three million years to develop the algorithm of the basic building block of the universe—the atom. Gradually, the molecules and later the stable elements developed. We will take a quick look at the chronology of events as they took place in order to create the human being.

EVOLUTION

According to the Big Bang theory, the universe was formed 13.8 billion years ago. The earth was born 4.5 billion years ago. The first signs of life were seen 4.1 billion years ago. No one really knows how or why nature took the quantum leap from inanimate to animate; the fact remains that it did. The early life forms were busy trying to establish the algorithm of survival. It took them almost two billion years; only then did organisms with complex cell structures appear. Nature took a better part of 1.2 billion years to fine-tune the algorithm of survival of complex cells. That is when the first multi-cellular life form made an appearance on earth; this was 0.8 billion years ago. Evolution gathered momentum from there on. Fish and proto-amphibians appeared 0.5 billion years ago. Reptiles appeared 0.3 billion years ago, and land plants were quick to follow. Dinosaurs first appeared on the scene 0.23 billion years ago, and mammals 0.2 billion years ago. Generations of these life forms helped nature to fine-tune the algorithm of survival, growth, and sexual reproduction, and, finally, 65 million years ago, the first primate made an appearance. Far later, just 2.5 million years ago, primitive human beings were born. To put things in the right perspective, dinosaurs ruled the earth for 135 million years; the human being has been around for only 2.5 million years. The point to be noted is that nature has taken almost four billion years to create the algorithm of the software of the human being. Until this point, all life forms have been running on the imperative software developed by nature, which is known as instinct. It was only after billions of years of software development that nature created an organism that has the free will to choose. The algorithm of survival, growth, sexual reproduction, and living in herds has been etched on our genes so that we are let free to put our free will to good use. All the progress, innovation, creation, science, art, and philosophy that one sees are the result of the free will of the human species, and so is the havoc and damage to ecology that the human being has meted out. But, of course, the human being is yet a child; just 2.5 million years old, but he is learning fast.

Evolution According to Eastern Philosophy: A Paradigm Shift

Eastern philosophy has always perceived the universe not as matter/energy but as mammoth software. The first to evolve were the algorithms of the five basic elements—the *panchamahabhuta* where *panch* means five, *maha* means principle, and *bhuta* means elements. The five mahabhuta are *Prithvi* (earth), *Aap* (water), *Tej* (light/fire), *Vayu* (air), and *Akash* (space). Everything in the universe is a combination of these five elements. Every substance carries the characteristics of each of the elements according to the proportion of the elements in its unique combination. The universe is seen as a hologram of algorithms within algorithms within algorithms *(Desai, C R)*.

The West sees the world as a continuous process of energy changing into matter and matter changing back into energy. The East has always perceived the universe as a software in which data is constantly changing according to the program. The formula of an algorithm reads: Data + Program = Changed Data. According to Indian philosophy, in the formula of the algorithm of the universe, Data is qualities known as Prakruti and Program is properties known as *Purusha*. The universe is an ongoing process of Prakruti changing according to the program of Purusha.

Thus, Data + Program = Changed Data. The human being can perceive Data (Prakruti) through his senses as qualities, known as *Gunas*. The program (Purusha) is not perceivable by the senses; it can be seen as the program according to which qualities change. It is only by observing the pattern of change that we can derive the role of Purusha, the program. The program or Purusha in each substance is known as its *Dharma*. Every entity, phenomenon, substance, plant, animal, and human being is a software, a bundle of *gunadharma*; qualities bound by properties. It is a *subset of* and *subject to* the universal software of Prakruti and Purusha. Each substance and life form is driven by its inherent dharma; at the same time, it is constantly interacting with the software of everything around it. The drama of constantly interacting and changing *gunadharma* is perceived as life.

Evolution, a Mammoth Software Development Program

To understand evolution and the way nature sustains and maintains life, we need to perceive life through the eyes of Eastern scientists. Every plant, microbe, animal, and individual is software. The chromosome is the motherboard. The software of survival, growth, maturity, and reproduction is etched on the genes. As life progressed from unicellular to multi-cellular organisms, new features were added. Various species of multi-cellular life forms were released with the new software. The new software was being tested through the very act of living of these organisms. With each generation, as information poured in, subtle changes were made in the software to make it more robust and sustainable. Every generation contributed to the knowledge bank of the universe through the very act of living. The knowledge gathered by each generation was passed onto the next generation in the form of advanced software.

At regular intervals, when the accumulated knowledge reached a critical mass, evolution took a quantum leap and introduced next-generation software. From unicellular to multi-cellular to coelenterates and further to vertebrates, evolution took major strides. The knowledge thus generated was accumulating in leaps and bounds. The process of evolution accelerated.

The initial form of reproduction was asexual. As the mother grew and matured, the knowledge gained by her was accumulated in the gene. When it was time to reproduce, the mother cell divided into two, and so did the chromosome. *It is said that these species 'divide in order to multiply'*. This process of reproduction is known as binary fission. The daughter cells continued to build on the knowledge bank as they went through the process of living. But there was a slight problem. The daughter cells had access to the knowledge gained from the experiences of the mother alone. Knowledge transfer was very slow. In order to overcome this obstacle, nature devised a brilliant method of hastening the process of knowledge transfer; sexual reproduction was introduced. By this method of reproduction, the offspring inherited the knowledge gained by the mother as well as the father. The process of knowledge accumulation and transfer gathered further momentum. Far before Charles Darwin proposed his Theory of Evolution, Eastern scientists had defined the four stages of evolution according to the method of reproduction. The four stages are *swedaja* (born of the sweat—binary fission), *udbhija* (seed born—plant life), *undaja* (egg born—reptiles and birds), and, finally, *jaraja* (born from the uterus—mammals).

It seems that accumulation of knowledge is the method as well as the purpose of evolution. Every life form gains knowledge through the very act of living. This knowledge is accumulated and processed to generate a species that can gain knowledge in a better way than the lesser evolved species. Insentient unicellular and multi-cellular life forms evolved into animals with senses. Fish collected knowledge from the ocean. Amphibians crawled onto the earth and started exploring it through their senses. Some life forms burrowed deep into the earth and others took to the skies. Knowledge was pouring in from multiple sources. The rate of knowledge transfer from generation to generation multiplied several times due to the method of sexual reproduction. Though sexual reproduction is a far less efficient system of reproduction, it was introduced in order to hasten the process of accumulation and multiplication of knowledge. The latest software developed by nature is the human being.

The human being is the first life form to know that it knows. The human being is aware of knowledge; he can say, 'I know'. The software of the human being has three special features. These comprise the three big Cs—curiosity, creativity, and communication. The human being can use the three Cs to gain knowledge through curiosity, use the knowledge to generate further knowledge through creativity and innovation, and pass on the knowledge to others through communication. Knowledge did not have to wait until it was passed on through genes. Accumulation of knowledge could be the method and the purpose of evolution.

The theory seems valid except for one missing link. Is there any evidence of an intelligent super server that accumulates the knowledge gained from all the varied sources by billions of life forms? In the years leading to the Second World War, and during the war itself, there was mass genocide. Millions of lives were snuffed out. Most of those who were killed were males. In the following decade, there was a sudden rise in the birth rate of male children as compared with female children. The question is, how did nature know that the male–female ratio had been disturbed? What is the intelligence that keeps count of the male–female ratio of the millions of sexually reproducing species? This intelligence should also have the capacity to decide the gender of the offspring before it is born; maybe there is a super server. It is well-known that at times when the food supply is abundant, a species multiplies at an alarming rate. As the numbers grow, the food is consumed at a faster rate and then it starts dwindling. And so does the rate of reproduction. In fact, some species became extinct when they ran out of food. However, it has not been seen that only the males of a particular species have survived. If survival of the fittest was the method of evolution, the stronger males should have outlived the females. Even in the wild, it is not seen that only the males of a certain species survive. Another point to ponder is that if the urge of the 'selfish gene' was to increase its own species, it should have followed the most efficient asexual method of reproduction. The sexual reproduction method is cumbersome, complicated, slow, and hit-and-miss; nature need not have evolved to sexual reproduction unless the purpose was accumulation and transfer of knowledge. This is the evidence that makes one think of the existence of a super server that accumulates and processes knowledge and has the capacity to create the next generation of software. We have seen that nature has mastered the art of maintaining the balance of the universe. Life seems to be able to maintain equilibrium away from equilibrium. Each cell maintains its temperature within a particular range; it repairs itself and regenerates its parts or organs. This phenomenon has perplexed scientists. We will now see how nature maintains the internal balance of the human being. The human body has two major nervous systems, namely, the central nervous system (CNS) and the autonomic nervous system (ANS).

Central Nervous System

The CNS consists of the brain, the cranial nerves, the spinal cord, and a network of nerves that connects every organ of the body to the brain. There are two main branches of the CNS—sensory and motor. Sensory nerves carry sensations to the brain and motor nerves carry instructions from the brain to the organs and muscles. The network of sensory nerves collects sensations from all the sensory organs (eyes, ears, nose, tongue, and skin) from all over the body and carries them to the brain. The brain compiles all the sensations and creates a complete picture. The picture is compared with the memory of past events and a line of action is decided upon. The brain then sends instructions to the organs of action through the network of motor nerves. All this activity happens at lightning speed. This is how all voluntary action takes place.

The CNS has two more components that are important for the protection and development of the individual—reflex action and conditioned reflex.

Reflex Action

Reflex actions are instantaneous actions that are hardwired into the system. They are like short-cuts that are not processed through the thinking process of the brain. They are instant actions that protect the individual from harm. And their purpose is to protect the body from sudden danger when there is no time to think. Sneezing, coughing, blinking of the eyes, and ducking when the eyes notice a fast approaching moving object are some of the most common examples of reflex actions.

Conditioned Reflex

As the child grows, it learns how to co-ordinate muscle action for crawling, standing, maintaining balance, walking, and running. Once the muscles learn these actions, they are relegated to deep muscle memory. These actions happen at the spinal level. For instance, there is no conscious thought involved in maintaining balance while standing and walking; the brain is not involved in these actions. They have almost become a reflex action. This is known as conditioned reflex.

Conditioned reflex played an important role in the hunter/gatherer stage of human evolution. Animals develop conditioned reflexes at a very early age. They prove to be crucial to escape from predators and also in hunting for prey. Conditioned reflexes do involve the brain but have become a default setting. With enough practice, swimming, cycling, or skating also become conditioned reflexes. One generally does not forget how to perform these actions. They are etched on the innermost part of the brain. The process of habit forming is an extension of the process of conditioned reflex. The process is not restricted to muscle memory alone. It goes further to the level of cell memory and even more subtly to the level of emotional habits. Mental habits like worry, anxiety, suspicion, mistrust, greed, irritability, and anger gradually become part of our nature. This is what it means when we say that by nature a person is short-tempered, irritable, suspicious, or mistrusting.

The Triune Brain

In 1962, Dr Paul MacLean proposed the Theory of the Triune Brain. He dissected and studied reptilian and mammalian brains and compared them to the structure of the human brain. His findings are very interesting and are particularly significant in understanding the way our CNS functions.

MacLean found that the brain as a structure has evolved in three layers, hence the name 'triune brain'. The layers seem to correspond with the stages of evolution of life on earth. The innermost layer is the brain stem and corresponds with the structure of the brain of reptiles. MacLean calls it the reptilian brain. The second layer is the limbic system. The limbic system covers the reptilian brain like a canopy; limbic means like a canopy. Together, the reptilian brain and the limbic system are quite similar to the mammalian brain seen in animals that live in herds. The third part of the brain, the neocortex, is a relatively recent layer. A thin layer of the neocortex can be

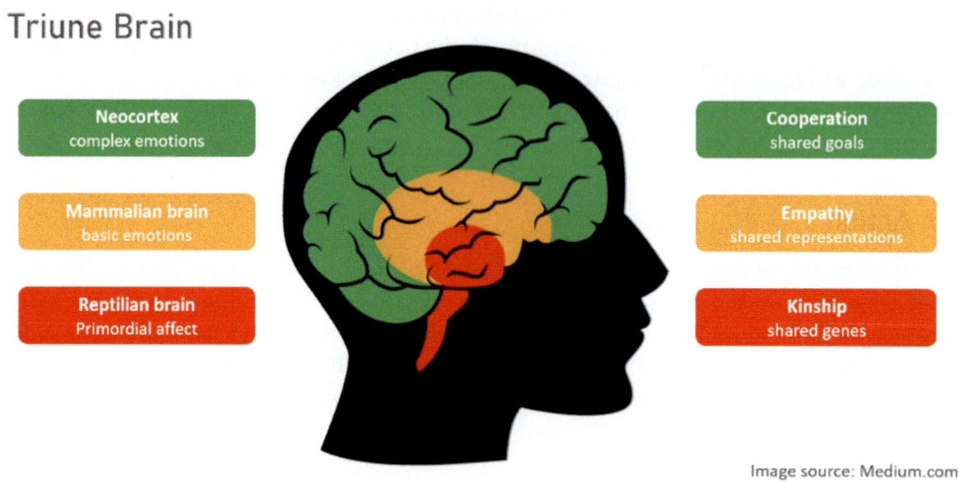

Figure 13.1 The triune brain.

seen in advanced mammals like chimpanzees, but in the human brain, the neocortex represents more than 60% of our brain. The triune structure of the brain can help us understand why we behave the way we do (Figure 13.1).

The Reptilian Brain

The reptilian brain has the responsibility of survival, protection, and procreation. It is aggressive, dominating, and persistent. Whenever the organism feels threatened, it is the reptilian brain that takes over with the fight or flight response; survival is at stake. Each one of us has reptilian streaks like aggression, domination, violence, and, at times, sly, slimy, and manipulative behaviour. Our strong sexual urge also finds its source in the reptilian brain. Nature needs the organism to procreate.

The Mammalian Brain

The mammalian part of our brain has the responsibility of ensuring that we perform all the functions that mammals do. It is responsible for the strong bonding between partners, the need to have offspring, and the love, care, and nurturing of the young ones. The mammalian brain is also programmed for protection, provision, and training of the next generation. In social animals like those that live in herds, and, of course, in human beings, the mammalian brain helps us understand our position in the herd, it helps us create social bonds, and gives us the feeling of belonging. On the flip side, the mammalian brain is responsible for our manipulative behaviour, the need to become the alpha male/female, possessiveness of our spouse and children, and greed for power, position, and possession. Many of the emotions and sensations that trouble us can also be traced back to the first two layers of the brain; fear, anxiety, worry, jealousy, envy, greed, one-upmanship, and, at times, shocking and shameful sexual urges. The first two layers of the brain have no idea of ethics, morals, social etiquette, or manners. They are primordial.

It is the job of the neocortex (the third layer of the brain) to recognize these sensations, understand where they come from, and over-ride the call for action if it is immoral, unethical, inappropriate, or antisocial. The main thing is that one need not feel guilty for getting these sensations or urges; they are natural. The primordial brain is just doing its job. We have to take care to see that the sensations of greed, aggression, and sex do not hijack our intellect and take us into the world of fantasy or worse still, make us act upon them. Actually, fantasizing about them is also action. The neocortex need not bend to the wishes of the primordial brain; it has a far more important role to play in our lives

Neocortex

Some mammals show a thin third layer that covers the first and second brain. This is the neocortex or the grey matter of our brain. In human beings, the neocortex constitutes more than 60% of the brain. Obviously, it must have a major role to play in our life. The neocortex is the seat of imagination, planning, projection, art forms, aesthetics, innovation, and creativity. It is the source of compassion, altruism, dedication, devotion, passion, and empathy. It is the source of our urge to break out of the shackles of 'I, me, and mine'. It is our natural urge of self-manifestation; the need to explore and go beyond the self-imposed limitations of our body, mind, and intellect. The neocortex is the source of evolution. The CNS is largely concerned with voluntary muscles and actions. The signals from and to the brain are largely transmitted by minute electrical currents. There are many other functions going on in the body to ensure existence and survival. Nature in its kindness has ensured that functions like respiration, circulation, digestion, and metabolism are involuntary. It has ensured that we do not have to invest conscious thinking time to run these routine activities. The involuntary functions of the body are governed by the ANS.

Autonomic Nervous System

As the name suggests, the ANS is an autonomous system, not under the direct control of the CNS. We can be thankful for nature that we do not have to invest conscious thought in running the house. The ANS controls blood pressure, body temperature, heart rate, digestion, metabolism, electrolytes balance like sodium, potassium and calcium, water balance, production of body fluids like saliva, tears and sweat, excretion of urine and stools, and also the sexual response of the animal.

The ANS has two main divisions:

- Sympathetic
- Parasympathetic

The autonomic nervous pathway has two nerve cells, one located at the base of the brain stem and the other in a cluster of cells known as a ganglion. A network of nerves from the ganglia reaches out to and surrounds each organ, gland, and blood vessel in that region. The ganglia of the sympathetic nervous system are mostly at the root of the spinal nerves as they leave the spinal cord at the level of each vertebra, on either side of the vertebral column. The ganglia of the parasympathetic division are mostly located near the organ that they are connected to. Together, the two systems control and balance all involuntary functions in the body.

The ANS constantly receives information of external changes through the senses and about internal changes through a wide network of sensors along the blood vessels and organs. The sympathetic and the parasympathetic systems work together to maintain the temperature of the body, and the blood supply to organs like the liver, spleen, kidney, and intestines to regulate their functions.

Sympathetic Nervous System

The function of the sympathetic nervous system is especially significant during a crisis. It is mainly responsible for the fight or flight response. This is known as the stress response and is especially significant when escaping from predators or hunting for prey. As a response to stress, the sympathetic nervous system raises the blood pressure, increases the heart rate, and dilates the airways, preparing the body for action. The hair stands on end, the palms start sweating, and the pupils dilate. Energy from the liver is released for the anticipated burst of action. Blood supply from the digestive system is diverted to the muscles. The whole system is put on red alert. The sympathetic nervous system uses norepinephrine as its neurotransmitter to relay its messages.

Parasympathetic Nervous System

The parasympathetic nervous system is mainly the peacetime nervous system. It conserves energy and restores normalcy. The heart rate is slowed down, blood pressure is reduced, and the blood supply is directed to the digestive system. It ensures a proper supply of digestive juices like saliva, gastric juice, intestinal juices, and bile for digestion. Nutrition absorbed from digestion is taken to the liver for processing and then carried to all the organs. The parasympathetic system aids the functions of renovation, rejuvenation, and reconstruction. The parasympathetic nervous system uses acetylcholine as its neurotransmitter.

Understanding how the ANS works helps us understand the role of stress in precipitating certain diseases. Today, we do not have to save ourselves from predators or go into the fight or flight response but, unfortunately, we have successfully replaced predators with other stressors. Our stress today stems mainly from excessive attachment to people, possession, or position. Fear and anxiety about the future and guilt and remorse about the past are our major stressors. Performance tension, job insecurity, and relationship issues add to the fray. Newspapers and TRP-driven news channels ensure that news about terrorism, wars, rape, riots, and natural calamities are flashed most dramatically and repeatedly. They make sure that the viewer never feels relaxed or safe.

The body cannot make out the difference between a real threat and a perceived threat. It just switches on the sympathetic nervous system. The blood pressure, heart rate, and respiratory rate increase. Blood flow is diverted from the digestive system and routed towards the major voluntary muscles. Since the threat is just a perceived one, it never really ceases to exist or to threaten the individual. One can never let his guard down. The whole body is on red alert indefinitely. Naturally, this leads to a whole range of NCDs. Constantly raised blood pressure leads to essential hypertension and cardiac disorders. Shallow thoracic breathing leads to inadequate oxygenation, muscle stiffness, and cramps, leading further to cervical and lumbar spondylitis, and arthritis. Since the digestive system is deprived of blood flow, digestion suffers, and nutrition is not absorbed well enough. It further leads to acidity, gases, and constipation. Anxiety leads to irritable bowel syndrome (IBS). Inadequate absorption of nutrition leads to nutritional disorders and deficiencies. Health goes spiralling downwards. Other factors that frustrate the efforts of the ANS to balance the system are junk food, over-eating, inadequate meals, irregular meal timings, irregular sleep timings, over-sleeping, lack of exercise and stretching, late nights, disturbed sleep, lethargy, and addictions. (We will be looking at the corrective measures later.) The CNS and the ANS together have been doing a great job of maintaining the balance of health. In addition, there is a third system that has a very important role in maintaining the health of an individual, which is the immune system.

THE IMMUNE SYSTEM

Large predators are not the only enemies of the human being. Smaller life forms like worms, insects, bacteria, and viruses are other enemies that the human being has to combat. Nature has pre-empted this need of the human being as it has for all life forms. It has created an immune system that makes it possible for the individual to live and thrive along with all other organisms.

A positive take home from the pandemic is the fact that literally hundreds of thousands of people who tested Covid-19 positive have recovered. A few did so with medical intervention but in most cases, their immune system bailed them out of the crisis. Nature has equipped the human being to protect itself from millions of known and unknown microbes. The immune system in every life form is designed to combat intruders like bacteria, viruses, and any toxic material like bee stings or scorpion venom that enters the body. The immune system identifies the pathogen and creates an antibody to combat it. After a raging battle, which may be seen in the form of swelling, fever, redness, and pain, the immune system overpowers the pathogen and cures the person. Most of us have experienced a number of infections like common colds, stomach infections, conjunctivitis, or sinusitis. Some of us have recovered from serious infections like pneumonia or bronchitis. A strong immune system is equipped to combat most pathogens. If a foreign material like a thorn or wood splinter enters the body, the immune system isolates it from the rest of the body and eventually expels it from the system. At times, when it fails to expel the foreign body, it sequesters the thorn or splinter and builds a tough layer around it, which, for all practical purposes, separates it from the body. Some of us have experienced this phenomenon in the form of a corn.

The beauty of the immune system is that it is intelligent; it does not indiscriminately destroy all bacteria that enter the system. There are many bacteria that are happily living within us. They are known as commensals. These bacteria do not harm the system. In fact, some of them, such as lactobacilli, have a symbiotic relationship with the individual. They live and thrive in the intestine and, in turn, create and provide the much-needed vitamin B to the individual. Other commensals live in the body and do the job of protecting us from pathogenic bacteria and fungi by not allowing them to take root or grow in their space. The immune system recognizes these friendly bacteria and does not harm them. The immune system is also equipped to identify and eliminate any aberrant cells in the body, such as cancer cells. It is only when the immune system gets weak that some cancer cells escape and start growing. We have to understand the immune system, and find out how it works, learns, develops, and becomes efficient. There are two types of immune system in the human being, namely, inherent and adaptive.

Inherent Immune System

The inherent immune system, as the name suggests, is an inherited pre-programmed immune system that is encoded in the genes. It provides non-specific defence against broadly classified stimuli and situations. This inherent immune system is a general immune system and is not designed especially for a specific pathogen. Its functions include the following:

- Acting as a barrier like the skin, intestinal lining, and the blood–brain barrier
- Attracting the attention of the white blood cells to the pathogen by producing specialized chemicals mediators like cytokines
- Identifying bacteria and removing dead cells and antibody complexes
- Activating the adaptive immune system

Adaptive Immune System

This is also known as the acquired immune system. It is a highly specific defence against any new pathogen that the body is exposed to. Its main components are white blood cells known as lymphocytes, B-cells, and T-cells.

The adaptive immune system performs the following functions:

- Generates specific antigens against the pathogen
- Retains memory of the organism and is in readiness in case of further exposure to it
- Learns from new experiences and makes the defence system wiser
- Plays a major role in making the immune system of the individual strong and efficient

At times, the adaptive immune system cannot differentiate between a pathogenic and a non-pathogenic substance and reacts strongly to a substance or chemical. This results in reactions like allergies, hay fever or asthma, and auto-immune diseases.

Sources of Immunity

Inherent immunity is encoded in the genes.

- Health of the parents during conception and the health of the mother throughout pregnancy decide how sturdy the immune system of the child will be.
- Breast milk of the mother and colostrum are two major sources of immunity. Good health of the mother, proper lactation, and insistence on breastfeeding are essential parts of immunity building.
- Exposure to small doses of common pathogens during childhood activates the adaptive immune system and makes it robust.

Recap

Nature protects the individual and maintains the balance of health through:

Central nervous system
- Protective reflexes
- Conditioned reflexes

Autonomous nervous system
- Sympathetic nervous system
- Parasympathetic nervous system

Immune system
- Inherent immune system
- Adaptive immune system

The CNS maintains balance at the physical level, ANS at the physiological level, and the immune system at the biosphere level, making it possible for the organism to continue living in harmony with other life forms. The three systems of natural defence can be loosely compared to the three humours in Ayurveda known as Tejas, Rajas, and Ojus. Tejas can be compared to the electrical activity of the CNS and the role of Rajas is similar to the ANS that governs all involuntary activities in the body. Ojus can be understood as the immune system. Ojus is said to be the final and most precious humour extracted from food. Wrong eating habits, malnutrition, excessive stress, and excessive obsession with sex and masturbation are said to reduce Ojus and compromise immunity. Nature has created an efficient system to ensure the balance of health. The system has been working efficiently for millions of years and has sustained and propagated millions of species of plants, fish, birds, and animals. However, the system needs active participation from the organism to maintain itself. It needs help in the form of air, water, food, and rest with regularity. These are the basic simplistic needs of the system. Animals are guided by natural instinct in their Circadian cycle. The body gives simple signals to indicate what it needs in the form of breathlessness, thirst, hunger, need to pass urine or defecate, and fatigue as the need to rest and sleep. Animals recognize these signals and follow them. They wake up naturally after they have had enough sleep, breathe regularly, drink when thirsty, eat when hungry, pass urine and stools when they get the signal, and sleep when tired. Nature, in turn, rewards them with a healthy life. The offspring of an animal learns to walk, run, or swim within hours of being born. It learns to protect itself through stealth, speed, or camouflage. It learns what to eat and what not to eat guided by its strong instinct and the parents. Within a short time, it learns to forage or hunt and becomes a self-sufficient adult. Human beings, on the other hand, take almost 12 years to come anywhere near becoming self-sufficient. Besides, the human being has never restricted himself to a habitat that can be called his natural habitat. We find human habitation near rivers and the sea and also high in the mountains. Humans live in tropical jungles and also in arid deserts. The human being is omnivorous-herbivorous, as well as carnivorous. He has been bestowed with the free will to choose, which means that he can overrule the dictates of his instinct. That is why the human being needs more training to judiciously choose to do the basic things that are necessary to support the CNS, ANS, and the immune system. To compound the issue, the human being has an emotive mind and a sharp intellect. The emotive mind generates strong desires and equally strong fears. These strong desires and fears hijack the intellect and cloud the decision-making capacity of the individual. It is clear that there are many things about healthy living that we can learn from animals but most others we have to work out for ourselves. This is where Indian philosophy and Ayurveda, the ancient Indian science of life, come to our rescue.

INDIAN PHILOSOPHY

Indian philosophy is based on the four Vedas—*Rigveda*, *Samaveda*, *Yajurveda*, and *Atharvaveda*. Ayurveda is a part of Atharvaveda. Ayuh means life and Veda means science; thus, Ayurveda is the science of life. We need to understand some of the basics of Indian philosophy in order to understand and appreciate the validity, consistency, and logical bases of Ayurveda. We will be visiting only the parts that are relevant to us in the context of physical, physiological, mental, social, and spiritual health.

Vedanta is the philosophical foundation of the *Vedas* and is found in the Upanishads, at the end of each of the Vedas. According to the Upanishads, the universe is a constantly changing and evolving algorithm. The formula of an algorithm is: Data + Program = Changed Data. In the universal algorithm, Data is known as Prakruti and the Program is known as Purusha. The universe is Prakruti that is Data changing according to a Program that is Purusha.

The universe is perceived as a hologram of an algorithm within an algorithm within an algorithm *ad infinitum*; every algorithm is a subset of and subject to the universal algorithm (Figure 13.2).

As can be seen in Figure 13.2, the algorithm of an individual is a subset of and subject to the algorithms that govern gender and age-related changes. These, in turn, are subject to the algorithm that governs humanity… and so on to the laws of biology and chemistry. Finally,

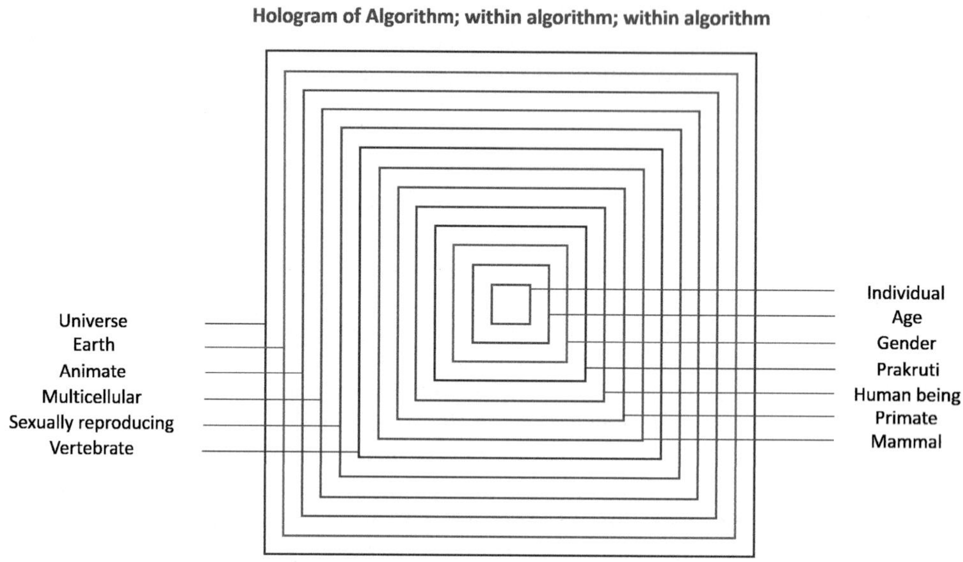

Figure 13.2 Hologram of an algorithm within an algorithm within an algorithm.

everything in the universe is subject to and a subset of the algorithm that governs the universe, such as the laws of gravity, electromagnetism, strong force, and weak force. A subset cannot break the laws or transgress the algorithms governing any of the sets above it. At the same time, with enough knowledge of the governing algorithm, it can transcend the laws to create the next-generation algorithm. This is precisely the way evolution takes place; knowledge accumulation in the super server leads to the next-generation algorithm. The process continues even today. All life forms run on the algorithm that governs their species. The algorithm is imperative and is etched on the genes of the organism; it is known as instinct. If the animal inadvertently or due to circumstances breaches the laws of any algorithm above it, the organism suffers or dies. This is true for all animals and also for human beings. If we break the laws of nature, we suffer; we are not allowed to transgress the laws of nature. Nature does not understand be-cause; it just understands cause and effect. Nature never bothers to find out why we fell, whether we slipped and fell or were pushed or wanted to commit suicide; if we fall, gravity takes over and we hurt ourselves. It is obvious that we have to understand the laws of nature and follow them, else, we suffer. Understanding the laws of physics helped human beings to learn to skate, ski, and sky dive. We could invent the wheel, the motor, and a battery and electricity. Accumulation of knowledge further led to the invention of aeroplanes and made space travel possible. The list is endless. In fact, humanity has just started. The fact remains that we can never transgress the laws of physics; but with understanding, we can transcend the laws to create the next-generation algorithms. It is time we understand the laws of nature and learn to follow them in order to maintain the balance of health. The algorithm that governs human behaviour is the latest creation of nature; the human being is endowed with free will. The algorithm that governs all our body functions and a large part of our behaviour is the same as other primates. It is imperative and we cannot transgress it. If we transgress, we suffer. However, nature has allowed us the leeway to experiment within the boundaries of these laws, understand them, and expand our limits. But if we want to transcend the laws and enhance our abilities, we have to study the algorithm that governs human beings. This is precisely what Eastern scientists have done. While the West was busy understanding the laws of physics and chemistry and dazzling the world with amazing inventions, Eastern scientists were busy trying to understand the algorithm that governs the human being and to enhance its scope and abilities. This effort has led to the development of Ayurveda and the most advanced technology of health enhancement, Patanjali Yogasutra.

The World through the Eyes of the East

The real world does not exist in the form of matter and energy, it exists in the form of algorithms. It is a world of infinite possibilities governed by the laws of probability. Eastern scientists had recognized something that quantum physicists were to find out much later. They realized that the moment human consciousness or an observer perceives the algorithm of any substance, it manifests itself as matter. When consciousness is withdrawn or there is no observer, the substance goes back into its algorithm form of existence. It is human consciousness that makes the universe manifest itself in the form of matter and energy. Only the manifest universe of the present moment appears to the observer in the form of matter and energy. The past exists as an imperative algorithm and cannot be changed. The future exists in the form of algorithms of infinite possibilities; it exists in the form of declarative algorithms. Every moment, the human being has the freedom to choose from the infinite possibilities. You choose what you want to see, feel, and think about this moment; that becomes your present. The choice is made by our action; action is known as *Karma*. Life is not happening to us; we are doing life. The aim of Indian philosophy and Ayurveda is to empower the human being to choose knowledgeably, consciously, and judiciously. Quantum physicists discovered that the quantum world is a world of infinite possibilities governed by the laws of probability. In Indian philosophy, the law of probability is known as the Law of Karma. It is your action that decides the algorithm that opens out as your present. If the scientist wants to see the world as a wave, he sees it as a wave; if he wants to see it as a particle, he sees it as a particle. When the observer is withdrawn, the universe goes back to its un-manifested algorithm form. The human being too is part of the universal algorithm. When a person wakes up and becomes aware, the universe appears in the form of matter and energy; when the person is in deep sleep, the universe goes back to its algorithm existence. The universe appears as matter and energy because that is the way our senses are designed. All human observation is subjective to the human species and appears the same to all of us because of the similarity of our sense organs. All our measuring instruments too are extensions of our senses. There is nothing known as universal objectivity. When quantum physicists saw this truth, it shook the very foundation of science. The human being is a part of the algorithm trying to understand the universal algorithm from within while living in it. It is like the fish trying to understand the ocean through its own eyes. Our sense organs pick up information or data in the form of qualities. We become aware of change in qualities as change in size, shape, colour, taste, sound, smell, or touch. Another change we observe is movement. Change makes us aware of the concept of time—past, present, and future; movement makes us aware of space and directions. Observation over a period of time makes us aware of cyclical changes and patterns of change, and we start perceiving a system. This we understand as knowledge. Pattern of change is knowledge; when we understand it, it becomes ***our*** knowledge. That is when we say, I know. According to the great management guru Peter Drucker:

> Knowledge is information in action.

Observing and understanding the pattern of change in information or qualities is the way to gain knowledge. Observation of the pattern of change followed by deep contemplation is the method of scientific enquiry followed by Eastern scientists. The aim is to derive the laws of probability that drive the world of infinite possibilities. They observed the pattern of change in Data to derive the Program that governs the change, based on the formula of an algorithm:

Data + Program = Changed Data

Prakruti or Data of each substance and phenomenon in the universe is perceived by the human being as qualities. We perceive qualities through our senses in the form of sight, sound, touch, smell, and taste. These qualities are known as Gunas. The human being can perceive qualities and changed qualities (Data and Changed Data). Purusha or the program is only an inference that is drawn by the individual by observing change. The inherent program of a substance is known as its dharma; we understand dharma as properties of the substance. Each entity, phenomenon, and life form is a unique bundle of qualities and properties or gunadharma—qualities bound by properties. It is a bundle of information (data) bound by inherent instructions (program). Each individual too is a software, a bundle of gunadharma that is constantly interacting with the software of everything around it. Information is gathered through the senses; instructions are understood through experience and observation. The only way the individual perceives the properties of any substance that he interacts with is through experience. That is why experience with total awareness has been given prime importance in Eastern philosophy.

We will try and see the universe through the eyes of an Eastern scientist.

Panchamahabhuta, the Basic Building Blocks of the Universe

According to Indian philosophy, each living and non-living entity and phenomenon in the universe is made of the five principle elements or Panchamahabhutas; Prithvi (earth), Aap (water), Tej (light/fire), Vayu (air), and Akash (ether/space). Each of the basic elements has certain basic qualities or gunas and properties or dharma. Prithvi represents solidity and storage, Aap—fluidity and transport, Tej—light, heat, and transformation, Vayu—movement and change, and Akash—space for movement and change.

These elements are present in every substance but in different proportions. Each element contributes its gunadharma to the substance in the proportion that it appears. The unique proportion of the constituent elements gives each substance its unique character of qualities and properties or gunadharma. Thus, each substance is a unique software.

Qualities like smell, touch, taste, shape, and sound of a substance are its gunas. The intrinsic changes that a substance undergoes over time like entropy in physical systems and ageing in life forms are due to their inherent properties or dharma.

The changes that take place in the world are due to the interaction of the gunadharma (software) of a substance with the gunadharma (software) of other substances and phenomena.

Every moment, the gunadharma of every substance is interacting with the gunadharma of everything around it. Every moment, the whole universe is evolving, changing the gunadharma of everything in it, giving rise to new gunadharma. These are known as emerging gunadharma; this is the basis of evolution, and it is happening every moment.

Scientists in the East observed something very important. Although the form, qualities, and properties of a substance change every moment, there is something of the substance that continues through all the changes that it undergoes. In Ayurveda, this basic unchanging character of a substance is known as its dosha or the basic tendency of the substance. The dosha of a substance is the inherent tendency that a substance brings to each interaction that it participates in. The dosha of each substance in an interaction contributes to the emerging gunadharma of the resultant.

Dosha (Desai, 2018)

The concept of dosha is a brilliant contribution of Ayurveda to science. We will invest some time in understanding the concept of Dosha.

Scientists found that each substance brings its inherent tendency or dosha to an interaction. The gunadharma of each participant in an interaction influences the gunadharma of the end product.

This phenomenon can be understood more easily in the process of cooking. Each ingredient comes with its dosha. The final product has a hint of the taste, colour, and smell of each of the ingredients. It is a combination of the doshas of each of the ingredients. The dish is not merely an addition of the gunadharma. It is a new substance that has its own gunadharma. Though the gunadharma of all the ingredients has changed, there is something of each substance that persists all through the changes and that is its tendency or dosha.

Earth, water, sun, wind, and space change with every season, yet each element retains its inherent character. Earth retains its solidity, water its fluidity, sun its heat, wind its movement, and space its capacity to envelop the world. The principal element Aap or water is seen in nature in different forms—water vapour, clouds, and flowing water or ice, yet it does not lose its wateriness. Here is another example. Sugar can be identified by its white colour, granular structure, sweet smell, and taste; these are its gunas. We know that it becomes sticky when it interacts with moisture, melts when heated, and gets caramelized when burnt. This is its dharma. In any interaction, sugar lends its sweetness and stickiness to the end product. This tendency is its dosha. The chemical structure of water in any form retains its H_2O-ness and sugar in any form remains a hydrocarbon; this could be understood as its dosha; a signature identity that persists through all change.

The brilliance of Ayurveda is that every substance, phenomenon, and even the human being is classified under the Tridosha System of Classification. In the case of an individual, the dosha or basic constitution is known as his Prakruti.

The Prakruti of an individual can be understood as his genetic profile. The form or gunadharma of the individual changes as age advances but his Prakruti, his individuality, remains the same throughout his life. In the individual, gunas are observable physical characteristics, and dharma dictates the process of growth, maturity, and ageing. The inherent tendency or Prakruti is beyond gunadharma. The Prakruti of the individual dictates how he responds and reacts to factors that he interacts with all through life.

> It is very important to be able to diagnose the Prakruti of an individual to understand how the intrinsic and extrinsic influencing factors impact him.

The Tridosha System of Classification

The Tridosha System of Classification classifies a substance or phenomenon according to the effect that it has on any interaction that it participates in. The three doshas are Vata, Pitta, and Kapha. The five principal elements, each with its gunadharma, combine to create three basic tendencies or dosha: Vata dosha, Pitta dosha, and Kapha dosha. Prithvi (earth) and Aap (water) combine to create Kapha dosha, Tej (light/heat) creates Pitta dosha, and Vayu (air) and Akash (space) together create Vata dosha. The gunadharma of the five principal elements are reflected in the dosha that they create. In Ayurveda, everything in the universe is classified under the three doshas. The dosha of a substance dictates the direction in which the substance tends to steer an interaction. Vata dosha has the characteristics of its basic elements Akash and Vayu. It contributes lightness, movement, and disruption to an interaction. Pitta dosha has mainly the characteristics of the Tej element, and contributes heat, metabolism, and transformation to an interaction. Kapha dosha has the characteristics of Prithvi and Aap, and brings fluidity, nourishment, and stability to an interaction. A substance classified as Vata increases the Vata dosha in an interaction; this is known as *vataja* or giving rise to Vata dosha. It is, the same with substances classified under Pitta and Kapha. Even a phenomenon like climate has been classified as vataja, pittaja, or kaphaja.

A dosha can also reduce the effect of another dosha in an interaction. For example, a Kapha substance reduces the Vata effect in an interaction. When it does so, it is said to have a *vataghna* effect (destroying or reducing Vata dosha). The first criterion of good health, according to Ayurveda, is samadosha, or balanced doshas. For a person to be in good health, the doshas in the body have to be balanced. The Tridosha System of Classification gives the physician a wide range of substances to combat the effects of a dosha that is in excess or to strengthen a dosha that is waning. For instance, when a patient goes to a physician for a symptom like acidity, the physician knows that Pitta dosha has increased. He then advises a *pittaghna* substance like milk to reduce Pitta dosha. But before treating the person, the physician has to diagnose the original Prakruti of the person so that he can find the perfect match of the corrective substance for the person.

Prakruti

The Tridosha System of Classification has defined the three basic doshas or tendencies: Vata (V), Pitta (P), and Kapha (K). Each individual is born with a unique Prakruti or combination of the three doshas. We can understand it as the basic constitution of a person. Since there are three doshas, mathematically there are ten possible combinations of Vata, Pitta, and Kapha. Three single dosha Prakrutis: Pure Vata (V), pure Pitta (P), and pure Kapha (K) are known as single dosha Prakruti.

Six combination Prakrutis: one dosha is dominant, the second dosha less so, and the last dosha is very low or recessive. For instance, the Prakruti of a person with dominant Kapha dosha, secondary Vata dosha, and weak Pitta dosha is read as Kapha Pradhan Vata or Kapha/Vata (K/V) Prakruti. In this way, there are six possible combinations, namely, K/V, K/P, P/V, P/K, V/K, and V/P. One equal dosha Prakruti: here all the three doshas, V/P/K, are equal. In practice, however, pure V, P, or K and equal V/P/K are rarely seen. Most individuals fall within the six basic Prakruti combinations K/V, K/P, P/V, P/K, V/P, and V/K. Over centuries, Ayurvedic physicians have drawn a ready reckoner of physical, physiological, and psychological gunas or characteristics that can be used to diagnose the Prakruti or basic constitution of an individual. Some physicians may use pulse diagnosis (Nadi Parikshan) to confirm the diagnoses. A person with Kapha pradhan (Kapha dominant) Prakruti is typically stocky, sedate, humble, trustworthy, perseverant, and tending towards obesity. He reflects the tendency of Prithvi (earth) and Aap (water) mahabhutas. A person with Pitta pradhan Prakruti is muscular, sharp, analytical, short-tempered, and tends towards acidity and high blood pressure. He reflects the tendencies of Tej (light/heat) mahabhuta. A person with Vata pradhan Prakruti is lean, flitting from one topic to another, open to new ideas, and has disturbed digestion and cracking joints. He reflects the tendencies of Vayu (air/wind) and Akash (space) mahabhutas. These attributes remain with the person right through life. We see these people every day. They are so different from each other and yet all of them are normal. Each Prakruti has its strengths and weaknesses, and every Prakruti is susceptible to and has a predilection for certain diseases. Ayurveda has classified the individual by his Prakruti and the factors influencing health with its dosha under one system of classification, namely, the Tridosha System of Classification. This empowers the physician to deliver the best form of personalized healthcare to each individual. Personalization is the core strength of Ayurveda and that is possible because of the Tridosha System of Classification. Every day, each one of us interacts with multiple influencing factors, often with many at the same time. Every moment, the balance of doshas is subtly disturbed. The ANS with its multiple strategically positioned sensors and sympathetic and parasympathetic systems is a self-correcting mechanism that constantly re-establishes the balance of doshas. This is known as homeostasis. The lesser the variations, the more stable is the health of the individual. If a person knows the dietary items and lifestyle that is best suited to his Prakruti and keeps his lifestyle as close as possible to what suits his Prakruti, he can actively ensure that his health remains stable. On the other hand, if he indulges in substances that do not suit his Prakruti, an imbalance of doshas is triggered, which, in turn, manifests as discomfort and pain. If the imbalance continues for a long period, the discomfort converts into a disease. Substances and lifestyles that suit your Prakruti are said to have *satmya* or compatibility with your Prakruti; those that do not suit your Prakruti are said to have *asatmya* or incompatibility. The Tridosha System of Classification makes it possible for us to understand the diet and lifestyle that suits our Prakruti the best. The branch of Ayurveda that defines the system of satmya and asatmya is known as Swasthavrutta. Swasthavrutta—*Swastha* means healthy and *vrutta* means regime.

AYURVEDA

Ayurveda has been developing and growing for millennia. It may be recalled that Ayurveda has identified ten major factors that influence the health of an individual. These include:

1. Ahar (diet)
2. Vihar (vocation)
3. Achar (habits, addictions, and hobbies)
4. Vichar (values, principles, and attitude)
5. Nidra (sleep pattern)
6. Maithun (sex life)
7. Dinacharya (lifestyle)
8. Rutucharya (changes in lifestyle with seasons)
9. Desh (infrastructure, facilities, and amenities)
10. Kaal (geo-political conditions and religious practices)

The Tridosha System of Classification has classified the multiple variables of each of the influencing factors into Vata, Pitta, and Kapha. For instance, if in an interaction a substance increases Vata dosha, it is said to be vataja; if it decreases Vata dosha, it is known as vataghna. This has made it possible for the physician to understand the impact of each variable of the influencing factors on the delicate balance of Vata, Pitta, and Kapha, and its impact on the health of an individual.

Generations of physicians have selflessly added to the humungous pharmacopoeia of Ayurveda. It is simply amazing to see the details to which the physicians have studied literally thousands of food items, herbs, and animal products in every region. There are volumes and volumes to be studied in the Ayurveda pharmacology known as *Dravyaguna*. There are detailed instructions on how to identify a herb and the effects of each herb on the doshas.

The scriptures define how a physician should prepare himself to collect the herb, the best time to collect it, and how to preserve it. Each herb has to be processed in a particular way to enhance its effects on the doshas when used as medicine; the processing is known as *Sanskar*. A lot of importance has been given to the attitude, frame of mind, and intention of the physician while preparing the medicine. Ayurveda physicians even today pay a lot of attention to these details while preparing the medicines that they use.

When one approaches an Ayurveda physician (Vaidya) with an ailment, he diagnoses the imbalance (*Vikruti*) by assessing the current proportion of doshas as compared with your Prakruti or original proportion of doshas. He then suggests carefully prepared medicines from his vast pharmacopoeia. These medicines have been prepared from herbs, animal products, minerals, or metals. The potency of the original herb or substance has been enhanced by following a strictly defined process, known as Sanskar. The process has been defined in the scriptures step-by-step and in minute details. The art of treatment of disease is known as *Kaayachikitsa* and is beyond the scope of this chapter. It is more important for us to understand what the Vaidya does after the treatment.

After treating the ailment, the Vaidya makes the patient aware that the reason for his illness is that he has transgressed certain rules of Swasthavrutta. The cumulative effect of having transgressed these laws for a long period has resulted in a sustained imbalance of doshas that has presented as a disease. He then suggests subtle corrections in the patient's daily routine in order to ensure that the balance of doshas is maintained. We will be well-advised to understand the laws of Swasthavrutta and follow them as closely as possible to remain healthy; this is active healthcare.

Swasthavrutta (Ranade et al., 2004) defines the best routine to be followed by an individual to ensure that the balance of doshas in the body is not disturbed too much through the day. General advice on best practices for the individual has been defined under the following parts:

- *Dinacharya*—Routine during the day
- *Ratricharya*—Routine for the night
- *Rutucharya*—Routine according to seasons
- *Sadavrutta*—Good or proper behaviour
- *Trayopastambha*—The three pillars of healthy routine, namely, diet, sleep, and self-restraint

Dinacharya: Daily Routine

Swasthavrutta gives a lot of importance to cultivating good habits or habits that are conducive to one's Prakruti. The daily routine that is best for maintaining good health should become a regular practice and should not be used as a detoxification or a weight loss program after which one can go back to malpractices. It should become a default arrangement practised every day unless something untoward happens to disturb the routine, after which one goes back to the regular practice.

Wake-Up Time

It is suggested that one should wake up at least one and a half hours before sunrise. This is known as the *Brahma-muhurta*. This time of the day is when the mind is fresh and most active. There are no outside disturbances to distract a person and the mind is open and receptive to new ideas and insights. It is the best time for meditation, contemplation, and a short prayer of gratitude to the Maker. A person is not rushed or hassled and can allow his mind to receive new insights; the antenna of the mind is sharp and receptive. This is the best time to calmly plan the whole day. It is Vata dosha time; Vata dosha represents movement, so it helps movement of the bowel. Healthy passage of urine, gases, and stools becomes easier.

Hygiene

In Dinacharya, a lot of importance has been given to the hygiene of the mouth, teeth, and gums. The toothpaste that we use should contain certain astringent herbs to keep the teeth tightly held together and the gums healthy. Most Ayurvedic toothpastes do contain these herbs. Cleanliness of the genitals and the anus has been given special attention. Use of water is far better than using toilet paper. There is an elaborate description of the care of all the sense organs with regular use of herbal oils and drops for eyes and ears for better vision and hearing. Gargling with a herbal mouthwash is suggested for oral hygiene and better taste. Special herbs for gargling have been suggested. Gargling thoroughly after every meal is definitely preferable to just wiping the mouth with a tissue. Applying oil to the whole body and keeping it on for ten minutes before taking a bath each morning is the best way to prevent wrinkling of the skin, dry skin, and itching. This is known as *Abhyanga*. It reduces Vata dosha and helps to keep the skin young and the complexion glowing. It nourishes the muscles, lubricates the joints, and increases body awareness.

Exercise

According to Swasthavrutta, exercise keeps the body light and nimble. From the latter half of October, up to the first half of March, one should exercise to half our strength. Mouth breathing, dryness of throat, and sweating at the brow and armpits are indicators that you have done enough exercise. In the other months of the year, exercise should be less than half strength. We are warned that exercise more than this decreases muscle power and causes the drying of joints. Subtle corrections will have to be made for people who have sedentary jobs. Nevertheless, over-exercising is definitely discouraged.

Six Ss of Exercise (Desai, 2020)

There are six important Ss in exercise, namely, strength, stamina, stretching, speed, skill, and spirit. All six aspects of exercise have to be given due attention. The best combination is a set of six Suryanamaskar followed by 25–30 minutes of aerobic exercise (preferably in the open air) like a racquet game, a jog or swim, and ending with a set of six Suryanamaskar. Walking mindlessly on a treadmill in a closed air-conditioned gymnasium reduces the benefits that one gets from exercise. The body is put on auto-pilot and the spirit or mind is drifting, especially if the TV in the gymnasium is loudly blaring the breaking news of the day.

Meal Timings

Having regular meal timings is especially encouraged in Swasthavrutta. If the meal timings are regular, the digestive juices like saliva in the mouth, gastric juice in the stomach, pancreatic juice, bile, and intestinal digestive juices start accumulating in their respective places just before mealtime. Smells of freshly cooked warm meals stimulate the juices, prepare them for digesting, and extract all the necessary nutrients from the food, with the appetite now well stoked. If one does not eat at that time or if one pacifies the digestive juices with a cup of coffee, one loses the chance to get the vital nutrients from the meal. Digestion is disturbed, leading to acidity, gases, and constipation, setting off a cycle of digestive disorders. Having fresh, warm, homemade meals at regular hours has been given prime importance. A small walk for ten minutes, followed by relaxation for about fifteen minutes after the afternoon meal, is said to be very good for health.

In the evening, one is encouraged to have a warm bath and a relaxed meal. A family that eats together and prays together stays together. Spending quality time with your near and dear is a necessary part of Dinacharya.

Ratricharya: Night Routine

The evening meal should be slightly smaller than the afternoon meal. The meal should be taken at about nine o'clock in the evening. This should be followed by a small leisurely walk for about ten minutes; it is known as *shatpavali*—100 steps. One should not sleep immediately after a meal.

One should avoid loud music or watching disturbing movies or programs before going to sleep (for obvious reasons). In the northern hemisphere, one should sleep with the head either to the east or north. On lying down it is best to lie on the back for eight breaths, on the right side for 16 breaths and then for 32 breaths on the left side; after that, one should allow the body to rest in its position of comfort.

Rutucharya: Seasonal Routine

One should remember that Ayurveda has grown in India and hence considers the seasons as seen in India. However, some of the principles defined in Swasthavrutta, with subtle modifications, hold true for most geo-climatic conditions. During the hot summer months, the influence of the sun is strong and body strength is low; hence, one should avoid heavy work or exercise. After mid-January, the effect of the moon increases, and this is the time when one can work for long hours and perform physically demanding activities.

The calendar of the year has been divided into six *rutus* or seasons. *Varsha* and *Sharad* rutu are the rainy season, *Hemant* and *Shishir* are the winter season, and *Vasant* and *Grishma* are the summer season. Swasthavrutta has outlined the best diet and the activities to be taken up during each of these seasons. Rainy season is Vata time, winter is Kapha time, and summer is Pitta time of the year. The diet has to change to ensure that the internal balance of the body is maintained during these periods. The festivals and special dishes prepared for each of these festivals have been traditionally designed to keep the doshas in balance.

Special emphasis is laid on the gradual changes in diet as the rutu changes from one season to the next. The changes cannot be dramatic; one has to gradually reduce the food items taken in one season and ease in the diet of the next. The changes in diet in the last 15 days of the previous season and the first 15 days of the next are especially important.

Sadavrutta: Good or Proper Behaviour

Proper behaviour at the physical and mental levels and responsibility in speech are considered to be habits that one needs to inculcate. Sanskar or upbringing of the child is very important because these habits are best inculcated at a young age. Violence, theft, jealousy, telling a lie, gossip, and maligning others are to be avoided. One should also avoid wishing ill for anyone, envying others, and disrespecting the Holy Scriptures. One should not stay in the company of people who indulge in such activities. Instead, one should inculcate the habit of wishing good for others and doing as much as one can to help them. Keep the senses in reign and do not indulge their demands for more and more gratification with excessive eating, loud sounds, and garish entertainment or pornography. Cultivate respect for elders, the wise, and the knowledgeable. Direct your excess energy and need for adventure towards challenging activities for the good of others. Be soft-spoken and kind. Avoid the use of foul language. The suggestions given in Sadavrutta seem to be simple common sense, but we shall see the importance of inculcating these good habits when we deal with the concept of Karma.

Trayopastambha: Diet, Sleep, and Self-Restraint

Trayopastambha, the three pillars of good health, are Ahar (diet), Nidra (sleep), and Brahmacharya (self-restraint).

Diet (Ahar)

The general impression is that Ayurveda is all about denial and depriving ourselves of all the tasty and exciting things that we love to eat, and that it is against the consumption of meat and alcohol. The truth is quite different. Ayurveda has studied the gunadharma of the meat of fish, crustaceans (prawns, crabs), amphibians, chicken, sheep, large animals, and even wild animals. It has studied the gunadharma of different types of alcoholic drinks prepared from a variety of ingredients like grain, honey, flowers, and fruit. Having studied the gunadharma of all these dietary items, Ayurveda suggests the rutu in which each of them is conducive to health. They suggest the type of wine to be consumed in each season, with, of course, a caution against over-indulgence. Having the same type of meat and wine all-round the year is discouraged as being incompatible with the body. Certain types of wine are best consumed in summer while harder forms of alcohol should be reserved for the winter. The diet should be designed according to one's vocation and daily activities to ensure that the body can tolerate the food items and yet remain healthy. The Ahar (diet) section in Ayurveda is particularly interesting, informative, indulgent, and yet scientifically beneficial to good health.

The diet section deals with the six tastes (*rasas*) that should be included in each meal and also the way a meal should be served.

- *Madhur ras* (sweet) like rice, wheat, *jowar* (sorghum), and *bajra* (pearl millet), and milk products are Kapha-based and are important for giving strength and energy; they should form the bulk of the diet and should occupy the centre of the plate.
- *Amla ras* (sour) taste present in lime and pickles increase the appetite and salivation, and add to the taste, making eating a good experience. They should be served in small quantities to the left of the staple food.
- *Lavan ras* (salt) should be served at the top of the plate and should be added to the food items as per taste; the tongue can be trusted to tell you how much salt you need. In a hot country like India, one loses a lot of salt through sweat. The salt needs to be replaced regularly, except in people suffering from hypertension.
- *Katu ras* (spicy) taste: The second most important dietary ingredients are pulses, legumes, and vegetables served in the form of curries. The spices that make Indian curries dear to most people belong mainly to katu ras. It is katu ras that makes pulses and legumes easier to digest and adds the yummy taste to the meal.

- *Tikta ras* (bitter): We generally tend to avoid anything with a bitter taste, but bitter food has the property of stimulating the taste buds, making the food easier to digest, and helping to mitigate the effects of any toxins in the food. *Tur dal*, *methi*, spinach, and bitter gourd are examples of tikta ras and should be included in a proper diet. These food items along with katu ras food items should occupy the upper portion of the plate.
- *Kashaya ras* (astringent) food items are slightly heavy for digestion and their use should be kept to the minimum. A meal should end with a small portion of rice and buttermilk (kashaya rasa); it facilitates digestion.

Most Indian middle-class families, even today, have at least one meal that has most of the ingredients as suggested in Swasthavrutta. Ordering a single food item, illogical diet of just salads or sprouts, only carbs, or heavy meat items plays havoc with digestion and absorption of food, and also disturbs regeneration of body cells. Energy levels steadily drop, leading to imbalance and eventually disease. Diet freaks, people who eat out often, or binge eaters be warned.

Some Basic Dos and Don'ts about Diet

1. **Water intake and meals.** Drinking a lot of water before or immediately after a meal should be avoided as it dilutes all digestive juices. One may have sips of water while eating.
2. **Excessive eating.** Eating within 3–4 hours of the previous meal does not allow the previously consumed food to digest well. One must wait until one is properly hungry before having the next meal
3. **Inadequate eating.** Avoid eating at the wrong time or eating far less than one needs and eating at odd times because it may not be possible to eat at mealtimes.
4. **Incompatible foods.** Having two food items that are not compatible with each other, such as alcohol and milk products or honey with warm water, should strictly be avoided.
5. **Fasting.** Illogical long periods of fasting cause weakness and reduce Ojus, resulting in diseases that are very difficult to treat.
6. **Best food.** The best food is what grows in that season in that region. Eating food that is out of season and imported from a different geo-climatic region should be avoided.
7. **Avoid:**
   a. Eating foodstuff that does not agree with the Prakruti of the individual, such as a Pitta Prakruti person having spicy food
   b. A person suffering from excess of Vata dosha having food items that increase Vata dosha
   c. Food items that have proven to be incompatible with your system
   d. Mixing contrasting food items like milk and fish, citrus fruits, and milk and sugar
   e. Eating food items that do not suit your age, such as excessive Vata foods in old age when the digestive system is compromised
   f. Eating half-cooked or undercooked food
   g. Eating food that one does not like or when one is depressed
   h. Eating unripe or over-ripe fruits or meat of a diseased animal
   i. Eating on the run or gulping food in a hurry
8. **Recommendations:**
   a. A meal should be had warm, in good company, and without talking too much while eating.
   b. It is best to have two full meals a day.

c. As far as possible, each meal must have all six tastes.
d. One must have a diet that is personalized to one's Prakruti, age, geo-climatic conditions, region, season, and current state of doshas.

As we dive deeper into the science of Swasthavrutta, we see that dietary items have been classified according to many different criteria. The traditional diet has been designed after taking into consideration all these factors.

1. The doshas the food item increases and decreases
2. Rasa (taste), *Veerya* (nutritive value and the tissue that it strengthens), and *Vipak* (metabolism of the food item)
3. Tastes, colour, shape, and size of the food item
4. Time taken for the food item to ripen; the shorter the period the lesser the nutritive value. Mushrooms have a far lesser nutritive value than coconuts
5. Process of preservation and time since harvest. Grains in the first year after harvesting have less value than in the second year
6. Preservatives used, such as oil, salt, and sugar for pickles, and neem leaves for grain
7. Processing: finer ground grain has more Vata producing properties. Maida (finely ground wheat increases Vata far more as compared with whole wheat)
8. Fermenting increases Pitta producing effects
9. Roasting a grain before cooking makes it easier to digest
10. Process of cooking such as steaming, shallow frying, deep frying, roasting, and baking
11. Cooking over an open fire or in a cooker
12. Condiments added, which increase or decrease the dosha producing qualities
13. Garnishing and embellishments that increase or decrease dosha
14. Additives that mitigate side-effects and make a food item easier to digest
15. Geo-climatic conditions and season when a particular food item is consumed
16. Time of the day that the dish is best suited for the body
17. Type of food items: millets, pulses, vegetables, fruits, dried fruits, condiments, meat of different animals, alcohol made of different base materials
18. Arrangement of food items in a meal, and the way a dish is served
19. The time, quantity, and way of having a meal (the when, how much, and how)

All these criteria of classification are qualitative and need to be given due importance. One realizes that there is far more thought invested in designing a diet than the calories, protein, carbohydrate, and fat content. Further, the diet needs to be personalized to the Prakruti, gender, age, vocation, and current health and disease status (state of doshas) of the individual as well as the rutu or season in which it is consumed.

The ideal way to create a diet plan is to superimpose qualitative over quantitative criteria and personalize the diet to one that gives the best possible benefits to the individual.

Nidra: Sleep

A human being spends about one-third of his life in sleep; hence, sleep is an important aspect of health. The age-old saying, *early to bed and early to rise makes a person healthy, wealthy, and wise* holds true even today. It is not easy to follow this advice in today's world, but it holds true all the same. The fact remains that the human being is not a nocturnal animal and needs to sleep at night. Barring a few emergencies, our aim should be to plan our day in such a way that we can sleep early and wake up early. In the long run, we pay a heavy price for our late-night parties, binge watching of

TV, and even studying until late at night. The requirement for sleep reduces as age advances—preschool age 10–14 hours, school age (6–13) 9–11 hours, teenage 8–10 hours, adults 7–9 hours (though six hours may be adequate), and senior citizens 7–8 hours (though five hours may be adequate). The best time to go to sleep is before 10 pm. It may seem impossible but still, it is the best in order to ensure that you wake up early and fresh. Mental concentration, grasping capacity, and ability to comprehend are at their peak early in the morning. Morning is the best time for contemplation, meditation, and getting 'Aha' moments of insights. That is what makes one healthy, wealthy, and wise. Maybe there is a lot of truth in what the elders have said. Having a good night's sleep ensures that the body recovers from the fatigue of the previous day. It resets the clock and lays the foundation for a bright new day. The quality of sleep depends a lot on how one leads towards bedtime. A person is encouraged to finish the evening meal early, go for a short stroll, and then sit for about ten minutes quietly and let the events of the day sink in and settle. This is the time one invests in going over the activities of the day, learning from the mistakes, and at the same time congratulating oneself for the work done well. This is the time to thank the Maker for having seen you through the day. This is the time to forgive anyone who has knowingly or inadvertently hurt you and apologize to some whom you may have hurt. Having settled the mind, one should approach the bed with a feeling of gratitude. This is the best frame of mind before going to sleep.

Brahmacharya: Self-Restraint

Brahmacharya is often translated as celibacy, but it is better understood as self-restraint and moderation in all our day-to-day activities, desire, fulfilment, and pursuit of pleasures. Even apparently healthy pursuits like exercise, dieting, and fasting should be done in moderation. The middle path (Madhya marg) or the path of moderation is the safest. Fulfilment of desires is the main motivation for most of our actions and plans for the future. Life has to be a fair balance between shouldering responsibility and self-gratification and enjoyment. Over-indulgence in eating and drinking, excessive entertainment, and spending hours on social media have deleterious effects on our physical and mental health. In *grahasthashrama* or the home-maker phase of life, the couple is encouraged to have intercourse with the purpose of propagating the species. In winter, there is no restriction to the number of times that one indulges in intercourse with the lawful partner, keeping the health of both in mind. In the hot season, intercourse should be restricted to about once a fortnight. Keeping the mind obsessed with the idea of sex, un-natural sex, masturbation, and pornography is strictly prohibited. The thumb rule of Swasthavrutta is *Ati sarvatra varjyate*—avoid excess in everything. Indian philosophy is not against enjoyment; it is only against excessive attachment to anything. Excessive attachment to person, object, or concept is the major source of stress, disease, and suffering. We have taken a brief review of Swasthavrutta. We have mainly seen the general advice that applies to everyone. The Ayurveda physician goes into detail and gives advice personalized to the individual, based on his Prakruti, age, gender, vocation, current health and disease status, dosha status, and family background.

Personalization is the core strength of Ayurveda.

We need to pay special attention to two points that are the foundation of Swasthavrutta:

- Classification
- Habit building

Classification

Ayurveda is based on the Science of Classification. In the section on diet, we have seen the extent to which food items are classified. The classification is mainly on qualities and most of the qualities cannot be quantified or graded; at the same time, they have more significance than calories that can be counted. It proves Einstein's words, 'Most things that count cannot be counted'. We have seen that Indian philosophy sees the world as a mammoth algorithm. As we know, the algorithm forms the base of computer technology. The form of mathematics used in computer science is known as the Set Theory. The components of an algorithm are classified into subsets, sets, supersets, and universal sets. The sets are then joined with syntax that defines the relationship of the sets with each other and finally states the action to be taken. If (this set) and (this set) not (this set) nor (this set) ... then do this. This is the way an algorithm is written.

This is precisely the way the science of Ayurveda functions. Human beings, as well as all influencing factors, are classified into subsets, sets, and supersets under the Tridosha System of Classification. The structure of an Ayurveda *shloka* or a statement in the Ayurveda scriptures is quite similar to that of an algorithm. If a Pitta Prakruti person has spicy (pittaja) food in the afternoon (Pitta time) in summer (Pitta season), he should be given milk (pittaghna) and taken to a shaded cool place (kaphaja). In Sanskrit, the language of the scriptures, all conclusive statements define action. Grammar and precise syntax have been given prime importance in Sanskrit. Panini, the father of Sanskrit grammar, is known as the first computer technologist. The science that Ayurveda is based on is the Science of Classification. The Science of Classification, along with the set theory, based on the foundation of classification, has the capacity to deal with multiple, multi-optional, qualitative, and quantitative variables. Computer technology is proof enough that this is the science of the future. It is amazing that Ayurveda physicians reached this level of excellence without the benefit of supercomputers, ML, and AI.

Habit Building

Swasthavrutta is not a detox program or a corrective measure; it is a way of life. Parents are taught to inculcate good habits in their children right from childhood. The importance of good habits is deeply rooted in the insightful concept of Karma in Indian philosophy. The literal meaning of Karma is action. Indian philosophy gives tremendous importance to the choices we make, our thoughts, emotions, and the actions that we perform every moment and throughout life.

It is common knowledge, and science has proven beyond doubt, that everything including the person himself is constantly changing according to the laws of physics, chemistry, and biology. Every action of every individual subtly changes the direction in which the world changes every moment. At the same time, every action, emotion, thought, and desire of ours changes us. This is the power of free will.

Desires, thoughts, emotions, and action of the individual leave an indelible mark on his personality. They say that an action done once is like a line drawn in thin air, almost as if it never existed; when the same action is repeated a few times, it is like a line drawn on water; the mark stays for a short time and vanishes. Repeated a few more times, it is like a line drawn in the sand, which stays till the next wave. But if the action is repeated over and over again, it is like a line etched on stone and stays for years. Scientists say that an action done 27–30 times becomes a trait; doing it 30–50 times makes it a tendency, 50–70 times makes it a habit, and 70–100 times makes it a part of your character. The good habits of Swasthavrutta will become part of your character; all it takes is about three months of being good every day.

The theory of Karma is based on this simple principle. When a certain action is performed repeatedly, it becomes a force. We know it as the force of habit. Every moment that you fail to take an active decision to perform a new action, harbour a different emotion, or nurse a fresh thought, this force of habit takes your decision for you. Even in moments when you feel that a particular action was taken after a lot of deliberation, the force of habit has influenced your action steering it in the very direction that you habitually take. The force of habit or Karma then starts shaping your future and your destiny. Karma is responsible for bias, mistrust, fear, anxiety, and worry because that is what you always did. Being aware every moment, being in the here and now is the only way to escape the force of your Karma and write your own destiny. That is why being in the here and now has been given so much importance in meditation.

An analogy will make it easier to understand the concept of Karma. Most of us use the Internet so often. When we start the Internet, there appears a list of the recent topics that you had browsed for as your oft-visited sites. Real life is like opening the Internet every morning. Your fears, anxiety, and worry start showing immediately as your oft-visited sites. When you meet a person, your previous biases have already brought a smile or a frown to your face. As Emerson would say, 'What you are shouts so loudly in my ears that I cannot hear what you say'. Your oft-visited sites dominate your thoughts, emotions, and, finally, actions. That is why addictions are so difficult to give up. They lurk behind the screen and catch you in your moment of unawareness and you are back where you started. We all know that we cannot just wipe off or change the order in which our oft-visited sites appear. The best way to do it is to consciously visit another site more often and stay on it for longer. Talking about your woes to people, constantly complaining about a thing, and reminding yourself of the insults and bad treatment that someone has subjected you to are like repeating an action over and over again; it becomes part of your character. Fault finding and complaining becomes you. Your default setting is such that whatever you are presented with, your eyes will first find fault with it. You may make a good journalist but surely not a happy one; people will know you as a complaint box. Complaining becomes your identity and victim becomes your status. And then you say, My Karma! How true; it is your doing. The same is true with good habits inculcated as Swasthavrutta; they become your default setting; your Karma. With practice, waking up early without an alarm is easy, the bowel moves regularly, and daily hygiene becomes second nature. Putting in an hour or two in praying, meditating, and studying is routine; an hour of exercise and you are off to work. You feel hungry at the right time. Your system is used to the meal that has been set according to your Prakruti, the food gets digested easily and you get all the nutrients that your body needs. You don't have to think; being healthy comes naturally to you. Sadavrutta makes you a likeable person and Brahmacharya keeps you on the Madhya marg, the golden mean. Mentally it keeps a person relaxed and upbeat. The mind is free to express its creativity and innovation. The path is open for you to become truly healthy, wealthy, and wise. You can be proud of it; after all, it is your Karma, your doing.

Too Clean Is Not Really Good

The coronavirus pandemic has taught us a few lessons. A positive take home from the pandemic comes from the fact that literally hundreds of thousands of people who tested COVID-19 positive have recovered; a few due to medical intervention but mostly because their immune system bailed them out of the crisis. Nature has equipped the human being to protect itself from millions of known and millions of unknown microbes. The death toll of Covid-19 was alarming but surprisingly the per million population death rate in developed countries was multiple times more than that in developing, over-crowded countries. This is because the normal person in developing countries is exposed to a far wider range of microbes than the normal individual in developed countries. He has a stronger immune system than his brethren from developed countries. People from the developing countries were saved not because of poor standards of hygiene, as some intelligent people would like us to believe, but because people here are earthy in their lifestyle and dietary habits. They understand that they are as much part of the ecosystem as every other organism; this way of thinking is built into their culture. They eat home-cooked fresh food without preservatives. Their children enjoy the rough and tumble of growing up, playing out in the open. There is limited use of cosmetics, antiseptics, and detergents. They are not driven by misguided standards of hygiene; at least not as yet, though they are getting there fast. The elite from cities who have adopted the western lifestyle and concepts of hygiene suffered a higher death rate than people living in crowded areas or hutments. People living in villages were affected the least. The reason is the excessive, almost obsessive, use of disinfectants, pesticides, detergents, chemical fertilizers, antiseptics, antibiotics, and preservatives, in the pursuit of paranoid ideas of hygiene. We have ended up replacing microbes with chemicals. A child that has grown up crawling on disinfectant, breathing in air laden with room fresheners and mosquito-repellents, given boiled, RO filtered or bottled water, fed processed food prepared from grain grown on chemical fertilizers, sprayed with pesticides, and preserved with chemical preservatives never got a chance to train its adaptive immune system to deal with bacteria and viruses. Instead, he has grown up with allergies to gluten, lactose, and even peanuts, along with hundreds of other substances. Imagine the chemicals and bactericides that are used in cosmetics, shampoos, body lotions, creams, face packs, hair dyes, anti-dandruff lotion, and deodorants; beautification comes at a heavy cost. A whole range of chemicals is used in plastic containers to store cooked or raw food. Cold storage of food items delays decay but doesn't stop it; the nutritive value drops. Chemicals used in paint, plywood, and building materials are harmful to health. The list is endless.

Non-Communicable Diseases

Among those who succumbed to Covid-19, patients had co-morbidities like diabetes, hypertension, heart disease, pulmonary disease, and other compromising conditions. Covid-19 infection was the last straw on the camel's back; the grounds were prepared by existing co-morbidities. All through the year 2020, the world was frantically trying to defend itself from Covid-19, and, in the frenzy, we forget that even today 70% of deaths are due to NCDs. NCDs are also known as lifestyle diseases and are precipitated by the wrong lifestyle, diet, junk food, lack of proper exercise, stress due to comparison and competition, and, of course, addictions. We need to sit back and take a good look at how we live. There is no way we can go back to the villages, but we need to redesign our ideas of hygiene, healthy diet, and lifestyle. We need to give good thought to our ideas of enjoyment and entertainment, and revisit our idea of a good life, of success, and our priorities in life. We have to become aware of the fact that we have a blessing known as free will and use it judiciously to take control of a whole range of factors that are under our direct control.

> Nothing other than wisdom can save the individual from himself.

The problem of NCDs opens a Pandora's Box of challenges. The aetiology of NCDs is not clearly understood. It is clear that there are multiple factors leading to NCDs. Many of the influencing factors are qualitative and cannot be graded or quantified. In fact, science has not yet succeeded in identifying the influencing factors and separating them from non-influencing factors. The role and mechanism of action of the factors influencing health have not yet been understood. The current medical system is just too busy combating disease. The strategy is simply to plug holes as they appear; there has been no effort to reinforce the structure. Confronted by a disease, there is a rush to identify the one most significant causative agent, create a molecule that will eliminate the causative agent, or suppress the symptoms and create a standardized medicine that will alleviate the symptoms of the majority of the patients. This strategy is proving to be consistently inadequate in treating NCDs. The strategy of *one cause, one disease, one standardized treatment* cannot be effectively used in the case of NCDs. We do not have the technology to deal with multiple simultaneously acting, qualitative influencing factors. The government and the medical system cannot deal with the choices made by the individual in diet, lifestyle, habits, and addictions. It is time to recruit the individual into taking care of his/her health. The individual is no innocent bystander; he actively participates in maintaining or ruining his health.

The coronavirus pandemic has taught us the following:

1. The first and last line of defence is robust health and an efficient immune system.
2. We cannot isolate ourselves from the rest of the world and live in an aseptic bubble.
3. Excessive use of bactericides, antiseptics, and chemicals is never enough to keep away infection. It harms the individual and leaves him/her handicapped and vulnerable.
4. The natural protection from infections is a strong immune system.
5. Individuals with co-morbidities or NCDs have a poor prognosis when struck by any infection.
6. We need to develop a comprehensive, multidimensional, proactive, and personalized healthcare system that empowers the individual to actively participate in enhancing his/her health.
7. The individual needs to be empowered to knowledgeably and actively participate in taking care of his or her health.

This is precisely what Ayurveda and Swasthavrutta give us.

> Be natural; eat natural.

One thing to learn from Ayurveda is the use of natural products like toothpaste, soap, body lotion, and shampoo for maintaining your hygiene. One can use natural products such as mouth wash, face packs, cosmetics, and deodorants. Preservatives like sugar, salt, and oil are preferable to chemical preservatives. Use of organically grown products that are not sprayed with pesticides are good for the health and do not produce allergies. Changing the *when* you eat, *what* you eat, and *how* you eat may be an enjoyable experience. Those of us who are lucky to be staying with our family can enjoy warm fresh meals with those who love and care for us. It gives a sense of belonging and a feeling of being wanted and loved.

Every individual needs to understand his Prakruti and should be guided to choose the right diet and lifestyle in order to be able to actively participate in maintaining his or her health.

BALANCE TO EXCELLENCE

We have had a brief look at Ayurveda and the treasure of knowledge offered to us by Swasthavrutta. We have learnt that it is possible for every individual to actively participate in maintaining the balance of health by making healthy choices. Achieving a state of balance and sustaining it over long periods is the first step towards healthy living. We will now move on to the next step where the individual can use his free will to enhance his health at the physical, physiological, mental, and spiritual levels. Indian philosophy offers us the scientifically designed technology of health enhancement—the Patanjali Yogasutra and Hatayoga.

The Yogasutra of Patanjali (Yardi, 1996)

Yoga is revered as one of the six principal philosophies in India. Sage Patanjali is known as the father of yoga since he wrote the Patanjali Yogasutra around the first century AD. The Yogasutra is a detailed exposition on the steps to be followed by an aspirant in pursuit of enlightenment or self-realization, written in the form of sutras or aphorisms.

The Patanjali Yogasutra has four steps (*Padas*).

1. *Samadhi pada*, where *samdhi* or sama means balanced and *adhi* means awareness. It deals with the importance of reaching the state of Samadhi.
2. *Sadhana pada* is the step of dedicated practice. It deals with the methodology to reach the state of Samadhi through the eight limbs of yoga, which is Ashtanga Yoga. The eight limbs are Yama, Niyama, Asana, Pranayama, Pratyahar, Dharana, Dhyan and Samadhi. The point to be noted here is that *the state of Samadhi is not the end of the journey; it is the beginning of a journey.*
3. *Vibhuti pada*, the third step, elaborates on the stages of evolution of a student (*sadhak*). It outlines the process and gives glimpses of the superhuman powers that a sadhak experiences as he advances in his study and practice of yoga. There is a clear warning to the student that though these powers are superhuman, the sadhak should not get distracted or entangled in the feeling of superiority if he wants to progress to step four.
4. *Kaivalya pada* is the fourth step. Kaivalya can be understood as *only-ness*. The concept of only-ness is similar to the concept of Advait (non-dualism or not-two-ness) from the Vedanta.

The four steps of Yoga are an arduous journey to be taken on by serious seekers of enlightenment. Significant to us in the present context is Ashtanga Yoga from step two, the Sadhana pada.

According to Indian philosophy, the five principal elements Prithvi, Aap, Tej, Vayu, and Akash are represented in the human being as five *koshas* or sheaths, from the gross (the earth) to the subtle (space).

- Prithvi—Earth—Annamayakosha—Physical
- Aap—Water—Pranamayakosha—Physiological
- Tej—Light/Fire—Manomayakosha— Mental
- Vayu—Air—Buddhimayakosha — Intellectual
- Akash—Space — Anandmayakosha — Spiritual

Ashtanga Yoga

Ashtanga Yoga has eight limbs or practices that need to be followed simultaneously and not in a series, as in the case of the four steps or padas. The aim is to elevate the potential of an individual in all the five koshas or levels of existence.

The eight limbs of Ashtanga Yoga are:

1. *Yama*: Abstinence
2. *Niyama*: Observance
3. *Asana*: Posture
4. *Pranayama*: Breath control
5. *Pratyahara*: Directing the senses inwards
6. *Dharana*: Commitment

7. *Dhyan*: Meditation
8. *Samadhi*: Balanced awareness

Yama: Abstinences

- *Ahimsa*: Non-violence
- *Satya*: Abstinence from falsehood in thought, action, and speech
- *Asteya*: Non-stealing
- *Brahmacharya*: Self-restraint
- *Aparigraha*: Non-acquisitiveness

It is important for the aspirant to cultivate these as part of his character so that there is no distraction that can interfere with the single-minded pursuit of excellence.

Niyama: Observances

- *Sauch*: Cleanliness of body and mind.
- *Santosh*: Contentment: this is important because a discontented mind is always longing for something and keeps distracting the disciple.
- *Tapah*: Austerities: this means cultivating the habit of patiently bearing discomforts like heat/cold, hunger/thirst, standing/sitting, and silence without getting restless or distracted. This is not an attempt at self-mortification; one just needs to build endurance to such discomforts.
- *Swadhyaya*: self-study of scriptures.
- *Ishwarapranidhana*: surrendering and dedicating all actions to God the supreme Guru. Surrender helps the disciple to keep the ego in check.

Yama and Niyama define the lifestyle of a sadhak or disciple. These are simple rules that keep distractions to a minimum and leave the individual physically and mentally free for the pursuit of higher ideals. Serious sportspersons and sincere students are commonly seen to follow most of these dictums.

Asana: Posture

Patanjali suggests a comfortable and steady posture, *sthirasukha asan*.

Pranayama: Control of Breath

Patanjali suggests external and internal regulation of breath and simple and steady breathing.

Hatayoga has taken Asana and Pranayama to another level. These are the Yogasanas that have gained tremendous popularity the world over. Today, the world is aware of the benefits of regular practice of Yogasanas under the guidance of a trained teacher. A simple practice of a set of 12 Suryanamaskara every day gives flexibility to the body and the spine. It improves blood circulation to all endocrine glands and establishes hormonal balance. The movement of the intestine is regulated, which improves appetite, digestion, and excretion.

The literal meaning of Pranayama is breath control (*Prana* means breath and *Ayam* means control). The significance of Pranayama goes far beyond. The *panchapranas* (five pranas) control all the involuntary activities of the body. Pranamayakosha is the physiological sheath of the body. The five pranas are *prana* (cognition, mentation, and thought), *udan* (intake of breath), *samana* (digestion), *vyana* (distribution of breath and nutrition), and *apana* (excretion). Control over these physiological functions is Ayam. Pranayama is control and regulation of the physiological sheath. Regular practice of Yogasanas and Pranayama fine-tunes the Annamayakosha (physical sheath) and Pranamayakosha (physiological sheath) of the individual. Doing so will improve appetite, digestion, and absorption and distribution of nutrition. The efficiency of the cardio-pulmonary system improves and can be seen as reduced resting pulse rate and increased lung capacity. The endocrine glands function efficiently, and the immune system becomes sharp and efficient. The flexibility of the spine and all the joints improves, thus improving performance in sports and athletics. The gait, stance, and posture improve, lending grace and poise to the personality of the individual. A person will be well-advised to build into his daily routine at least 30 minutes of Yogasanas and Pranayama practice.

Pratyahara: Withdrawal of the Senses

Following the rules of Yama and Niyama and regular practice of Yogasanas and Pranayama fine-tune the Annamayakosha and the Pranamayakosha. These are the external aids to health enhancement. The next step is to practice conscious contemplation.

The five senses are constantly running after their objects of gratification and do not allow the mind to concentrate or contemplate. Withdrawing the senses and looking inwards help gain control over the senses and remove the major impediments to contemplation

The first five limbs of Ashtanga Yoga, namely Yama, Niyama, Asana, Pranayama, and Pratyahar are known as Bahyakriya—external activities. The next three limbs Dharana (fixed attention/commitment), Dhyan (meditation), and Samadhi (balanced awareness) are known as Antarkriya—internal activities.

Dharana: Commitment

Dharana is commitment to the pursuit of excellence. One needs tremendous, consistent, and sustained effort to reach excellence in any field. Every great sportsperson and athlete knows that training the mind to keep up the practice through thick and thin in spite of physical discomfort and mental distraction is the key to success and excellence. Every day you are competing with yourself towards becoming a shade better than what you were yesterday. This is known as Dharana or single-minded commitment.

Dhyan: Meditation

The world over, people have realized the importance of meditation in reducing stress and maintaining mental balance in these difficult and trying times. There are more than 100 different types of meditation and a lot has been written about meditation. At the same time, there is a lot of confusion about the subject. It is said about meditation that those who know don't talk and those who talk don't know. This is true about the second phase of meditation, but we can talk about the first. There are two phases of meditation; the doing phase and the happening phase.

Phase One: The Doing Phase

There are three steps in the doing phase of meditation.

1. **Coming to the present**. The human mind has an inherent tendency to constantly drift into the past or into the future. Reminiscing about the past, regretting lost opportunities, reliving past insults, slights, and mistakes, and thinking about what one could have, should have, or would have done in a particular situation keep the mind occupied for hours on end. On the other hand, projecting oneself into the future and thinking about what all could go wrong—the pain, disappointment, problems, and sorrow—will drag the mind in other directions. Both these distractions take the mind away from the

present. Staying in the past generates regret, guilt, and remorse. Thinking about the future generates fear, worry, anxiety, and stress. The safest place to be in at such a time is the present. The first step of meditation is known as escaping to the present, away from the guilt and remorse of the past and worry and anxiety of the future.

There are many techniques of coming to the present. *Anapan*—concentrating on the incoming and outgoing breath, and Silva Mind Control—counting backwards from 100 to zero, or saying the alphabet backwards are a few techniques of bringing oneself to the present.

2. **Staying in the present**. Those of us who have tried meditation will vouch for it; coming to the present may be easily possible but staying there is very difficult. The mind slips out like an errant brat in the blink of an eye. It not only escapes your vigil but also drags you helplessly, as if by the nose ring, back into the past or the future. You only realize it far later when you are trapped once more, away from the present. Staying in the present needs constant vigil. Concentrating on an object, a picture of the deity or a flame are some of the methods suggested. Time and time again, however, the mind escapes. Or worse, it drags the intellect along with it to its favourite past time in the past or the future; away from the present. At this time, one realizes that it is very difficult to reign in the mind without the help of the intellect. This is the time to recruit the intellect.
3. **Harnessing the intellect**. The main problem with most of us is that we consider our intellect as our identity. Separating our intellect from our self is a matter of understanding. Imagine the time we are leaving for work occupied with thoughts of what we are going to do at the office when we suddenly realize that we don't have our car keys. At that time, you tell your intellect to drop all thoughts of the office and urgently think about where your keys could be. This self that takes control of the intellect directing it to do what you want it to do is your 'Self'. This is the captain of the ship; the intellect, mind, and body are important, but they are under the command of the 'Self'. This is the self that has to take command of the ship. With the help of the intellect, the self has to take control of the mind that keeps drifting into the past and the future, instigating a mutiny.

The intellect and mind have to be kept together in the present, involved in an activity that the Self decides is important and meaningful.

This is not exactly part of meditation but for people like us who have not dedicated themselves to the path of meditation (Dhyan marg), it is very important to understand this step of meditation. We all have dreams and aspirations and will go a long way to fulfil them. Harnessing the intellect and keeping the body, mind, and intellect working together 100% in the present is the best way to achieve whatever we want, and to make our dreams come true.

Phase Two: The Happening Phase

The sincere few who ardently follow the path of meditation manage to reach a stage where meditation happens. This stage of meditation is an experiential stage, and each has a different experience according to his beliefs, upbringing, and mental state. This is the stage about which they say that those who know don't talk and those who talk don't know. We will not talk about it.

Samadhi: Balanced Awareness

Sama means balanced and Adhi means awareness. Samadhi is the aim and final stage of Ashtanga Yoga. This is a state of total awareness, without any bias, likes, dislikes, desires, or fears polluting awareness. We know that very often most of our decisions are swung in one direction or another because of our fears or desires. Our emotions hijack our decision-making capacity, and our intellect supports the decision because the intellect too is hijacked along with the self. Many people who have tried giving up an addiction and have failed will identify with the power of the mind to direct our decisions. The mind more often than not swings the decision towards the addiction. On a subtle level, each decision is marred by our biases that have become part of our Karma or force of habit. It is in the state of Samadhi or balanced awareness that our decisions will be unbiased and make us do whatever the situation demands rather than what our biased mind demands. With Swasthavrutta, we have ensured that our weaknesses do not obstruct our progress. With yogasanas and Pranayama, we have enhanced our strengths. With meditation, we have come to a stage where our decisions are not swung too much by our biases. We now have a finely tuned and sharpened potent tool.

The question is, what do we aim this potent instrument at?

We all know that an empty mind is the devil's workshop. If we do not give our body, mind, and intellect something meaningful to do, they are going to gravitate towards their old habits of drifting into the past or the future; or worse, drift towards self-defeating or destructive activities. We come back a full circle and end up struggling with life and trying to fulfil the childish demands of the mind.

What should we do? What is the purpose of life? There is enough evidence in science and philosophy that point a finger towards the purpose of our life.

That is going beyond balance and being truly human.

GOING BEYOND BALANCE: BEING HUMAN

As we know, everyone that is born will die someday. What we die of is not so important. What is really important is how we live the life that we have been given; but then what is life?

Life is nothing but time between birth and death. How we spend this time gives meaning to life.

It is what one does with robust health and the time between birth and death that will make life meaningful and worth living.

The Finger Pointing to the Moon

We have seen evidence that there could be a very meaningful purpose to our birth as the human being, which is like the finger pointing to the moon. We will now see some other indicators that prove to us that our birth as a human being has far more significance than we ever imagined.

Maslow

Abraham Maslow, the well-known American psychologist, raised this question about 60 years ago and tried, in his own way, to answer it. He proposed his much-discussed theory called the Pyramid of the Hierarchy of Psychological Needs of a human being. At the bottom of the pyramid is the basic need of survival, security. Next comes the need for belonging, love, and acceptance. The third is the need for respect and appreciation. According to Maslow, the final need of the human being is self-actualization. Self-actualization, according to him, is the desire to express oneself and manifest his unique destiny.

Maslow interviewed a few people who had reached the heights of self-actualization. Each of them narrated a different story that had led them on the path of their destiny but there were some points common to all. All of them said that they were pursuing a dream that was larger than the person himself. And all of them spoke about experiencing some form of ecstasy and bliss that they had never experienced before.

Maclean

At around the same time as Abraham Maslow, anatomist Dr Paul Maclean proposed his Theory of the Triune Brain. He studied the structure of the brain of reptiles, mammals, and human beings. In his theory, he shows the stages of evolution of the brain from reptiles to mammals and further to the human brain. The neocortex of the brain is responsible for creativity, innovation, compassion, love, and altruism. The question is, can the functions of the neocortex point a finger towards the purpose of life of the human being as a species?

Genetics

Geneticists, in their study of the genetic structure of human beings as compared with other animals, came across a very interesting fact. Sixty per cent of the human genes are the same as unicellular animals; let us call them amoeba genes. Of the remaining 40%, 38.4% are the same as the chimpanzee. We will call them monkey genes. Only 1.6% of our genes are purely human. The genome of the human being is like a three-layered cake in the form of a pyramid. The broad base of the pyramid, holding 60% of our genes, resembles the amoeba genes. The second layer comprising 38.4% of our genes resembles mammals, and the thin crust of 1.6% of genes are the genes responsible for free will. There is a definite purpose behind this proportion.

Our 1.6% human genes represent our free will and govern the functions of the neocortex. This is the power that we have to participate in and give direction to the constantly changing universe. We can imagine that as the human being evolves and becomes more responsible with his free will, the proportion of purely human genes will steadily increase.

This is more evidence that will make us aware of the investment that has gone into creating each one of us. It will help us appreciate the sanctity of being born as a human being. It will help us to grow out of our petty concerns, and value our life and each moment that we have been blessed with. Sixty per cent of genes are dedicated to fulfilling the needs of survival and security. They look after immunity and govern all the involuntary activities of the body. The second layer of 38.4% genes looks after our needs that resemble those of a monkey, growth, maturity, finding a partner, reproduction, and nursing the young ones. These genes help us find our place in the hierarchy and co-exist with the rest of the members of the herd.

The third layer of just 1.6% genes is responsible for our free will, creativity, and innovation. It is also responsible for the typical human traits like compassion, sense of duty, responsibility, and altruism. They are designed to help the individual to evolve to the next level.

Eastern Philosophy

Eastern philosophy has always been seeking the higher goal in life. Inner exploration has led to great philosophies like Advaita philosophy of the Vedanta, Buddhism, Jainism, Sankhya philosophy, Nyaya philosophy, and Yoga. Each individual is born with a unique set of qualities and a given time of his lifespan. He is advised to use this time to hone his skills and explore the treasure house of knowledge in the world through experience and seek his own destiny that is far beyond material gains, power, position, and possession.

Eastern philosophy is not against enjoyment; it is against getting attached to the source of enjoyment at the cost of the higher purpose of life. The emphasis is on doing and experiencing rather than having and possessing.

Eastern philosophy believes in rebirth and gives us the assurance that this life is just one more run in the eternal relay of life. It urges us to do our best in this lifetime. Our actions in this lifetime will be stored in the form of Karma, and we can pick up the threads where we left them, in the next life. We are warned to take each step in this lifetime with care because we are laying the grounds for our next life through our Karma in this life. Vedanta philosophy takes this concept a few steps beyond, but it is out of the scope of this chapter.

Evolution

In the section on evolution, we have seen that evolution took place with the accumulation of knowledge leading to more advanced software. The latest product of evolution is the human being—you and me. The human being is the only life form that can say, 'I know'. It is the only life form that has free will, with the help of which he can participate in change and give direction to change. This is another pointer that tells us that gaining knowledge through experience and using it to give proper direction to change may be the purpose of life. This may be the path one may choose to follow in order to evolve to the next stage of evolution.

Marga: The Path

Indian philosophy clearly says that each one has to find his own destiny. Knowing that each person is unique and that all cannot follow the same path, the individual is given a choice. Indian philosophy suggests four different pathways to self-realization; *Karma marga*—the path of selfless action; *Bhakti marga*—the path of devotion *Dhyan marga*—the path of meditation; and *Dnyana marga*—the path of knowledge. An individual can choose the path that suits his Prakruti and natural inclination. The foundation of the journey is experience and surrendering all actions to the supreme power.

Choice

Since Eastern philosophy has always been following the Science of Classification, philosophers have classified all actions and experiences into three categories. This is known as the Triguna classification (Chinmayananda, 2006). The three gunas are Satva, Rajas, and Tamas. Satva signifies purity, knowledge, and Karuna or compassion; Rajas signifies activity, competition, and effort; and Tamas signifies lethargy, arrogance, and greed. All the factors influencing the life of an individual have been classified under the Triguna System of Classification, based on whether they increase or decrease a particular guna. Food items, lifestyle, daily routine, emotions, thoughts, and, finally, actions are classified as satvic, rajasic, and tamasic. The individual is encouraged to choose the satvic option each moment. This makes it easier for him to stay on the path of his higher destiny. If one chooses rajasic or tamasic, he just makes it that much more difficult for himself. God does not punish him for his misdeed; the individual punishes himself by choosing the path full of pain and suffering; the choice is ours.

The Journey

In the pursuit of our destiny, we have two important aids, namely, passion and reason. According to Kahlil Gibran, reason and passion work together. Reason is the keel of our ship and passion the wind in the sails. Reason without passion leaves the ship drifting around with the tide; passion without reason will crash the ship onto the rocks. Meditation strengthens reason but there has to be a passion in life that gives power to our sails.

The question is how do we find our passion?

Each one of us is unique. We have our strengths and our weaknesses. In childhood, we all invest time in a lot of play. In this period, most of us find out something that comes naturally to us. Some are good at athletics and sports, some at craft, some at art, and yet others at maths and science. These are indicators of our strengths. They define the area in which we should be seeking our passion. We then try doing more things in this field, and our destiny urges us on by showing the beauty of our path to our mind and revealing secrets of knowledge to our intellect. The more time we spend in that particular field, the more exciting becomes the journey because it involves us, body, mind, and intellect. We will discover our passion through our play.

The Secret of Happiness

According to Aristotle, happiness is the only thing that we do for nothing else; every action of ours is otherwise done for happiness. Nature has been using the *carrot and stick* principle very effectively to sustain all life forms. Right from bacteria all the way to human beings, every life form moves away from pain towards pleasure. Bacteria use chemo-tactic movement, plants grow towards sunlight, animals move towards greener pastures, and human beings have surpassed all other life forms in their pursuit of happiness. Nature has endowed the human being with four happiness hormones that will encourage the individual to stay on the right path. These four hormones are endorphin, dopamine, oxytocin, and serotonin. Endorphin or endogenous morphine is a happiness hormone that is released while doing physically challenging exercise. This encourages the individual to do exercise more often in order to keep himself fit. Dopamine is a hormone that is released with every big and small achievement in life. The exhilaration one feels on learning how to swim or ride a cycle is a classic example. Dopamine encourages the individual to hone his skills and steadily move towards excellence.

Oxytocin is a hormone that is released when we hug someone dear. Giving a hug to your children, spouse, and parents increases the bonding and gives you a feeling of being loved, wanted, and needed, fulfilling one of Maslow's hierarchy of needs. Research has proven that having a close-knit family keeps away the danger of cardiac illness.

Serotonin is released when we do a good turn to another, help others, and do something good for society. It is almost as if nature knows the purpose of life and is encouraging the individual to keep himself fit as he gets his dose of endorphin. While he explores his strengths, scales them, and fine-tunes them, he gets his dose of dopamine. Nature shows us that we are social animals; living together for each other has a synergistic effect. It encourages us with oxytocin to value and love each other. Finally, knowing that the purpose of life is beyond 'I, me, and mine', nature encourages us to do things for the progress of humanity and rewards us with serotonin for our efforts. After that, we are given total freedom to follow our passion.

THE SCIENCE OF LIVING

We have seen that the human being is designed and destined to achieve great heights in life. The way to do it is to first understand our unique design or Prakruti and align all our choices in diet, lifestyle, and vocation to suit our Prakruti with the help of Swasthavrutta. We should keep ourselves fit with daily exercise. Yogasanas and Pranayama help us to enhance our strengths. Our mental balance is very important and the practice of meditation every day helps us to maintain this balance. Finally, we have to realize that life is the time between birth and death and that we are at the steering wheel of our life. We have to be aware of each moment and make satvic choices in our day-to-day and moment-to-moment thoughts, emotions, and actions because every emotion, thought, and action contributes to the force of habit or our Karma. Our Karma shapes and designs our destiny.

Our birth as a human being is a blessing; we must respect its sanctity. We must aim to make our life meaningful, and, in the process, understand the meaning of life through experience because each one of us is destined for scaling new heights.

This is the science of life.

HEALTHCARE

Being healthy and living a productive, happy, and meaningful life is the birthright of every human being. It is possible for each one of us to achieve good health with the help of Swasthavrutta. Each one of us should have the means and the know-how to enhance our health with the help of exercise, proper diet and lifestyle, yogasanas, Pranayama, and meditation. Each one of us has to be made aware that evolving as a human being is the purpose of life and be encouraged to follow the call of our destiny.

We need a comprehensive, multidimensional, personalized, and proactive healthcare solution.

We have the Science of Enhanced Living and the philosophy to support it. We have computer and information technology at our fingertips.

We need a system that can reach the science of enhanced living to each and every individual on this planet. We have created an intelligent search engine that can diagnose the Prakruti and current health status of each individual. The search engine can personalize the healthcare solution to the Prakruti, age, gender, vocation, geo-climatic conditions, and the current health and disease status of the individual.

Being an intelligent search engine, it will improve the level of personalization with every user over a period of time. The improvement will happen with the help of AI and ML. It is only a question of time before this system empowers each individual, community, and government to take care of health for the betterment of humanity. It will be possible for every individual to live a healthy, happy, productive, and meaningful life.

REFERENCES

Desai, Chandrashekhar (2018, September); *Transdisciplinary Education*, Talk delivered at University of Trans-Disciplinary Health Sciences and Technology, Bangalore.

Desai, C. R. (2020, March 8); Presentation at IMA, Pune.

Ranade, S., Paranjpe, G. R., Sathye, B. V. (2004); *Swasthavrutta*, Anmol Prakashan, India.

Swami, Chinmayananda (2006); *Vivekachoodamani*, Chinmaya Prakashan, India.

Yardi, M. R. (1996); *The Yoga of Patanjali*, Bhandarkar Oriental Research Institute, Poona.

Chapter 14

Role of Homoeopathy in Prophylaxis and the Symptomatic Management of Influenza-Like Illnesses (COVID-19) Patients

Srijan Goswami* and Chiranjeeb Dey

CONTENTS

INTRODUCTION

The back-to-back waves of the COVID-19 pandemic have made a devastating impact globally. The conventional healthcare system is going through serious pressure as cases of the disease continue to spread and the numbers of hospitalizations are increasing every moment. It is becoming hard and challenging because the hospital resources are limited in number as compared with the rate of daily hospitalizations. There are significant shortages of patient care facilities and medical care providers, and on top of that, conventional healthcare systems do not have any proven treatments for COVID-19 patients. Experimental drugs like hydroxychloroquine, followed by remdesivir, ritonavir/lopinavir, and favipiravir are being administered under emergency use authorization (EUA). There is evidence that these experimental medications are causing adverse drug reactions, thus claiming the lives of the hospitalized COVID-19 patients. And those patients who survive the EUA medications and hospitalizations are left with iatrogenic immunosuppressive states leading to increased susceptibility towards secondary life-threatening infections like fungal diseases. In this scenario, complementary and alternative medical systems (CAMS) are providing commendable results with negligible adverse effects or iatrogenic issues in patients with COVID-19. There are several clinical cases recorded and published by various independent homoeopathic doctors and researchers worldwide. But unfortunately, because of a biased medical model and greed for monopolies, these effective treatment methods are not

DOI: 10.1201/9781003178514-17

given equal opportunity as their conventional counterparts (Goswami & Gupta Bakshi, 2020; Hegde, 2014; World Health Organization, 2020; Jian et al., 2020; Yuki et al., 2020).

In this chapter, the authors have tried to compile the fundamental concepts that help in understanding the role of the homoeopathic system of medicine in the prevention, treatment, and management of patients having influenza-like illnesses or COVID-19. This chapter is intended for scientists, academicians, educators, and professionals who are not at all familiar with the subject of homoeopathy. The concepts of homoeopathy in relation to the ongoing pandemic are presented in a way that is easily understandable for a common person as well as a professional.

HOMOEOPATHY: A BRIEF OVERVIEW OF FUNDAMENTAL PRINCIPLES

Homoeopathy is a system of medicine that treats diseases with remedies, which, if given to a healthy person, would develop symptoms like those of the disease. Homoeopathy and homoeopathic preparations are recognized by the World Health Organization and are legally practised under government regulations worldwide. Dr Christian Friedrich Samuel Hahnemann, a German physician founded and established the system of homoeopathy in 1796 and thus is known as the Father of Homoeopathy. Dr Hahnemann has provided the fundamental working principles of homoeopathy in his scholarly work titled "The Organon of Medicine", which has six editions and 294 aphorisms. In order to understand the science behind the homoeopathic system, one must understand the 294 aphorisms of the Organon of Medicine in depth. The term homoeopathy is derived from two Greek words *homoios* and *pathos*. The words *homoios* means "similar" and *pathos* means "suffering". The backbone of homoeopathy is based on *Similia Similibus Curentur*, which means "like cures like". The fundamental principles of Homoeopathy are presented as follows (Hahnemann, 1833; Venkateswara Homoeopathic Medical College and Hospital, 2020; Organon and Philosophy, 2021):

1. **Law of Similia**. It is the most fundamental law. It states that the symptoms experienced by the sick are not the disease but are reactions of the defence mechanism of the body, which mobilizes its resources to counteract the morbific influence. Symptoms are the basic reaction of an organism under stress. In order to help the organism, these symptoms act like individualistic clues that will help select the appropriate remedy. Therefore, the choice of the remedy is based on the principle of *Similia Similibus Curentur*. The drug must have the capacity to produce most symptoms similar to that of the disease when given to a healthy person (Hahnemann, 1833).
2. **Law of Simplex**. This law states that only one single, simple medicinal substance is to be administered at a time. As the medicines are proved singly, we are aware of their individual action. The action of multiple drugs will cause confusion for a second prescription and determining the direction of disease. Some drugs are antidotes to each other, or they may interact with each other, which may affect the patient adversely (Hahnemann, 1833; Venkateswara Homoeopathic Medical College and Hospital, 2020; Organon and Philosophy, 2021).
3. **Law of Minimum**. This law states that the minimum dose should be prescribed at a given time. The minimum dose is the quantity of medicine that is capable of bringing about curative action (Hahnemann, 1833; Venkateswara Homoeopathic Medical College and Hospital, 2020; Organon and Philosophy, 2021).

4. **Drug Dynamization and Potentization**. A process in which a crude medicinal substance is reduced to its sub-physiological state and its latent medicinal properties are unfolded by the method of potentization or dynamization. Homoeopathic medicines are based on the principle that high dilutions of potentially active molecules retain a memory of the original substance. Hence, the starting materials, the homoeopathic stocks, and/or mother tinctures are subjected to a process of serial dilution and succussion in order to potentize the product with an inert carrier material. Originally, Hahnemann employed this process to diminish the toxicity of potentially hazardous substances. The name potentization to characterize this process was given by him later (Hahnemann, 1833; Venkateswara Homoeopathic Medical College and Hospital, 2020; Organon and Philosophy, 2021).
5. **Totality of Symptoms**. According to Dr Felix James V, the concept of the "totality of symptoms" is characteristic of holistic medical sciences and thus a characteristic feature of the homoeopathic system. Homoeopathy treats the patient who has the disease, thus all the signs and symptoms presented by the patient from the former healthy state to the now diseased condition are considered before selecting a remedy. Dr J.M. Kanjilal explains the totality of symptoms as a combination of certain groups of symptoms in definite settings with a definite background and certain individualizing characteristics set appropriately on the symptom complex, so that it can point to the drug having a similar peculiar symptom complex. The totality of symptoms helps distinguish one clinical presentation from another on a subtle level (Venkateswara Homoeopathic Medical College and Hospital, 2020; Organon and Philosophy, 2021).
6. **Individualization and Personalized Treatment**. Homoeopathic medicines are prescribed on the basis of individualization, which is tailoring the remedy according to the individual's needs. It means every individual is different from others in some way; be it stature, talking, choices, behaviour, or susceptibility to diseases (Venkateswara Homoeopathic Medical College and Hospital, 2020; Organon and Philosophy, 2021).

The fundamental principles underlying the homoeopathic system of treatment is as vast as the ocean. It requires knowledge, skill, and holistic understanding of how the human body and nature are related and the influential effect on each other. It is not possible to include every concept in a single chapter, so the authors recommend thorough reading and proper understanding of the *Organon of Medicine* along with the subjects of conventional medical sciences, chemistry, and material and energy physics. Then one can realize the true science of homoeopathic treatments. This section is only presented to provide a context for the sections that are going to follow.

MECHANISM OF ACTION OF HOMOEOPATHIC MEDICATIONS

For planning a treatment regimen, it is important to understand the mechanism of action of the concerned system of medicine. It is known that the fundamental principle of homoeopathy is *Similia Similibus Curentur* or like cures like but rarely do we realize the actual mechanism by which like cures like functions. Homoeopathic medicines when administered in higher potency work at an energy level because they do not contain materialistic substances. The energy signature of the homoeopathic medicine acts on the nervous system of the individual consuming it. When one or two drops of a selected remedy are administered on the tongue of an individual, the energy signature is sensed by the nerve endings present on the tongue. The energy signature of the selected remedy is then carried forward by the nervous system as a signal (therapeutic stimulus) to the brain. The brain and the nervous system sense the signal and mount a response by triggering the complete neuroendocrine system, thus creating a chemical composition inside the body that is similar and of slightly higher intensity in relation to the disease the individual is experiencing. Through stimulation of the neuroendocrine system, the body initiates protective responses similar to responses given in the case of natural disease. The activated healing mechanisms of the body neutralize the pathological derangements by the action of various homoeostasis restoring mechanisms natural to the body. This process heals the individual from the natural disease. After the natural disease is healed, the chemical effect of the medicinal substance remains in the system, which will be inactivated automatically when its period of action is over. The mechanism of action is based on neuroendocrine-immunology (NEI) in which the energy signature is converted to chemistry with the help of the neuroendocrine system. This makes homoeopathy an individualized or personalized system of medicine as compared with the conventional system. It is not possible to understand and appreciate the scientific basis of homoeopathy just by judging the discipline from the reductionistic viewpoint of conventional allopathic systems if *Contraria Contrariis Curentur*. According to *Organon of Medicine*, aphorism 2, the highest ideal of cure is rapid, gentle, and permanent restoration of health, or removal and annihilation of the disease in its whole extent in the shortest, most reliable, and most harmless way, on easily comprehensible principles. The mechanism by which homoeopathic medicine shows its curative properties is much safer as compared with industrially synthesized chemical drugs that are known to create iatrogenic complications (Hahnemann, 1833; Venkateswara Homoeopathic Medical College and Hospital, 2020; Organon and Philosophy, 2021) (Figure 14.1).

HOMOEOPATHY FOR COVID-19: CLINICAL TRIALS

As COVID-19 is a new disease, the scientific community is working tirelessly to discover treatment methods that may help address the situation. The researchers and physicians of homoeopathy are also involved in identifying and standardizing treatment protocols for patients suffering from COVID-19. Every country has mandated a strict set of rules for clinical trials to be performed related to COVID-19 treatment. Any candidate drug that does not fit in with the conventional clinical trial guidelines is non-accepted. This is one of the fundamental mistakes that we make when we deal with complementary and alternative systems of treatments. Our mindset is conditioned with the ideology that the "reductionistic approach is the only way of performing scientific studies" and "conventional medicine is the gold standard of healthcare". But in reality, this is not the case. Homoeopathy, or any complementary and alternative medicine system, is a personalized system of treatment. This means homoeopathy does not address the disease in an isolated manner, it aims in healing the patient who has the disease. In short, the approach of homoeopathic treatment (complementary and alternative systems of medicine) is "patient-centric" and "not disease-specific". This specific section is intended for scientists and academicians who are not familiar with the differences between homoeopathy and conventional medicine. Having a sound understanding of basic differences will help in planning, designing, and assessing medicinal substances and clinical trials. Table 14.1 points out some fundamental differences between homoeopathy and conventional medicine.

Since the pandemic started, several clinical trials have been performed using candidate homoeopathic medicines to find out remedies based on the ideology of "one drug fits all" in order

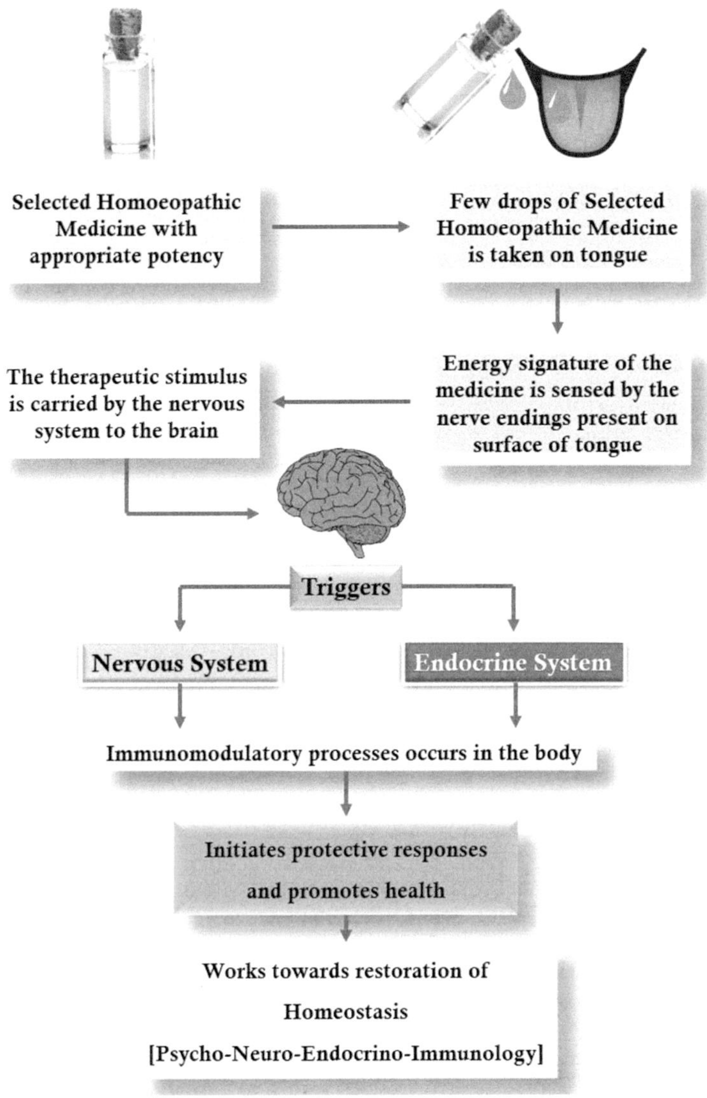

Figure 14.1 General mechanism of action of homoeopathic potentized medication.

to receive approval from the authorities regulating clinical trials. This is as illogical and unscientific as "asking a fish to climb up a tree". Forcefully manipulating scientific studies to receive approval for treatment will not help in the long run. Instead, the scientific community needs to be more open-minded and logical in understanding that the conventional reductionistic system is not the only way. Most importantly, homoeopathic researchers need to hold on to the fundamental principles based on the *Organon of Medicine*. The homoeopathic system and other complementary and alternative systems of medicine have their own set of guidelines and principles that need to be applied, monitored, and regulated if the intention is to find remedies that satisfy

TABLE 14.1 BASIC DIFFERENCES BETWEEN THE HOLISTIC SCIENCE OF HOMOEOPATHY AND THE REDUCTIONISTIC SCIENCE OF CONVENTIONAL MEDICINE

	Homoeopathy	Conventional Medicine
1.	*Similia Similibus Curentur* – like cures like.	*Contraria Contrariis Curentur* – opposites cure opposites.
2.	Patient-centric or personalized system of treatment.	Disease-specific or generalized system of treatment.
3.	Every individual is constitutionally different, their response to the same disease varies and thus treatments cannot be generalized.	One drug fits all approach.
4.	Holistic approach (see Chapter 3)	Reductionistic approach (see Chapter 3)
5.	Acts at the energy level and thus works in tune with the healing mechanisms of the body.	Acts at the physical level and thus works by suppressing the normal healing mechanisms of the body as it sees symptoms as disease.

the therapeutic principles of the concerned system of medicine (in this case, homoeopathy). It is not appropriate to look for statistical averages or the statistical normal in cases of personalized forms of treatment. It is the uniqueness of the homoeopathic system that one specific medicine can be used to treat multiple diseases, also, many patients with the same disease may require different individualized medicines, and this simple aspect (among many) is indicative of why the "one drug fits all" ideology cannot be applied to homoeopathy (Kurd et al., 2021; Manchanda et al., 2021; Mukherjee et al., 2021; Adler et al., 2021; Takacs et al., 2021; Ministry of AYUSH, Government of India., 2020).

HOMOEOPATHY FOR COVID-19: INDICATED MEDICINES ACCORDING TO SYMPTOM SIMILARITY

COVID-19 patients present a broad spectrum of symptoms from being completely asymptomatic to mild-moderate to severely critical. Fever (98%), cough (82%), shortness of breath (55%), fatigue (70%), myalgia (44%), and sputum production (33%) are the most common symptoms reported, whereas less common symptoms include headache (13%), diarrhoea (10%), nausea and vomiting (10%), and haemoptysis (5%) (see Chapter 1 for detailed signs and symptoms). Homoeopathic medicines are selected as per the individualized need of the patient (Figure 14.2).

Taking the psychological makeup of the individual, physical symptoms, characteristic particulars, age, occupation, previous illnesses, and life circumstances unique to the individual irrespective of the disease which he/she is suffering from are taken into consideration. After the selection of the appropriate remedy, deciding the potency, dosage, and frequency are very much critical in initiating the optimum response and achieving faster healing. Decimal or centesimal potencies are used for the treatment of acute conditions. The selection of a similar remedy (as per the totality of symptoms) and appropriate homoeopathic potency is key and are dependent on factors like susceptibility of the patient (high or low), type of disease (acute/chronic), seat/nature and intensity of the disease, stage and duration of the disease, and the previous treatment of the disease. The medicines given here are suggestive based on their use and studies in the past in

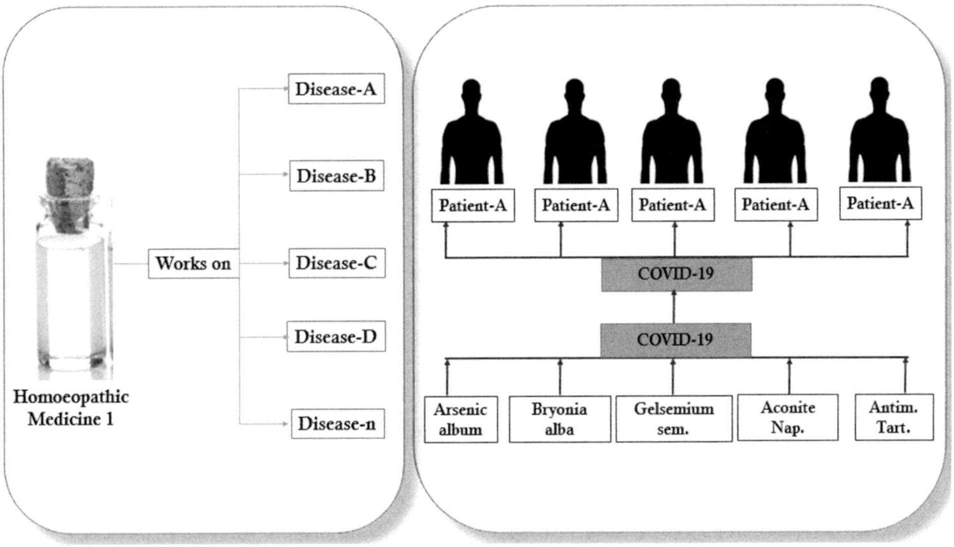

Figure 14.2 Homoeopathy as a polychrest as well as an individualized system of treatment.

diseases of similar presentation to COVID-19 (Ministry of AYUSH, Government of India., 2020; World Health Organization, 2009).

The Ministry of AYUSH, Government of India, indicated a few homoeopathic medicines to be implemented as adjuvant to standard management guidelines for mild cases (symptomatic amelioration and mitigation approach) that includes *Aconitum napellus*, arsenicum album, *Bryonia alba*, *Gelsemium sempervirens*, *Rhus toxicodendron*, *Eupatorium perfoliatum*, ipecacuanha, Belladonna, and Camphor depending upon the totality of symptoms. Also, medicines like phosphorous, Chelidonium, *Veratrum viride*, Iodum, *Cinchona officinalis*, Lycopodium, arsenicum iodatum, antimonium arsenicicum, stannum metallicum can be administered if the symptoms match with the medicine (Ministry of AYUSH, Government of India., 2020; World Health Organization, 2009).

It is to be understood that the homoeopathic system of medicine works in tune with the body's immune system and normal healing mechanisms. Thus, the medicine to be selected must be based on the guidelines presented in the *Organon of Medicine* and *Homoeopathic Materia Medica* and strictly not on the reductionistic ideology of "one drug fits all" just to win the race for approval.

HOMOEOPATHY FOR COVID-19: THE MYTHS, MISINFORMATION, AND CONCERNS

The wrong formation is very dangerous, especially in this pandemic situation. And with access to social media, myths, misinformation, and fake news spread like wildfire. Lots of myths and misinformation are circulating regarding homoeopathy in relation to COVID-19 and may cause harm if not checked at the proper time. A lack of proper education about the homoeopathic system of medicine is the main reason behind the spread of misinformation.

After the announcement that arsenicum album 30CH can be used as a preventive treatment or as an overall immune booster for protection against COVID-19, people started buying and consuming the medicine like they consume any cough syrup or health tonic. Instead of taking the medicine as per the dosage guidelines issued by the Ministry of AYUSH, Government of India, they started consuming the medicine as they would consume any other allopathic medicine. People have the idea of more is good (conventional ideology) which is not the case with homoeopathic medicines. These kinds of actions will lead to homoeopathic aggravation and may worsen the situation. Also, due to competition and overwhelming profits, pharmacies intended to sell conventional medicines (having no knowledge of homoeopathic preparations) started selling arsenic album 30 CH. Several non-government organizations started donating arsenic album for free without any formal homoeopathic physician training or any prior knowledge of the mechanisms by which homoeopathic medicine work. This resulted in misuse and overuse of arsenic album, which is dangerous for long-term health.

Aspidoperma Q, is another such medicine that is linked to COVID-19. Through social media, misleading information was spread that homoeopathic aspidosperma Q increased oxygen levels in COVID-19 patients. False information like this is more dangerous than the pandemic itself. In the absence or lack of oxygen cylinders and hospital facilities, people out of desperation started buying bottles of aspidosperma Q and started depending on it to work on severe COVID-19 patients (requiring hospitalized life support).

In times like this, information is a very sensitive resource. False information holds the potential to add fuel to the already ongoing pandemic.

CHALLENGES AND FUTURE RESEARCH POSSIBILITIES

Forget coronavirus, homoeopathy cannot cure anything.

This statement is a very common perspective about the homoeopathic system of medicine projected by individuals through word of mouth, print mediums, and online social media. These adhominem statements are the result of a half-hearted understanding of science, biased knowledge of the subject matter, greed for a medical monopoly, and a dogmatic mindset. Homoeopathy is not a conventional system of medicine (or allopathy) and thus underlying principles of treatment are also different. So trying to make sense out of the holistic science of homoeopathy by applying the reductionistic ideology of conventional medicine is completely illogical and unscientific as "judging a fish by its ability to run on land". If anyone wishes to determine whether the homoeopathic system of medicine is effective or not, then a proper understanding of the principles mentioned in *Organon* and their relation to conventional sciences are crucial. Also, one needs to understand that homoeopathy is a personalized system of medicine while conventional medicine follows the one drug fits all approach. So statistical analysis and assumption of the mean value is applicable for drugs used in the conventional system, but this methodology will not hold true for personalized systems. In short, homoeopathy is a patient-centric approach while the conventional system is a disease-specific approach. This is exactly what the Father of Medicine, the Great Hippocrates, and the Father of Modern Medicine, Sir William Osler, taught us, that is, "It is much more important to know what sort of patient has a disease than what sort of a disease a patient has. The good physician treats the disease, the great physician treats the patient who has the disease" (A–Z Quotes, n.d.a). The conventional system addresses symptomatic management, but homoeopathy treats the patient who has the disease.

Another false notion associated with homoeopathy is that "it acts as a placebo". A placebo is defined as a medicine or procedure prescribed for the psychological benefit of the patient rather than for any physiological effect. When viewed from the aspect of reductionistic conventional medicine, this would seem illogical because according to conventional ideology, "visible matter" is everything and "invisible energy" is of no consequence. So, any component that is meant to impact invisible psychology in no way should have a visible physical impact. Thus, the notion that homoeopathy is a pseudoscience came into existence. But we need to understand that "matter is made out of energy" or invisible energy controls the visible matter. So, medicines used in homoeopathy act at the energy levels, and the psychological aspect (or mind) is an invisible intangible aspect composed of energy that is present outside and regulates the physical body (see Chapter 3). Homoeopathic medicines (present in the form of energy signature) act on the invisible life force or the natural healing force (the invisible energy regulating the physical body) and the signal generated is transferred through the neuroendocrine system of the physical body, thus creating changes at the chemical level (curative modifications). The entire process falls under a branch of advanced evidence-based science called psychoneuroendocrinoimmunology (PNEI), which states that psychology (invisible energy) impacts the physical body (visible matter) through the neuroendocrine system. Also, even if homoeopathic medicines were true placebos (as some individuals claim) and patients receiving those were cured of a disease condition (just because of their belief), then what is the problem if those medicines are implemented? The ultimate aim of medical science is to address the disease condition with fewer adverse reactions, if that is the case, then we should be open to providing any treatment or combination of treatments that are suitable for our patient under consideration. And if a patient is cured just by using a "placebo", then why do we even need industrially synthesized chemical drugs, which have evidence of creating adverse reactions inside the body creating iatrogenic conditions? Because the Father of Medicine, the Great Hippocrates, and the Father of Modern Medicine, Sir William Osler, stated that "the person who takes medicines has to recover twice, once from the disease and once from the medicine. Keep your drugs in [the] chemist's pot, if you can heal your patients with substances natural to them" (A–Z Quotes, n.d.b).

The third important challenge is the dedicated involvement in the research and development of homoeopathic treatment protocols. The majority of the homoeopathic physicians are not involved with scientific research, and this is the reason behind the lack of data about treatment procedures. Also, this system of medicine is not profitable for the industry, this is why organizations performing research and development do not receive the proper amounts of financial support that their conventional counterparts receive. It is high time that not only the homoeopaths but also the pharmacologists, conventional medical professionals, and other allied science personnel need to come forward and involve themselves in the collaborative development of the homoeopathic system and establish its authenticity instead of blindly calling it out as fake. It is to be understood that the approach we take to study science determines the outcome and thus making the right choice is important.

REFERENCES

(2021, October 19). *Notes on Organon of Medicine & Philosophy – I.* Homeopathy Resource by Homeobook. Com. Retrieved November 24, 2021, from https://www.homeobook.com/notes-on-organon-of-medicine-philosophy-i/

Adler, U. C., Adler, M. S., Hotta, L. M., Padula, A. E. M., de Toledo Cesar, A., Diniz, J. N. M., Mestre, C. A. A., Spiller, K. R., Soares, L., de Freitas Santos, H., & Martinez, E. Z. (2021). Homeopathy for Covid-19 in primary care: A structured summary of a study protocol for a randomized controlled trial. *Trials*, *22*(1). https://doi.org/10.1186/s13063-021-05071-5

A–Z Quotes. (n.d.a). *Top 25 Quotes by Hippocrates (of 158).* Retrieved March 8, 2022, from https://www.azquotes.com/author/22138-Hippocrates

A–Z Quotes. (n.d.b). *Top 25 Quotes by William Osler (of 135).* (n.d.). Retrieved March 8, 2022, from https://www.azquotes.com/author/11160-William_Osler

Goswami, S., & Gupta Bakshi, U. (2020). Understanding classical naturopathy: The Hippocratic way of healing. In A. Sharma et al. (Ed.), *Herbal Product Development Formulation and Applications* (1st ed., pp. 293–320). Apple Academic Press. https://doi.org/10.1201/9781003003182

Hahnemann, S. (1833). *Organon of Medicine.* (5th ed., 1833). B Jain Publishers.

Hegde, B.M. (2014) *What Doctors Don't Get to Study in Medical School.* Paras Medical Publisher.

Kurd, R., Freed, Y., Jarjoui, A., Izbicki, G., Levin, P., Helvitz, Y., Sherr, J., & Oberbaum, M. (2021). Homeopathic treatment for COVID-19-related symptoms: A case series. *Complementary Medicine Research*, 1–6. https://doi.org/10.1159/000517924

Manchanda, R. K., Miglani, A., Gupta, M., Meena, B. S., Chadha, V., Joseph, F., Kalsi, A., Konthembath, P., Sharma, K., Rama, K. N., Kaur, P., Thavarayil Kannoth, J., Nagrath, C., Jethani, A., Nellikka Aniyeri, S., Chawla, A., Ray, M. K., Ghuliani, M., Kudiyarasu, R. K., . . . Sharma, B. (2021). Homeopathic remedies in COVID-19: Prognostic factor research. *Homeopathy.* Published. https://doi.org/10.1055/s-0041-1725989

Ministry of AYUSH, Government of India. (2020). *Guidelines for Homoeopathy Practitioners for Prophylaxis and Symptomatic Management of Home IsolatedCOVID-19 Patients.* https://www.ayush.gov.in/docs/CCRH-%20Revised%20Guidelines%20for%20Homoeopathy%20Practitioners%20for%20Prophylaxis%20and%20Symptomatic%20Management%20of%20COVID-19%20Patients%20in%20Home%20Isolation.pdf

Mukherjee, S. K., Ganguly, S., Das, S., Chatterjee, K. K., Naskar, K. K., Dey, S., Choudhury, S., Paul, A., Sarkar, S. S., Bhattacharyya, S., Sengupta, S., Alam, S. M., Bhattacharya, P., Naskar, S., Mukherjee, S., Shamim, S., Mandal, D., Sardar, S., Sarkar, S., . . . Saha, S. (2021). Homeopathic medicines used as prophylaxis in Kolkata during the COVID-19 pandemic: A community-based, cluster-randomized trial. *Homeopathy.* Published. https://doi.org/10.1055/s-0041-1734026

Shang, J., Wan, Y., Luo, C., Ye, G., Geng, Q., Auerbach, A., & Li, F. (May 2020). Cell entry mechanisms of SARS-CoV-2. *Proceedings of the National Academy of Sciences*, *117*(21), 11727–11734. https://doi.org/10.1073/pnas.2003138117.

Takacs, M., Frass, M., Walder, G., Fibert, P., Rottensteiner, M., Glück, W., Lechleitner, P., Oberbaum, M., Leisser, I., Chandak, K., Panhofer, P., & Weiermayer, P. (2021). Adjunctive homeopathic treatment of hospitalized COVID-19 patients (COVIHOM): A retrospective case series. *Complementary Therapies in Clinical Practice*, *44*, 101415. https://doi.org/10.1016/j.ctcp.2021.101415

Venkateswara Homoeopathic Medical College and Hospital. (2020, June 16). *Organon of Medicine and Homoeopathic Philosophy.* Retrieved November 24, 2021, from http://www.venkathomoeo.org/departments/organon-of-medicine-and-homeopathic-philosophy

WHO Clinical Care Severe Acute Respiratory Illness (SARI) Training, & World Health Organization. (2020). Retrieved from https://openwho.org/courses/severe-acute-respiratory-infection on 22nd June, 2020.

World Health Organization. (2009). *Safety Issues in Preparation of Homoeopathic Medicines.* World Health Organization.

Yuki, K., Fujiogi, M., & Koutsogiannaki, S. (2020). COVID-19 pathophysiology: A review. *Clinical Immunology*, *215*, 108427. https://doi.org/10.1016/j.clim.2020.108427

Homoeopathic Practice in the Midst of COVID-19

A Physician's Clinical Experience

Shyamali Guha*

In this chapter, an experienced homoeopathic physician, Dr Shyamali Guha, shares her experiences in dealing with patients having influenza-like illnesses (possibly COVID-19) during this pandemic period. Susceptibility to cold, slow healing, frequent infections, extreme tiredness, and gastrointestinal derangements are the hallmarks of a weak immune system. Individuals suffering from mentioned symptoms require treatment that will help restore immune system functioning. In the present pandemic situation, it is important to have a proper diet, a sufficient amount of clean water and appropriate exercise as these are essential for the restoration of immunity. Chronic illnesses like diabetes, cardiac complications, hypertension, high cholesterol, renal complications and pulmonary complications are indicative of long-term immune system dysfunction and increase the risk of being infected by opportunistic pathogens like SARS-CoV-2. COVID-19 is a completely new influenza virus. The most common symptoms of this virus are dry cough, fever, tiredness, diarrhoea, anorexia, anaemia and debility.

- **Incidence 1:** Many patients visited the clinic with symptoms such as tiredness, debility and mild grade fever (some of them had RT-PCR tested positive for COVID-19). Along with these basic symptoms, patients were showing symptoms similar to *Gelsemium sempervirens*. Based on the principles of homoeopathy, patients were given *Gelsemium sempervirens* in appropriate potency, dose and repetition (as per the requirement of the individual patient). Patients started feeling better within a few hours and the physical complications healed within seven to ten days. The RT-PCR test for those patients came negative for COVID-19 after 14 days of treatment.
- **Incidence 2:** A patient complained of severe headache, throat pain, body aches and restlessness, along with symptoms similar to Belladonna. The patient was administered Belladonna in appropriate potency, dosage and duration. The complications were healed within a few days and the RT-PCR report was negative for COVID-19 within ten days after homoeopathic treatment.
- **Incidence 3:** A female patient already under treatment with conventional medicine was advised to go for homoeopathic treatment by conventional physicians. The patient had a recurring mild grade fever. With prominent symptoms of COVID-19, the patient showed

DOI: 10.1201/9781003178514-18

similarity to *Cinchona officinalis* and thus was given the same medicine in appropriate potency, dosage and duration. The symptoms resolved within ten days of treatment.

- **Incidence 4:** A patient arrived with an oxygen level below 90%. After assessing the condition, the patient was administered with *Arnica montana*. *Arnica montana* is indicated as a prophylactic for pus infection, tissue degeneration and septic conditions, with a marked effect on the blood. The patient was kept under observation, and within one to two hours, the oxygen level increased to 97%.
- **Incidence 5:** A patient had a low-grade fever, muscular cramps, a headache and was thirsty. Along with possible COVID-19 like symptoms, the patient showed similarities with *Bryonia alba*. The patient was administered with "Bryonia" several times, becoming free of all symptoms. Only anosmia was present. After a few days, he was totally free from COVID-19.

Chapter 15

Solving the Mystery of COVID-19

Holistic Medical Nutrition Therapy

Biswaroop Roy Chowdhury*

CONTENTS

INTRODUCTION

The author and his team have had the rare privilege of treating and curing more than 5000 patients, indeed, this was at the peak of the pandemic between June 5, 2020, and July 14, 2020. This was possible with the help of a network of more than 200 influenza experts spread all across the country (and also a few outside the country).

The author and his team of experts achieved a cure with zero medication and zero percent mortality, with more than 80% of patients resolving their symptoms in 72 hours following a three-day flu diet (details of which are given in the chapters that follow) and 75% of patients (among those who went for a second RT-PCR test for SARS-CoV-2) testing negative for SARS-CoV-2.

These results may be baffling and may look manipulated and over-exaggerated for common people as well as conventional doctors with a mindset of treating influenza/Covid-19 patients with the medicine protocol set by WHO, where they are used to 3-4% mortality with an average hospital discharge rate of 14 days, but for the author and his team, the mystery was something else.

Out of the 5000 plus patients with classical influenza-like illness (ILI) symptoms as defined by the CDC, about 1000 patients came to the author and his team with a SARS-CoV-2 positive test

DOI: 10.1201/9781003178514-19

reported through RT-PCR, and the rest arrived without going for an RT-PCR test for Covid-19. This means, out of 5000 ILI patients, 1000 were Covid-19 patients and 4000 were non-Covid-19 ILI patients.

If we go by the guidelines of issuing death certificates released by ICMR (Indian Council of Medical Research), if any person dies with the classical symptoms of ILI, then the cause of death should be mentioned as Covid-19 even if the RT-PCR test for SARS-CoV-2 is negative before or after death. This means that ICMR believes that 100% of ILI patients have a single causative agent and that should be SARS-CoV-2, although this theory of ICMR does not have any evidence in the medical literature (NCDIR-ICMR, 2020). Going by the guidelines of "How to Report in Death Certificates" by ICMR, technically, I should say that in the last 40 days, we have cured 5000+ Covid-19 patients. However, the causative agent of the symptoms of flu or ILI can be among more than 200 identified viruses and could be other pathogens including bacteria, fungi, and even non-parasite causes including side effects of drugs and so on.

The mystery for the author and his team while treating these 5000 plus patients was that they could not find any particular symptoms among the ILI patients with a Covid-19 positive status that were unique to them (1000 patients with a positive RT-PCR report) and which could be distinguishable from the rest of the 4000 patients (surely many out of them might have a different causative agent than SARS-CoV-2).

UNFOLDING THE MYSTERY: OUT OF THE BOX OBSERVATION

Symptomatically, Covid-19 patients are identical to other ILI patients with no unique signs or patterns of recovery. To unfold the mystery rather than solve the puzzle called Covid-19, the author and his team wish to take the readers to the first week of January 2020 (around January 4–7) with the headline in most of the newspapers across the world "Cause of Wuhan's mysterious pneumonia cases still unknown, Chinese officials say" (Belluz, 2020), which even the WHO acknowledged on January 5, 2020, on their website (WHO, 2020a).

As per the WHO, on January 3, 2020 (WHO, 2020a), 44 patients with pneumonia of unknown etiology were reported by the national authorities of China.

Knowing that each year more than 2.5 million (Dadonaite, 2018) people die of pneumonia and around 450 million people suffer from pneumonia or ILI, the intriguing question is how the health authorities distinguished those reported 44 patients as pneumonia with unknown etiology. Let's have a look at the following facts:

1. In more than 60% of the cases of ILI, no virus could be detected (Yu et al., 2018).
2. In more than 20% of the cases of pneumonia, no causative agent could be detected (Ali et al., 2016)

All across the world, including our neighborhood, for every ten patients with ILI (symptomatically), at least six will not be detected with any virus known for ILI.

For every ten patients with pneumonia, at least two will not be detected with any known causative agent.

Meaning that more than 60% of patients with ILI can be called ILI patients with unknown etiology (cause), and 20% of pneumonia patients with unknown etiology can be called mysterious pneumonia.

Here, the author and his team wish to emphasize that symptomatically, the COVID-19 patients do not show any unique characteristics or signs or patterns that are distinguishable from other

ILI/pneumonia patients. In addition, it is not possible to rule out all the known causes of pneumonia as there are thousands of causative agents which may lead to pneumonia. Diagnostically, the best tool available to science is the PCR test (which is known as the gold standard), but with high false positives, which means that when PCR tests are conducted for more than 200 viruses known to humans to be the causative agent of ILI/pneumonia, statistically (on average), it will show positive for at least two of the 200 viruses, even in the absence of any of the 200 viruses, since the specificity of the PCR test, by design, cannot be more than 99%, which translates to showing two viruses as a causative agent, even if none of them may be present.

There are virtually no means to know whether the positive test is a TRUE positive or a FALSE positive.

Conclusively, the positive result (even though it is false positive) could be accepted as a causative agent of the ILI for a particular patient.

Hence, the question is "what was the basis of deciding that the causative agent of pneumonia among the 44 patients is of unknown etiology?" I tried to refer to the WHO website at the link but the matter does not exist (Figure 15.1).

Since the WHO and the Chinese health authorities have not given any data or evidence or study of proof, how can they rule out the possibility of all known causes of pneumonia? And how did they conclude that SARS-CoV-2 may be the causative agent of pneumonia among those 44 patients? Even if it is the causative agent, it may not be a new virus to humans, it rather may be one of the causative agents of pneumonia among those 20% of patients for whom the causative agent could not be detected earlier.

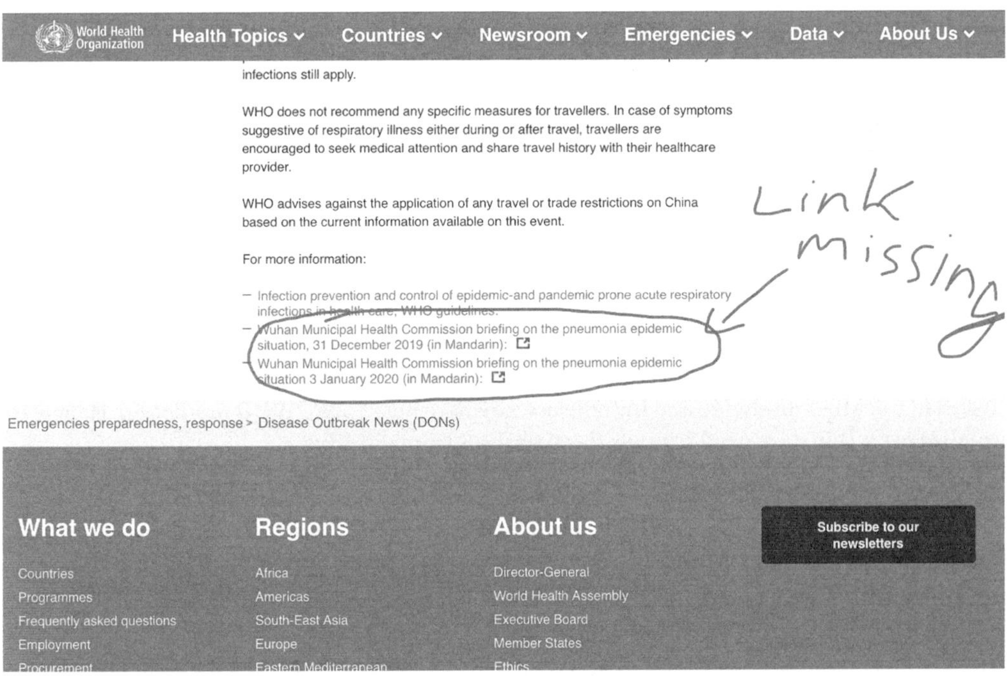

Figure 15.1 A screenshot representing missing links.

In simple language, SARS-CoV-2 may have been causing ILI/pneumonia for a long time, but it is only now that we have devised a method to detect the virus.

UNFOLDING THE MYSTERY: ANALYZING THE OBSERVATIONS

Based on my experience of treating more than 5000 patients, and with the previous evidence, we can conclude that SARS-CoV-2 is not a new virus, with no unique illnesses/symptoms, especially when the WHO or China have not given any evidence to prove it to be a new virus.

Hence, announcing a pandemic is technically wrong, as, by definition, a pandemic means a worldwide spread of a new disease. If we talk of India, the Epidemic Act 1897, as implemented by the Government of India, is unconstitutional and unwarranted since, by the WHO definition, epidemic means the occurrence of an illness clearly in excess of normal expectancy. For India, the average number of deaths due to pneumonia is 1.5 lakh per year. Deaths due to Covid-19 by July 13, 2020, were 22,000 which may not be true Covid deaths, rather deaths with SARS-CoV-2 due to experimental medical procedures and co-morbid conditions (as explained in the later chapters).

We must remind ourselves that the basis of lockdown and social distancing with the announcement of a pandemic and the implementation of the Epidemic Act was a prediction by the WHO in March 2020 (WHO, 2020a, b).

Prediction Number 1

Prediction for the world. If no lockdown or social distancing or other preventive measures are taken, then nearly 40 million people will die worldwide. Even if all prevention and lockdown measures are followed, then 20 million people will die worldwide in the next few months.

Prediction Number 2

Prediction for India. If no lockdown or social distancing or other preventive measures are taken, then up to 6,096,359 people will die, and if all the WHO guidelines of lockdown or social distancing are followed, then about 2,375,803 people will die due to Covid-19 in the next few months. Now, with a serology survey by ICMR, it was established that the case fatality rate (CFR) of Covid-19 was 0.08% (Online, 2020; WHO, 2020a, b), which is lower than seasonal flu, and the rate of transmission (RO) is 1.15, which is less than the common cold, meaning that Covid-19 is neither deadly nor infectious as has been predicted and projected. Fortunately, with a very low CFR and RO, deaths worldwide and in India are nowhere near to the WHO prediction. Hence, to normalize everything, we need to erase three phrases from our lives:

- It is not a mysterious virus
- No epidemic
- No pandemic

Through the media, you are made to believe that it is a mysterious deadly virus causing a high number of casualties, but with no supportive evidence. As by now, we know that it is just a regular flu (ILI), which is presented as COVID-19, so we decided to treat our patients with the same three-step flu diet that we used successfully to cure our flu patients since 2016.

IMPLEMENTING THE FOOD AS MEDICINE: THE THREE-STEP FLU DIET

The three-step flu diet works and is based on the evidence from more than 167 research papers from the last 100 years.

The following is the three-step flu diet.

Day 1 (Liquid)

Consume citrus fruit juice and coconut water in the quantities specified below:

- Your body weight (kg)/10, glasses of fresh citrus fruit juice + body weight (kg)/10 glasses of coconut water.
- Let us say your body weight is 60 kg so 60/10 = six glasses of citrus fruit juice and six glasses of coconut water.

Do not consume packed juice, instead, have fresh juice and take it without sieving. Take the juice and coconut water alternately every hour, sip by sip, spending at least 15 minutes on each glass. This will keep the temperature under control. Vitamin C in citrus fruit juice supports immunity and helps in getting rid of the virus.

Coconut water helps hydration. It is the best mineral water in the world made by God.

Day 2 (Fluid)

Consume citrus fruit juice and coconut water in the quantities specified below:

- Your body weight (kg)/20, glasses of citrus fruit juice + body weight (kg)/20 glasses of coconut water + your body weight (kg) × 5 g of cucumber and tomatoes.
- Let us say your body weight is 60 kg so 60/20 = three glasses of citrus fruit juice and three glasses of coconut water, as well as 60 × 5 = 300 g of cucumber and tomatoes.

You will be surprised to see that by the end of day 2, you start feeling better and your temperature is under control. You will have regained some strength.

Day 3 (Solid)

For breakfast, consume the following:

- Your body weight (kg)/30 glasses of citrus fruit juice + body weight (kg)/30 glasses of coconut water.
- If your body weight is 60 kg so 60/30 = two glasses of citrus fruit juice and two glasses of coconut water.

For lunch, consume the following:

- Your body weight (kg) × 5 g of cucumber and tomatoes.
- If your body weight is 60 kg, so 60 × 5 =300 g of cucumber and tomatoes.

By evening, you will be surprised to find yourself fit. You can have normal home-cooked food with less oil and salt, leaving animal protein for dinner.

If you follow this simple diet, you will be back to work on the fourth day.

Step Three

Usually, people try to manage the flu with medicines, and sometimes, there are chances for the virus to move down from the upper respiratory tract to the lower respiratory tract. As a result, breathing difficulty occurs and if checked with an oximeter, the oxygen level will be $\leq 90\%$. In such situations, the doctor will advise a ventilator because the lungs are full of water. What you have to do in such a situation is avoid going to the hospital because you will be put on a mechanical ventilator. You have to make your own ventilator at home. This is called prone ventilation (Guerin, 2014).

CONCLUSION

It should be noted that by July 14, 2020, we cured more than 5000 flu/Covid-19 patients with more than 200 experts, and at the time of submitting this chapter, the total count of patients went to more than 50,000 with around 650 experts, while maintaining zero mortality.

REFERENCES

Ali, A., Akhund, T., Warraich, G. J., Aziz, F., Rahman, N., Umrani, F. A., Qureshi, S., Petri, W. A., Bhutta, Z., Zaidi, A. K. M., & Hughes, M. A. (2016). Respiratory viruses associated with severe pneumonia in children under 2 years old in a rural community in Pakistan. *Journal of Medical Virology, 88*(11), 1882–1890. https://doi.org/10.1002/jmv.24557

Belluz, J. (2020, January 20). *Wuhan, China, pneumonia outbreak: A new virus may be the cause.* Vox. https://www.vox.com/2020/1/9/21058069/wuhan-pneumonia-outbreak

Dadonaite, B. (2018, November 4). *Pneumonia.* Our World in Data. https://ourworldindata.org/pneumonia

Guerin, C. (2014). Prone ventilation in acute respiratory distress syndrome. *European Respiratory Review, 23*(132), 249–257. https://doi.org/10.1183/09059180.00001114

NCDIR-ICMR. (2020). *Guidance for appropriate recording of COVID-19 related deaths in India.* https://ncdirindia.org/Downloads/CoD_COVID-19_Guidance.pdf

Online, F. E. (2020, June 12). *Coronavirus infection: Around 1 crore Indians were exposed, Sero-Survey finds.* The Financial Express. https://www.financialexpress.com/lifestyle/health/coronavirus-infection-around-1-crore-indians-were-infected-sero-survey-finds/1988886/

World Health Organization. (2020a, January 30). *Pneumonia of unknown cause: China.* https://www.who.int/csr/don/05-january-2020-pneumonia-of-unkown-cause-china/en/.

World Health Organization. (2020b, March 12). *What is a pandemic?* https://www.who.int/csr/disease/swineflu/frequently_asked_questions/pandemic/en/.

Yu, J., Xie, Z., Zhang, T., Lu, Y., Fan, H., Yang, D., Bénet, T., Vanhems, P., Shen, K., Huang, F., Han, J., Li, T., Gao, Z., Ren, L., & Wang, J. (2018). Comparison of the prevalence of respiratory viruses in patients with acute respiratory infections at different hospital settings in North China, 2012–2015. *BMC Infectious Diseases, 18*(1). https://doi.org/10.1186/s12879-018-2982-3

Chapter 16

Immunonutrition Therapy for COVID-19

Understanding the Immunomodulatory Effect of Vitamin D

Srijan Goswami*, Ushmita Gupta Bakshi, and Dona Khamaru

CONTENTS

INTRODUCTION

Medical conditions like pneumonia, severe acute respiratory distress syndrome (SARDS), myocarditis, thrombosis, and cytokine storm resulting from underlying uncontrolled inflammatory processes are linked to increased severity of COVID-19. It is known that T lymphocytes play a central role in the regulation of the body's inflammatory response and provide protection from viral infections (The Centre for Evidence-Based Medicine, 2020; Weir et al., 2020). Several studies have shown that an increase in vitamin D levels in the body not only creates a positive regulation of cell-mediated immune responses (Konijeti et al., 2016) but also helps decrease the disease severity of COVID-19 (Jain et al., 2020). Vitamin D possesses the ability to provide a positive immunomodulatory effect during both initial viraemic phases and subsequent hyperinflammatory phases associated with COVID-19 (Martineau & Forouhi, 2020). Lower levels of Vitamin D in the blood are found to be associated with COVID 19 patients who are hospitalized (Biesalski, 2020; Karahan & Katkat, 2020; Baktash et al., 2020). Several studies have shown that low levels of Vitamin D are associated with longer time on a ventilator because of cardiopulmonary complications associated with COVID-19 (Brenner et al., 2020; Williamson et al., 2020; Ilie et al., 2020; Radujkovic et al., 2020; Entrenas Castillo et al., 2020). Lower vitamin D levels are associated with higher SARS-CoV-2 positive PCR related to infectivity (D'Avolio et al., 2020; Merzon et al., 2020). Lower vitamin D levels are associated with elevated C-Reactive Protein (CRP) and fibrinogen-dimer levels in COVID-19 patients. These are all acute-phase reactive proteins or inflammatory mediators (Jain et al., 2020; Daneshkhah et al., 2020). Lower vitamin D levels are associated with a decreased clearance of

DOI: 10.1201/9781003178514-20

the SARS-CoV-2 virus (D'Avolio et al., 2020; Merzon et al., 2020). Low vitamin D levels are associated with an increased risk of developing or progressing chronic heart failure (CHF), coronary artery disease, diabetes, and hypertension (Kheiri et al., 2018; Berridge, 2017; Judd & Tangpricha, 2009; Office of Dietary Supplements – Vitamin D, n.d.). The scientific community does not have a huge amount of data on the actual mechanism of how vitamin D is particularly helping in respiratory tract infections with COVID-19, but it is documented that vitamin D has been shown to be effective against viral respiratory tract infections like Respiratory Syncytial Virus (RSV), influenza, and rhinovirus (Martineau et al., 2017). The present chapter discusses the impact of vitamin D in COVID-19 and possible mechanisms through which vitamin D expresses its immunomodulatory effects.

VITAMIN D, BASIC CHEMISTRY, AND METABOLISM

In order for us to really understand how vitamin D is helping the body to modulate our immune system and play roles in the prevention of COVID-19, we have to go through the basics like the metabolic pathways of vitamin D, build our foundation, and then we will study immune-modulation of the cascades involved. Vitamin D is a fat-soluble vitamin and is an essential component of the body's immune system. Milk, egg yolks, yoghurt, liver, and mushrooms are some of the natural sources of vitamin D. When vitamin D is consumed through food, it is ingested and moves down to the gastrointestinal tract. Being a fat-soluble vitamin, vitamin D requires binding with fats and cholesterol in order to be absorbed. This form of vitamin D is known as cholecalciferol. This is one of the ways vitamin D is obtained. Another way we can obtain vitamin D is through exposure to sunlight. The skin contains a special type of chemical (cholesterol) called 7-dehydrocholesterol. When exposed to sunlight, 7-dehydrocholesterol present in the skin is converted into cholecalciferol, which is a type of fat-soluble hormone. Cholecalciferol requires a transport protein called the vitamin D binding protein to be transported to target organs (Office of Dietary Supplements – Vitamin D, n.d.). When vitamin D (cholecalciferol) enters the liver, an important enzyme, integral for vitamin D metabolism, called 25-hydroxylase adds the hydroxyl group to the 25th carbon of cholecalciferol and converts it into 25-hydroxycholecalciferol; 25-hydroxycholecalciferol then gets transported to other organs, including the kidneys. The proximal convoluted tubule, of the kidneys, contains a special enzyme called 1α-hydroxylase. The enzyme 1α-hydroxylase helps add the hydroxyl group to the first carbon of 25-hydroxycholecalciferol. This reaction by the renal enzyme converts 25-hydroxycholecalciferol into 1,25-dihydroxycholecalciferol, commonly known as the active form of vitamin D (see Figure 16.1) (Office of Dietary Supplements – Vitamin D, n.d.).

VITAMIN D AND ITS IMMUNOMODULATORY EFFECTS

The most common effect of vitamin D is that it regulates calcium levels in the blood. However, in this section, we will try to understand the role of vitamin D in immune function. The immune system cells perform several functions. Like the kidneys, macrophages also contain the enzyme 1α-hydroxylase. Similar to the kidneys, 1α-hydroxylase helps convert 25-hydroxycholecalciferol to 1,25-dihydroxycholecalciferol, which is the active form of vitamin D. The immune system cells can then express the 1α-hydroxylase molecule, therefore converting provitamin D to vitamin D (see Figure 16.2). Vitamin D is a kind of steroid hormone and

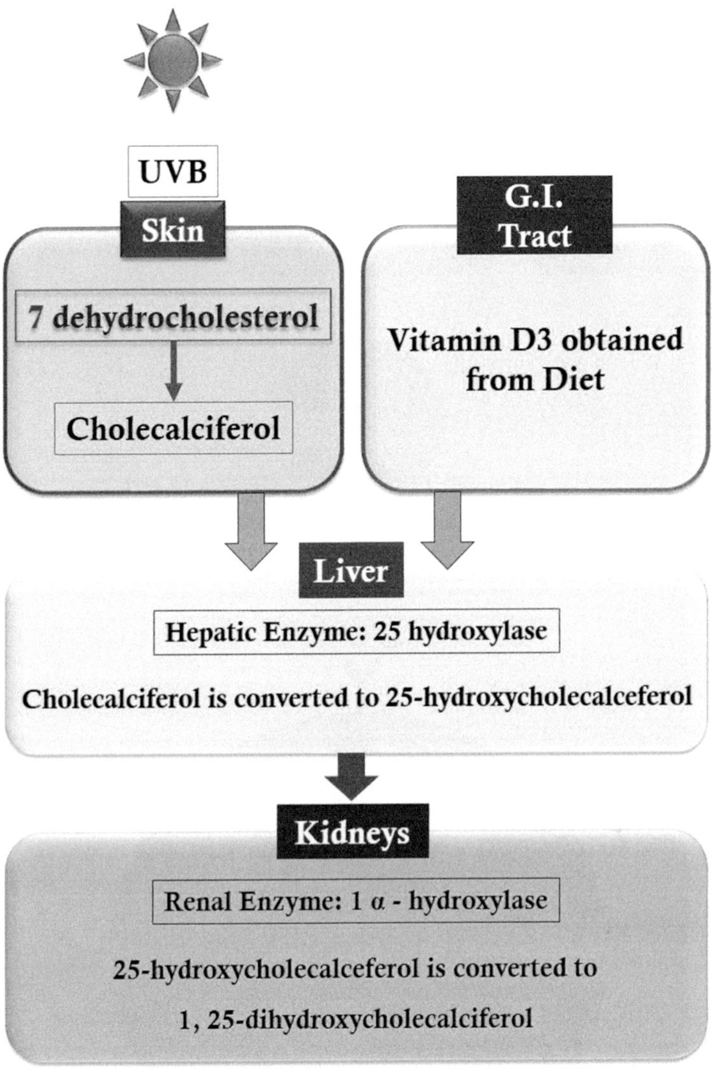

Figure 16.1 Schematic representation of active vitamin D formation.

thus can pass through the macrophage cell membrane directly (Rak & Bronkowska, 2018; Turrubiates-Hernández et al., 2021).

As vitamin D enters the cytoplasm, a protein called vitamin D receptor protein (a cytoplasmic protein) binds to it, transports it inside the nucleus, and activates specific gene expression. These gene expression events activate the production of two major groups of proteins having antimicrobial properties, one is cathelicidins and the other one is called β-defensins (see Figure 16.3). β-Defensins shows its antimicrobial activity primarily by destroying the viral (in this case SARS-CoV-2) cell membrane or envelope which is composed of a phospholipid bilayer. So, Vitamin D potentially leads to the destruction of viruses by increasing the expression of β-defensins (see Figure 16.4) (Martineau et al., 2017; Cutolo et al., 2020).

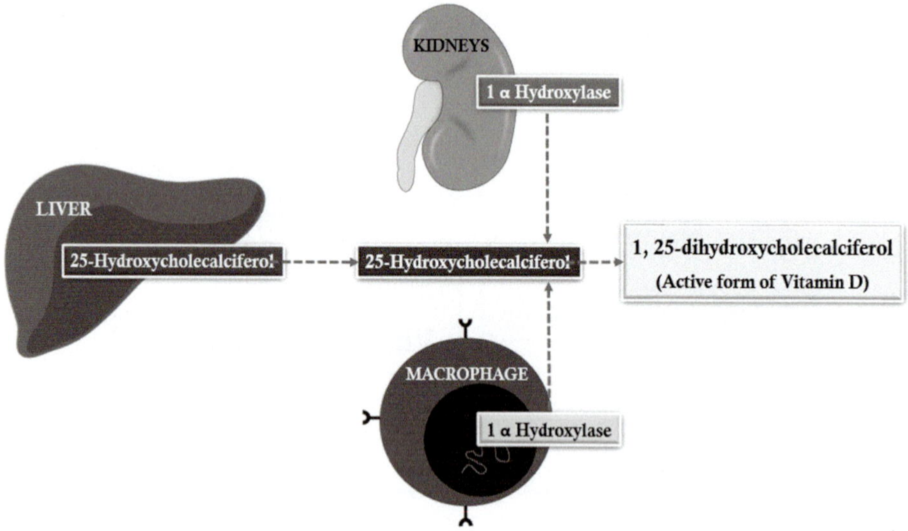

Figure 16.2 Active vitamin D formation and involvement of the liver, kidneys, and immune cells.

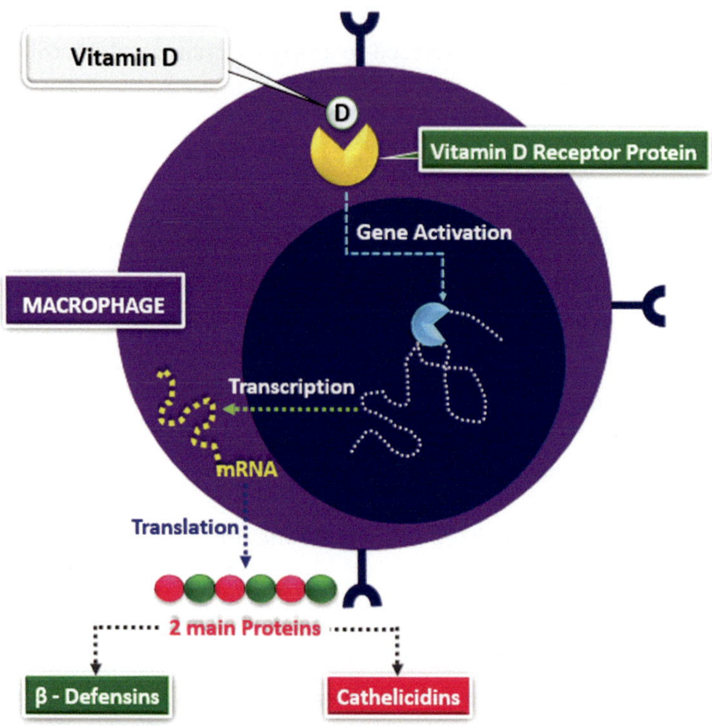

Figure 16.3 Vitamin D and secretion of β-defensins and cathelicidins.

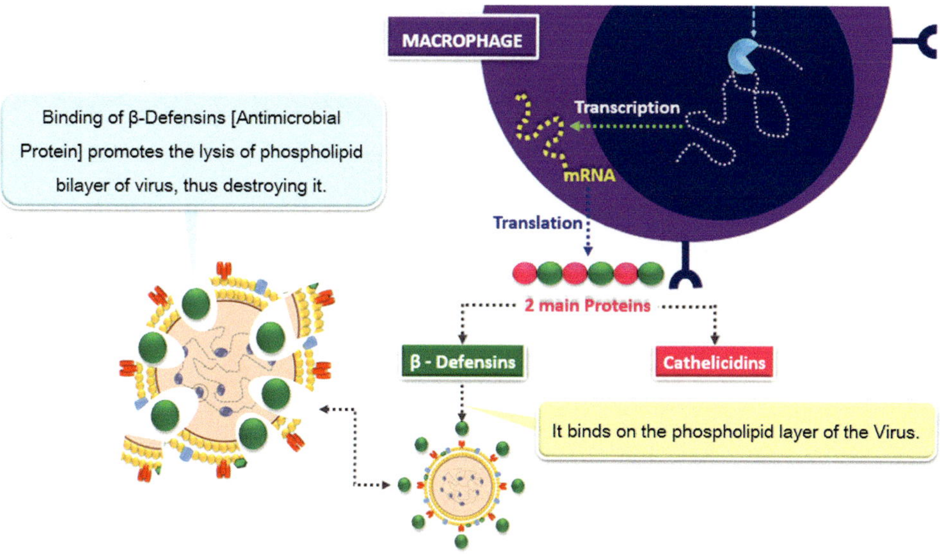

Figure 16.4 Vitamin D potentially leads to the destruction of viruses by increasing the expression of β-defensins.

Cathelicidins, are antimicrobial peptides that destroy viruses by cleaving viral envelope proteins through proteolysis. Cathelicidins also help in the stimulation of macrophages. Cathelicidins increase vascular permeability at the site of infection and cause more macrophages to infiltrate into the area where the pathogen is and subsequently activate the proliferation and recruitment of macrophages. This antimicrobial peptide regulates the movement and action of the macrophages towards the viruses by the process of chemotaxis (see Figure 16.5). Activated macrophages engulf the viruses by the process of phagocytosis. After digestion of the viruses in the phagolysosome of the macrophages, it then expresses a piece of that viral peptide (S-peptide) on the Major Histocompatibility Complex (MHC) class II molecule (see Figure 16.6).

The T helper cell binds to the MHC class II–antigen complex. The binding antigen is recognized by the T-cell receptor (TCR), MHC class II, and $CD4^+$ surface molecules (see Figure 16.6). Once this interaction happens, naïve T-cells have the opportunity to go two ways. If the reaction has interleukin-4, it convents the naïve T-cells to TH-2 cells. These TH-2 cells then start releasing more cytokines that activate B-cells. When B-cells are stimulated by interleukin-4 and interleukin-5, they proliferate and differentiate into plasma cells. The plasma cell once it is primed by these cytokines, starts secreting specific antibodies directed towards the spike protein of SARS-CoV-2. Once these antibodies are bound to the viral peptide, they enhance the complement-mediated destruction of the virus (see Figure 16.7). The other thing that it can do is increase the phagocytosis process through macrophages. The third factor is neutralizing the virus because antibodies neutralize by competitive inhibition. TH-2 cells release a particular cytokine called interleukin-10, which tries to inhibit the (second) pathway to make sure the naïve T-cells choose the TH-2 pathway. Thus, vitamin D also has the ability to support the anti-inflammatory pathway (see Figures 16.7 and 16.8). Thus, TH-2 pathway is a safe pathway.

Now let us understand the second pathway. In order for the naïve T-cells to go on the second pathway, a cytokine called interleukin-12 is needed. Interleukin-12 converts the naive T-cell into

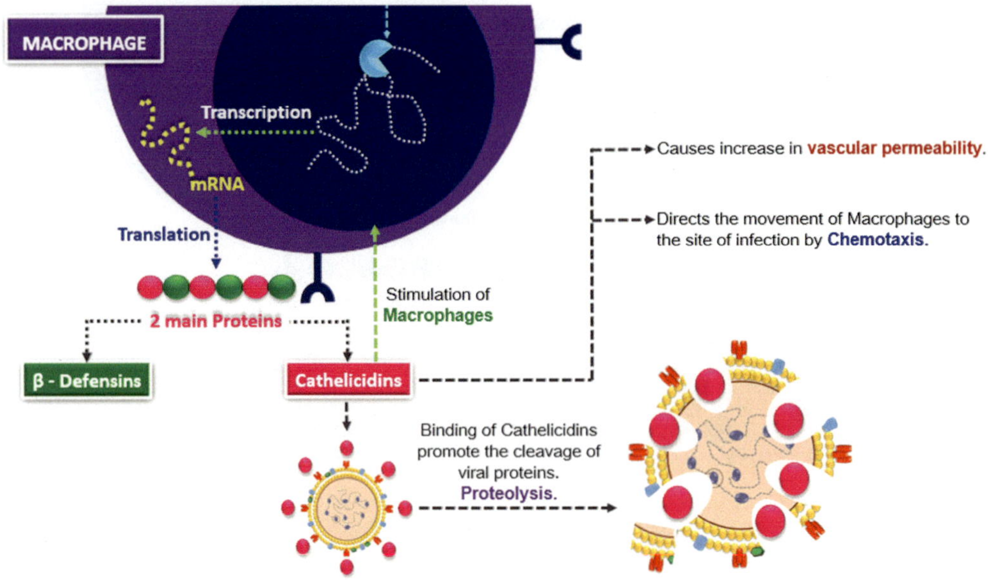

Figure 16.5 Vitamin D and cathelicidin induced immune response.

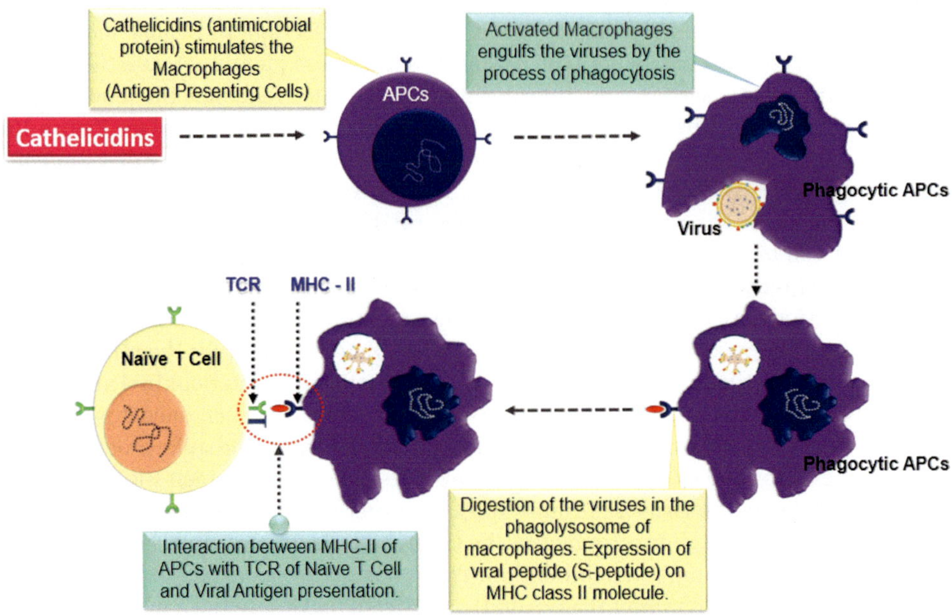

Figure 16.6 Cathelicidin induced macrophage activation, phagocytosis of the viral particle, and antigen processing and presentation to naïve T-cells.

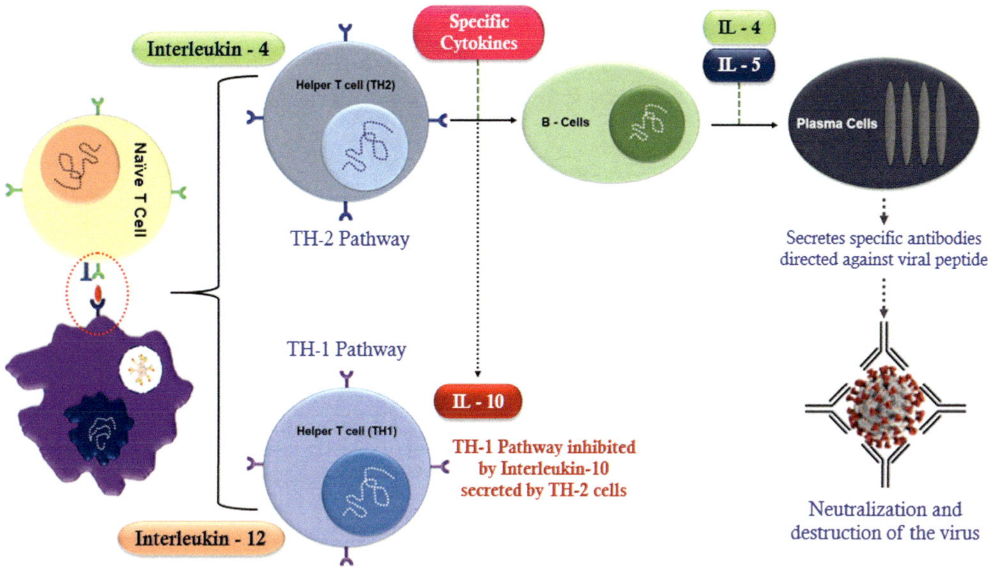

Figure 16.7 Selection of the TH-2 pathway.

another type of T-cell called the TH_1 cell. When it stimulates this process, the TH_1 cells start releasing high levels of interferon-gamma (IFN-γ) that increase the inflammatory cascade. IFN-γ activated macrophages start releasing a wide range of cytokines (IL-1, TNF-α, IL-6, and IL-8 and chemokine-CXCL). The major cytokine responsible for SARS-CoV-2 related complications is IL-6. These inflammatory cytokines together produce an uncontrolled cytokine storm leading to multisystem organ failure. These cytokines infiltrate the heart and induce cardiac failure (myocardial infarction). Cytokine infiltration of the lungs induces acute respiratory distress syndrome. When acting on the kidneys, it induces severe acute kidney injury. When the cytokines reach the liver (IL-6, IL-1, TNF-α), the production of different types of acute-phase reactant proteins is triggered. All these acute-phase reactant proteins increase the inflammatory pathways of the body. C-reactive protein promotes the inflammation of blood vessels by binding onto endothelial cells and inducing the generation of reactive oxygen species (ROS) and inflammatory chemicals, resulting in atherosclerotic plaque, leading to endothelial cell dysfunction. These inflammatory chemicals increase the risk of thrombosis or the state of hypercoagulation. These are the major reason for the worsening of the co-morbid conditions in COVID-19 patients. So now we have an idea of how these pathways may worsen the clinical condition. Let us now understand how vitamin D possesses the potential to reduce the risk of worsening co-morbidities by decreasing the levels of acute-phase reactant proteins (decreasing thrombotic state), thus decreasing the high mortality rate associated with all these complications from multisystem organ failure (see Figure 16.9).

VITAMIN D DEFICIENCY INDUCED IMMUNE DYSFUNCTION

Low vitamin D leads to decreased synthesis of antimicrobial proteins like β-defensins and cathelicidins. Decreased β-defensins leads to decreased attacks on the viral envelope and consequently

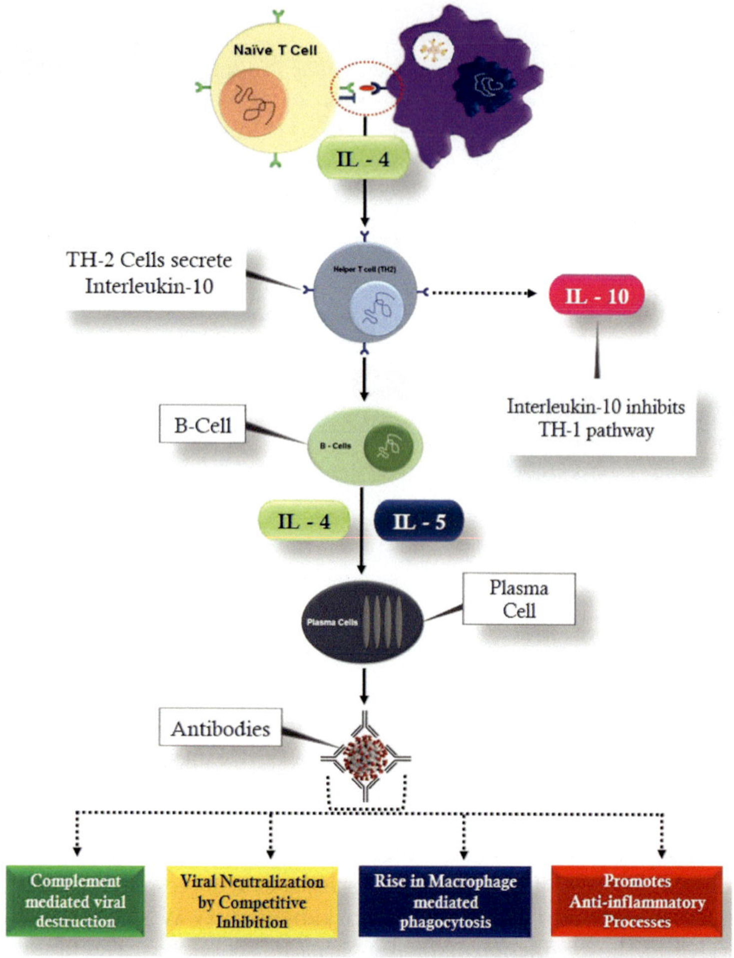

Figure 16.8 Selection of the TH-2 pathway.

the decreased destruction of the virus. Also, decreased cathelicidins leads to decreased macrophages activation, chemotaxis, and movement of the macrophages into the area of pathogen infiltration. The destruction of the virus induced by proteolysis or cleavage of the viral peptides is decreased and thus viral load increases. Decreased vitamin D in the blood not only leads to the decreased phagocytic activity of macrophages (decreased interleukin-4 production) but also leads to the suppression of the TH-2 pathway (decreased B cell activation, decreased plasma cell activation, decreased antibody production, decreased neutralizing of the virus, decreased complement system, activation of virus, and decreased phagocytosis of the virus). Suppression of the TH-2 pathway leads to a decreased production of interleukin-10. Decreases in the interleukin-10 level cause activation of the TH-1 (pro-inflammatory) pathway. If the TH-1 pathway is not suppressed, more inflammatory cytokines (like IFN-γ, IL-6) lead to increased production of acute-phase reactant protein causing multisystem organ failure, and thrombotic and hypercoagulatory states (see Figure 16.10).

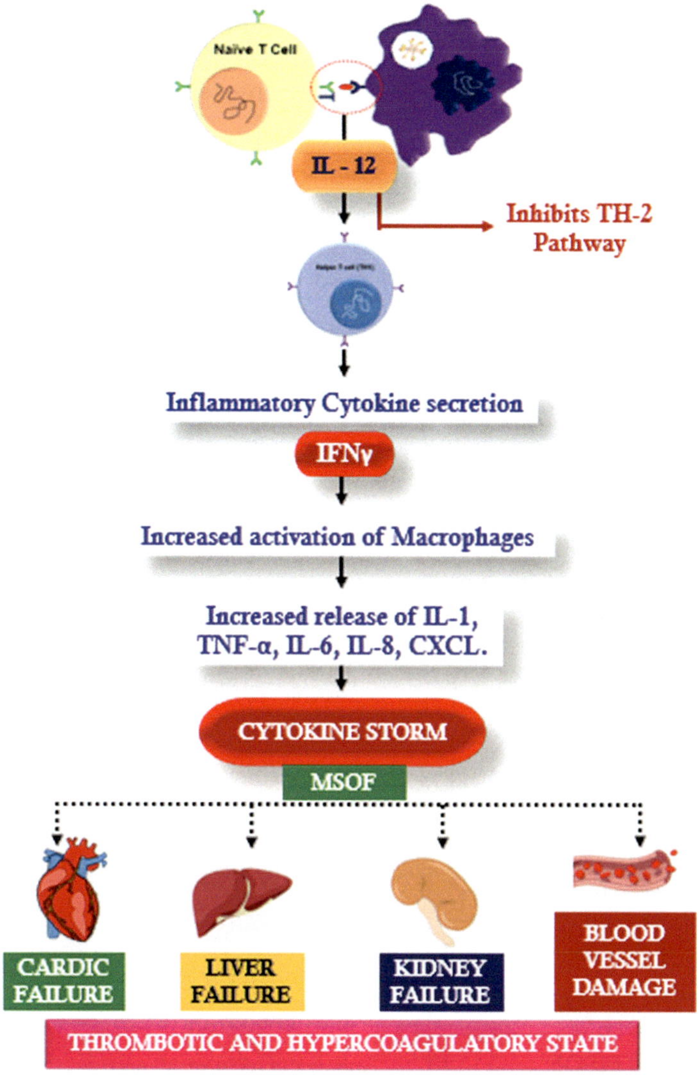

Figure 16.9 Selection of the TH-1 pathway.

IMMUNOTHERAPEUTIC EFFECT OF VITAMIN D

Increased level of vitamin D in the the blood increases the expression of β-defensins and cathelicidins. Increased β-defensins means increased destruction of the virus by proteolysis of the viral envelope. An increased level of cathelicidins leads to increased stimulation of macrophage activity, phagocytosis, and expression of the viral antigens on the MHC-II complex. If there is more vitamin D, the TH-2 (the anti-inflammation) pathway is stimulated and activated. This increases antibody production, an enhanced complement system, and phagocytosis. Also, increased vitamin D leads to an increase in the production of IL-10 (by the TH-2 pathway) which

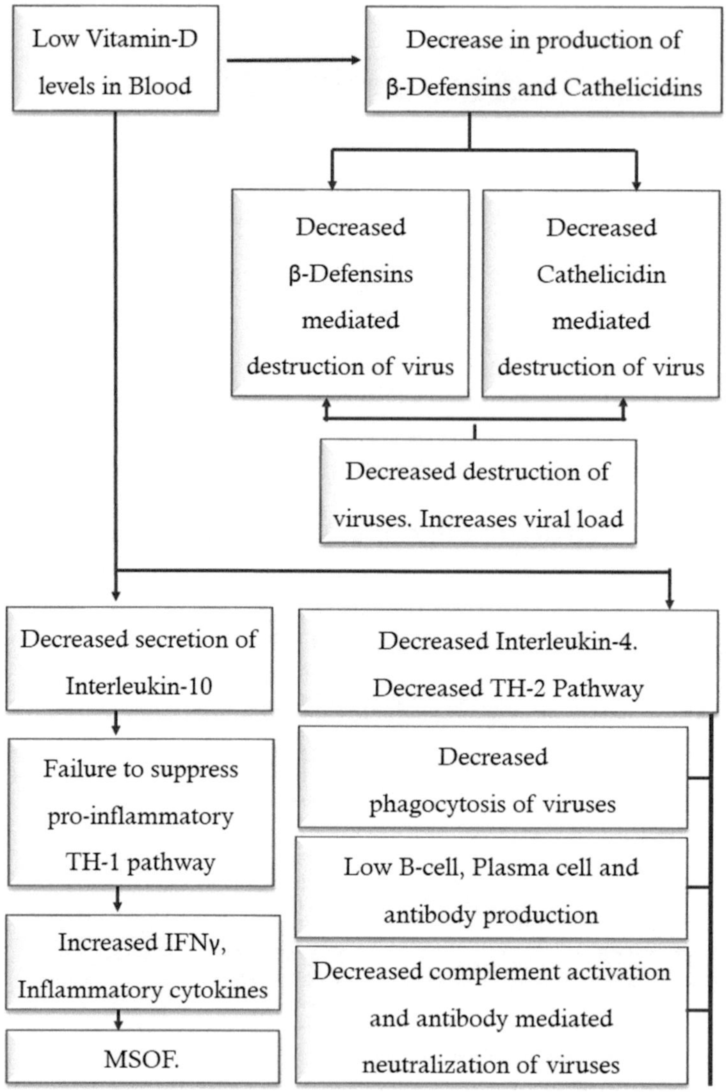

Figure 16.10 Vitamin D deficiency induced immune dysfunction.

inhibits transition to the TH-1 (pro-inflammatory) pathway, thus decreasing the cytokine storm, multisystem organ failure, inflammatory thrombotic states, and worsening of co-morbid states in COVID-19 (see Figure 16.11).

IMMUNOTHERAPEUTIC EFFECT OF VITAMIN D AND ACE-2–ANGIOTENSIN CASCADE

The immunotherapeutic effect of vitamin D on ACE-2–angiotensin cascade is an important aspect to consider. Angiotensinogen (AGT), an α2-globulin synthesized by the liver, is a precursor

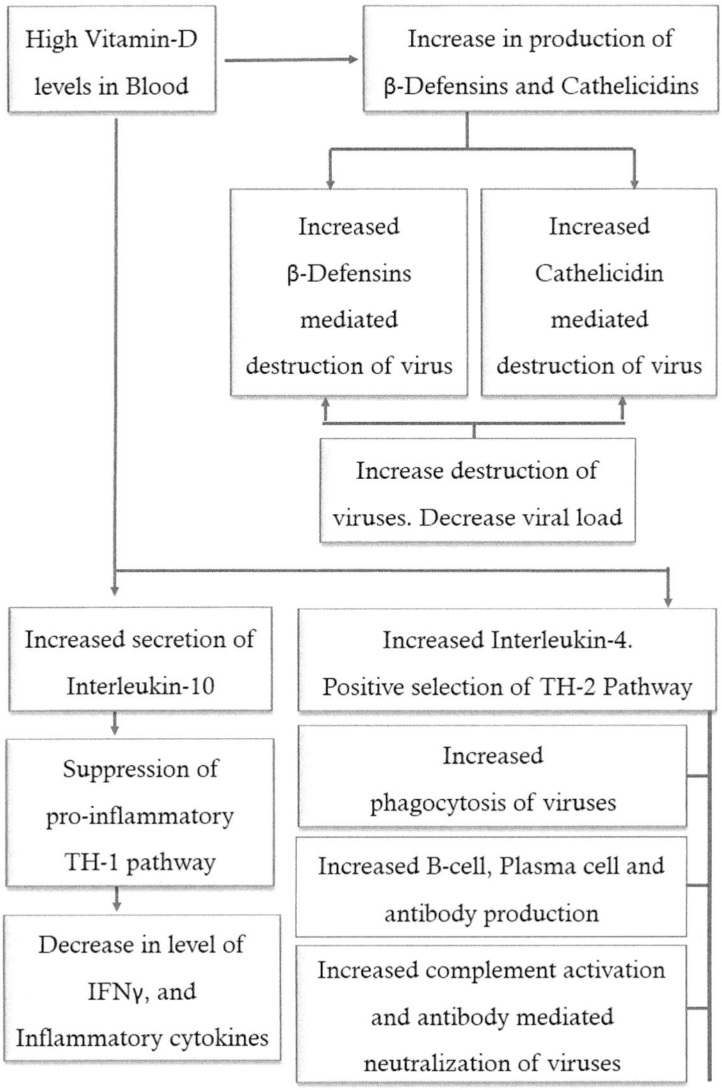

Figure 16.11 Immunotherapeutic effect of Vitamin D.

for all types of angiotensin peptide molecules (like angiotensin type-I) with the help of an enzyme called renin (secreted by the kidneys). So, renin helps stimulate the conversion of angiotensinogen to angiotensin type-I (AT1). Again, another enzyme called angiotensin converting enzyme (ACE), secreted by the kidneys and lungs, converts angiotensin type-I to angiotensin type-II. An increased level of angiotensin type-II is particularly known to increase the chances of lung injury. When the concentration of angiotensin type-II increases in circulation, it binds to the angiotensin receptor and stimulates vasoconstriction and increases in pressure, inflammatory processes, and fibrosis. All these factors contribute to lung injury. Vitamin D is known to inhibit

TABLE 16.1 THE RECOMMENDED DIETARY ALLOWANCE FOR VITAMIN D

Age of Individual	Recommended Dietary Allowance (IU/day)	Upper Level Intake (IU/day)
Infants 0–6 months	~400 (10 mcg)	~1000 (25 mcg)
Infants 6–12 months	~400 (10 mcg)	~1500 (37.5 mcg)
Children 1–3 years old	~600 (15 mcg)	~2500 (62.5 mcg)
Children 4–8 years old	~600 (15 mcg)	~3000 (75 mcg)
Individuals 9–70 years old	~600 (15 mcg)	~4000 (100 mcg)
Individuals above 70 years	~800 (20 mcg)	~4000 (100 mcg)
Pregnant and lactating females 14–50 years old	~600 (15 mcg)	~4000 (100 mcg)
Obese individuals: recommended dietary allowance of vitamin D × 3 = actual dose.		

Note: Values can be expressed in both international units (IU) and micrograms (mcg): 1 mcg of vitamin D is equal to 40 IU.

excessive secretion of renin from the kidneys, thus minimizing the conversion of angiotensinogen to AT1. A decrease in the level of AT1 means decreased production of angiotensin type-II, and consequently, less binding with the angiotensin receptor, less vasoconstriction, inflammation, fibrosis, and lung injury.

Angiotensin type-II (ATII) is associated with another pathway that involves angiotensin converting enzyme-2 (ACE-2) receptors. ACE-2 converts ATII into angiotensin 1-7 (AT1-7). As a part of the normal lifecycle, SARS-CoV-2 binds to ACE-2 receptors, thus decreasing its concentration. An optimum level of Vitamin D is known to stimulate the activity of ACE-2. When the expression and activity of ACE-2 increase, the conversion of ATII into AT1-7 also increases. This conversion leads to increased vasodilatory effects, decreased pressure in cardiopulmonary circuits, decreased inflammation, and fibrosis and lung injury. Vitamin D stabilizes respiratory membranes and capillaries.

SERUM CONCENTRATION OF VITAMIN D

It is very important to understand the causes of vitamin D deficiency because studies have shown that individuals deficient in vitamin D are more susceptible to infectious diseases like COVID-19. Vitamin D deficiency may occur due to common reasons like inadequate consumption as per recommended dietary intake values, decreased exposure to sunlight, obesity, ageing, and colour of skin. The deficiency may also occur due to underlying conditions like progressive chronic liver diseases (PCLD), chronic kidney disease or renal failure (CKD), CHF, hypertension (HTN), coronary artery disease, and diabetes mellitus (DM). All these diseases are co-morbid conditions associated with COVID-19. There are several groups of pharmacological substances such as laxatives, steroids, cholesterol-lowering drugs, seizure control drugs, anti-tuberculosis medications, and weight loss medications (to name a few) that are known to create vitamin D deficiency. Having a clear understanding of the threshold of low vitamin D, which potentially increases the risk of infection, are critical for treatment purposes. It has been observed that small daily doses of vitamin D are much more beneficial as compared with a large one-time dosage. Organizations like the Food and Nutrition Board and the Endocrine Society recommend the reference ranges presented in Table 16.1 as the appropriate dosages of vitamin D depending on age and sex.

The expert committee of the National Academies of Sciences, Engineering, and Medicine (NASEM) decides the dietary reference intake values for vitamin D and other nutritional substances. The dietary reference intake is a general term indicating a set of reference values implemented for the planning and assessment of nutrient intakes by healthy people based on physiological parameters (age, sex, body weight, etc.). The dietary reference intake includes parameters like recommended dietary allowance (RDA), adequate intake (AI), estimated average requirement (EAR), and tolerable upper intake level (UL). According to the Endocrine Society, toxicity caused by an excess amount of vitamin D is extremely rare.

REFERENCES

Baktash, V., Hosack, T., Patel, N., Shah, S., Kandiah, P., van den Abbeele, K., Mandal, A. K. J., & Missouris, C. G. (2020). Vitamin D status and outcomes for hospitalised older patients with COVID-19. *Postgraduate Medical Journal, 97*(1149), 442–447. https://doi.org/10.1136/postgradmedj-2020-138712

Berridge, M. J. (2017). Vitamin D deficiency and diabetes. *Biochemical Journal, 474*(8), 1321–1332. https://doi.org/10.1042/bcj20170042

Biesalski, H. K. (2020). Vitamin D deficiency and co-morbidities in COVID-19 patients: A fatal relationship? *NFS Journal, 20*, 10–21. https://doi.org/10.1016/j.nfs.2020.06.001

Brenner, H., Holleczek, B., & Schöttker, B. (2020). Vitamin D insufficiency and deficiency and mortality from respiratory diseases in a cohort of older adults: Potential for limiting the death toll during and beyond the COVID-19 pandemic? *Nutrients, 12*(8), 2488. https://doi.org/10.3390/nu12082488

Centre for Evidence-Based Medicine. (2020, November 2). *What is the role of T cells in COVID-19 infection? Why immunity is about more than antibodies.* The Centre for Evidence-Based Medicine. Retrieved June 19, 2021, from https://www.cebm.net/covid-19/what-is-the-role-of-t-cells-in-covid-19-infection-why-immunity-is-about-more-than-antibodies/

Cutolo, M., Paolino, S., & Smith, V. (2020). Evidences for a protective role of vitamin D in COVID-19. *RMD Open, 6*(3), e001454. https://doi.org/10.1136/rmdopen-2020-001454

Daneshkhah, A., Agrawal, V., Eshein, A., Subramanian, H., Roy, H. K., & Backman, V. (2020). Evidence for possible association of vitamin D status with cytokine storm and unregulated inflammation in COVID-19 patients. *Aging Clinical and Experimental Research, 32*(10), 2141–2158. https://doi.org/10.1007/s40520-020-01677-y

D'Avolio, A., Avataneo, V., Manca, A., Cusato, J., de Nicolò, A., Lucchini, R., Keller, F., & Cantù, M. (2020). 25-Hydroxyvitamin D concentrations are lower in patients with positive PCR for SARS-CoV-2. *Nutrients, 12*(5), 1359. https://doi.org/10.3390/nu12051359

Entrenas Castillo, M., Entrenas Costa, L. M., Vaquero Barrios, J. M., Alcalá Díaz, J. F., López Miranda, J., Bouillon, R., & Quesada Gomez, J. M. (2020). Effect of calcifediol treatment and best available therapy versus best available therapy on intensive care unit admission and mortality among patients hospitalized for COVID-19: A pilot randomized clinical study. *The Journal of Steroid Biochemistry and Molecular Biology, 203*, 105751. https://doi.org/10.1016/j.jsbmb.2020.105751

Ilie, P. C., Stefanescu, S., & Smith, L. (2020). The role of vitamin D in the prevention of coronavirus disease 2019 infection and mortality. *Aging Clinical and Experimental Research, 32*(7), 1195–1198. https://doi.org/10.1007/s40520-020-01570-8

Jain, A., Chaurasia, R., Sengar, N. S., Singh, M., Mahor, S., & Narain, S. (2020). Analysis of vitamin D level among asymptomatic and critically ill COVID-19 patients and its correlation with inflammatory markers. *Scientific Reports, 10*(1). https://doi.org/10.1038/s41598-020-77093-z

Judd, S. E., & Tangpricha, V. (2009). Vitamin D deficiency and risk for cardiovascular disease. *The American Journal of the Medical Sciences, 338*(1), 40–44. https://doi.org/10.1097/maj.0b013e3181aaee91

Karahan, S., & Katkat, F. (2020). Impact of serum 25(OH) vitamin D level on mortality in patients with COVID-19 in Turkey. *The Journal of Nutrition, Health & Aging, 25*(2), 189–196. https://doi.org/10.1007/s12603-020-1479-0

Kheiri, B., Abdalla, A., Osman, M., Ahmed, S., Hassan, M., & Bachuwa, G. (2018). Vitamin D deficiency and risk of cardiovascular diseases: A narrative review. *Clinical Hypertension, 24*(1). https://doi.org/10.1186/s40885-018-0094-4

Konijeti, G. G., Arora, P., Boylan, M. R., Song, Y., Huang, S., Harrell, F., Newton-Cheh, C., O'Neill, D., Korzenik, J., Wang, T. J., & Chan, A. T. (2016). Vitamin D supplementation modulates T cell-mediated immunity in humans: Results from a randomized control trial. *The Journal of Clinical Endocrinology & Metabolism, 101*(2), 533–538. https://doi.org/10.1210/jc.2015-3599

Martineau, A. R., & Forouhi, N. G. (2020). Vitamin D for COVID-19: A case to answer? *The Lancet Diabetes & Endocrinology, 8*(9), 735–736. https://doi.org/10.1016/s2213-8587(20)30268-0

Martineau, A. R., Jolliffe, D. A., Hooper, R. L., Greenberg, L., Aloia, J. F., Bergman, P., Dubnov-Raz, G., Esposito, S., Ganmaa, D., Ginde, A. A., Goodall, E. C., Grant, C. C., Griffiths, C. J., Janssens, W., Laaksi, I., Manaseki-Holland, S., Mauger, D., Murdoch, D. R., Neale, R., . . . Camargo, C. A. (2017). Vitamin D supplementation to prevent acute respiratory tract infections: Systematic review and meta-analysis of individual participant data. *BMJ*, i6583. https://doi.org/10.1136/bmj.i6583

Merzon, E., Tworowski, D., Gorohovski, A., Vinker, S., Golan Cohen, A., Green, I., & Frenkel-Morgenstern, M. (2020). Low plasma 25(OH) vitamin D level is associated with increased risk of COVID-19 Infection: An Israeli population-based study. *The FEBS Journal, 287*(17), 3693–3702. https://doi.org/10.1111/febs.15495

Office of Dietary Supplements: Vitamin D. (n.d.). National Institutes of Health, Office of Dietary Supplements. Retrieved June 19, 2021, from https://ods.od.nih.gov/factsheets/VitaminD-HealthProfessional/

Radujkovic, A., Hippchen, T., Tiwari-Heckler, S., Dreher, S., Boxberger, M., & Merle, U. (2020). Vitamin D Deficiency and Outcome of COVID-19 Patients. *Nutrients, 12*(9), 2757. https://doi.org/10.3390/nu12092757

Rak, K., & Bronkowska, M. (2018). Immunomodulatory effect of vitamin D and its potential role in the prevention and treatment of type 1 diabetes mellitus: A narrative review. *Molecules, 24*(1), 53. https://doi.org/10.3390/molecules24010053

Turrubiates Hernández, F., SánchezZuno, G., GonzálezEstevez, G., HernándezBello, J., MacedoOjeda, G., & MuñozValle, J. (2021). Potential immunomodulatory effects of vitamin D in the prevention of severe coronavirus disease 2019: An ally for Latin America (Review). *International Journal of Molecular Medicine, 47*(4). https://doi.org/10.3892/ijmm.2021.4865

Weir, E. K., Thenappan, T., Bhargava, M., & Chen, Y. (2020). Does vitamin D deficiency increase the severity of COVID-19? *Clinical Medicine, 20*(4), e107–e108. https://doi.org/10.7861/clinmed.2020-0301

Williamson, E. J., Walker, A. J., Bhaskaran, K., Bacon, S., Bates, C., Morton, C. E., Curtis, H. J., Mehrkar, A., Evans, D., Inglesby, P., Cockburn, J., McDonald, H. I., MacKenna, B., Tomlinson, L., Douglas, I. J., Rentsch, C. T., Mathur, R., Wong, A. Y. S., Grieve, R., . . . Goldacre, B. (2020). Factors associated with COVID-19-related death using OpenSAFELY. *Nature, 584*(7821), 430–436. https://doi.org/10.1038/s41586-020-2521-4

Chapter 17

Role of Biochemic Cell Salts in Prophylaxis and Complementary Nutraceutical Therapy of Influenza-Like Illnesses or Respiratory Tract Complications (COVID-19)

Srijan Goswami*, Ushmita Gupta Bakshi, and Chiranjeeb Dey

CONTENTS

INTRODUCTION

The biochemic system of medicine is a form of treatment that uses simple inorganic cellular minerals as a therapeutic component for the prevention, treatment, and management of several acute and chronic health conditions. The biochemic system is based on the principles of biochemistry and nutritional sciences. This system of treatment with inorganic minerals is approved by the World Health Organization (WHO) as well as recognized by several medical councils worldwide. Like any other nutritional substance, inorganic minerals (both in free form and in complex form) perform crucial functions in maintaining life processes and the state of health. Thus, in this system, the inorganic mineral salts are implemented for the prevention, treatment, and management of a wide range of acute and chronic disease conditions. Among the wide range of inorganic minerals that are critical for cellular functioning, the 12 most abundant salts are used as primary medicines in this system. There are no adverse reactions to these medicines because the 12 inorganic salts are actually the natural chemical components that make up the body and are available in nature. Abnormalities in cellular functioning can be restored by administering appropriate combinations of inorganic minerals in adequate concentrations, potency, and duration. Since the therapeutic substances used in this system are nutritional substances that are available in nature, this makes biochemic medicines suitable for children to old-aged persons (Goswami, 2019; Carey, 1924; Nasri et al., 2014; Mandala', 2010).

DOI: 10.1201/9781003178514-21

Dr. Wilhelm Heinrich Schuessler in the year 1973 introduced the biochemic system of medicine. Dr. Schuessler found that the perfect balance of nutritional substances is very much essential for the normal regulation and coordination of all the biochemical reactions occurring inside the human body. If under any circumstance the balance between nutritional substances is disturbed, homeostasis is disrupted, and as a result, the disease takes over. Correcting the nutritional imbalance will restore cellular homeostasis and help maintain the state of health. Biochemic medicine is grouped as a complementary system of treatment, meaning that it can be used along with conventional as well as alternative systems of medicine as a supportive therapy or it can be used as a standalone treatment in minor illnesses. Also, the biochemic system can be classified as a nutraceutical therapy because the term "nutraceutical" can be generalized as the use and implementation of nutritional substances found in nature, which are generally acquired through food, as a pharmaceutical substance. Substances that are food or a part of food not only have health benefits but can also prevent and heal disease conditions are termed nutraceuticals. This mode of treatment connects basic nutritional sciences with core medical practices. In short, they have extra-medicinal value along with their normal nutritional values (Goswami, 2019; Carey, 1924; Nasri et al., 2014; Mandala', 2010). Thus, the biochemic system can be classified as a complementary nutraceutical therapy that can be implemented for maintaining proper health, preventing susceptibility to a disease, and curing ailments by filling up the deficiency of the required nutrient by administering it in the perfect size, amount, and duration. The vast science of the biochemic system is presented briefly for ease of understanding. This chapter provides only the fundamental idea about the biochemic system of medicine specifically in relation to the prevention, treatment, and management of influenza-like illnesses (ILI) and respiratory tract complications.

THE BIOCHEMIC SYSTEM OF MEDICINE: A BRIEF OVERVIEW OF FUNDAMENTAL PRINCIPLES

First and foremost, it is important to understand that the biochemic system of medicine is not homoeopathy. The fundamental principle of the biochemic system of medicine is "filling up the deficiency" while the fundamental principle of homoeopathy is "Similia Similibus Curentur" (see Chapter 14 for basic ideas about homoeopathy). So, considering the biochemic system and homoeopathy as the same is scientifically incorrect. The biochemic system of medicine should be included as a specialized aspect of existing nutritional and dietary sciences and strictly not as homoeopathy. The only aspect of the biochemic system of medicine that has any similarity with homoeopathy is the technique of trituration. The Father of Medicine, Great Hippocrates, mentioned that "Let food be thy medicine", following the same ideology, a German physician, Dr. Wilhelm Heinrich Schuessler introduced the biochemic system of medicine in 1873 and laid the foundation of the effectiveness of nutritional therapy or using nutritional substances as medicine (nutraceuticals) for the treatment of deranged physical conditions. The evidence-based science of biochemistry is the basis for the biochemic system of treatment. The basic modus operandi of inorganic minerals can be realized by understanding the relationship between blood and the human body. Blood regulates the homeostasis of the body by maintaining an equilibrium between parameters such as fluid balance, temperature balance, glucose balance, amino acid balance, fatty acid balance, vitamin and mineral balance, enzyme balance, pH balance, electrolyte balance, and oxygen–carbon dioxide balance. The continuous flow of blood in the blood vessels helps to maintain a constant environment for the cells, thus maintaining the state of health. The relationship between circulating blood and the human body is the same as that of a plant and soil. Blood contains organic and inorganic substances. Although inorganic minerals are present in small amounts, they are crucial components because they act as workers and use water and organic substances for building and maintaining the normal structure and function of cells. The evidence-based science of biochemistry has revealed that biochemical pathways occurring inside cells are regulated by inorganic minerals. If, at any given point of time, the inorganic minerals become deficient in the body, the biochemical pathways falter, thus leading to disturbed homeostasis (the state of disease). Every disease that affects one's body is due to the deficiency of one or more of these inorganic minerals in the blood. In this system, the deficiency of inorganic minerals in the patient's body (that have disturbed homeostasis) is identified, and the homeostasis is restored by administering the required inorganic minerals in the proper combination, amount, and duration. The nutritional substances present in the blood are transported to all the cells of the body through circulation, thus helping them perform their physiological functions. Biochemic medicines (which come in tablet form) are taken orally, chewed, and swallowed. Like any other food substance, the therapeutic inorganic minerals present in the tablet are transported to blood circulation by absorption through the intestinal wall. The inorganic minerals present in blood circulation are assimilated into the surrounding tissue through capillary walls guided by the signaling mechanism of the brain and nervous system. The organic and inorganic nutritional substances must be present in sufficient quantity and form in order for the maintenance of cellular and overall homeostasis. The inorganic minerals administered in the biochemic system stimulate the natural, self-healing powers and enables the human system to address the disease state in a natural manner. Observation of the patient after administration of the appropriate remedy in proper potency and dose is important because, based on these observations, the subsequent action in the further treatment of the case under consideration will be performed (Goswami, 2019; Carey, 1924; Nasri et al., 2014; Mandala', 2010).

THE 12 FUNDAMENTAL INORGANIC CELL SALTS

Knowledge of the properties and mode of action is very much important when the symptom of any given case is considered. The following section contains a brief idea about the importance of the 12 tissue salts. For detailed knowledge about cell salts, it is advised to consult *Biochemic Materia Medica* and *Biochemic Practice of Medicine*:

- **Calcarea Flouricum:** Calc Flour is known to provide the characteristics of elasticity to cells or tissues by combining with organic substances like albumin. This salt is a constituent of elastic tissues and is present in blood vessel walls, muscular tissues, connective tissues, bones, and teeth. Deficiency of this salt results in loss of elasticity and a decrease in the contractile capability of elastic tissues. Any disease state that can be traced to an underlying loss of elasticity, this salt can be thought of. Calc Flour is effective in conditions similar to ILI or respiratory tract complications like conjunctivitis, cough and cold, coryza, tickling and burning sensation near the larynx, dryness and hoarseness of voice, asthmatic tendency with shortness of breath, nausea and vomiting, gastrointestinal complications (due to loss of elasticity), severe weakness, fever and body aches, and eczematous conditions of the skin (Goswami, 2019; Carey, 1924; Nasri et al., 2014; Mandala', 2010).

- **Calcarea Phosphoricum:** Calc Phos is critical for the proper growth and nutrition of the body and is present in blood plasma, saliva, gastric juices, connective tissues, and soft and growing tissues. This salt not only promotes normal cellular growth and regeneration and restoration but also plays an important role in blood coagulation. In the absence of Calc Phos, the body's normal regenerative and restorative capability becomes compromised. It acts as an important intercurrent remedy in relation to acute diseases either directly or preparing the way for other remedies by stimulating the system to action. Calc Phos is effective in conditions similar to ILI or respiratory tract complications like headache, excessive dryness and inflammation of the eyes, congestive state of the nasopharynx, numbness of tongue, nausea and vomiting, suffocative cough with soreness at the clavicular and sternal region, severe weakness with anxiety and palpitation, sharp pains around the heart during inspiration, and neuralgias. It helps with digestion and the assimilation of nutrients. The restorative power of Calc Phos is known to speed up recovery and replenish the body's reserves of strength (Goswami, 2019; Carey, 1924; Nasri et al., 2014; Mandala', 2010).
- **Calcarea Sulphuricum:** Calc Sulph acts as a blood purifier and restorer by removing waste products from circulation and maintaining cleansing influence throughout the system. The non-functional organic matter is thrown off by the action of Calc Sulph, thus protecting the tissues from being decayed. This inorganic salt is indicated in conditions arising from impurities in the bloodstream and has a complementary relationship with Kalium Muraticum. Calc Sulph is effective in conditions similar to ILI or respiratory tract complications like headache with nausea and vertigo, inflammation of the eyes, coryza and cold, diarrhea, cough with bronchitis-like conditions associated with fever, neuralgia, severe weakness, and skin complications (Goswami, 2019; Carey, 1924; Nasri et al., 2014; Mandala', 2010).
- **Ferrum Phosphoricum:** Ferrum Phos is a biochemic remedy for the first stage of inflammation. Iron and its salts are an essential component of hemoglobin and has the property of attracting oxygen and thus helping with carrying oxygen from the lungs to the blood vessels. Ferrum Phos helps in conditions with pain, heat, swelling and redness, quickened pulse, and increased circulation, all febrile and inflammatory conditions at their onset. Ferrum Phos is effective in conditions similar to ILI or respiratory tract complications like headache with nausea and vomiting, inflammation of the eyes with a burning sensation and retinal congestion, first stage of all cold and catarrh, diarrhea associated with inflammatory conditions, respiratory complications like rhinitis, laryngitis, tracheitis bronchitis, pneumonia, shortness of breath, malaise, weariness, severe weakness, and hemorrhage from any part of the body. This remedy is highly effective in all catarrhal and inflammatory fevers during the chilly or initiatory stage, rigor, heat, quickened pulse, and myalgia (Goswami, 2019; Carey, 1924; Nasri et al., 2014; Mandala', 2010).
- **Kalium Muraticum:** Kali Mur is present in blood cells, muscle tissues, nerves, and brain cells, and is a remedy indicated for the second stage of inflammation. This salt is complementary to the action of Calc Sulph as both are involved in the cleansing and restoration of blood. Kali Mur is effective in conditions similar to ILI or respiratory tract complications like headache with nausea and vomiting, inflammatory conditions of the eyes, catarrh and coryza, bronchitis, pneumonia with a rattling sound in the chest, thromboembolism, fever, and skin infections (Goswami, 2019; Carey, 1924; Nasri et al., 2014; Mandala', 2010).

- **Kalium Phosphoricum:** Kali Phos is present in all body fluids and tissues, mainly the brain, nerves, muscle tissues, and blood cells. This salt expresses marked action on vasomotor nerves, sensory nerves, motor nerves, and sympathetic nerves. Deficiency of this salt disrupts the nerve signaling processes, thus resulting in neurodegenerative conditions. Kali Phos is effective in conditions similar to ILI or respiratory tract complications like headache with vertigo, loss of sensory capabilities (taste or smell), neuralgia, myalgia, nausea and vomiting, painless diarrhea with severe fatigue, acute failure of pulmonary functions, pulmonary edema, progressive shortness of breath, sluggish circulation, confusion, loss of speech, and mobility (Goswami, 2019; Carey, 1924; Nasri et al., 2014; Mandala', 2010).
- **Kalium Sulphuricum:** Kali Sulph is essential for the third stage of inflammation. This salt is responsible for cellular respiration. It also acts as a lubricant and aids in the smooth functioning of all organs, thus designated as an anti-friction salt. Kali Sulph is effective in conditions similar to ILI or respiratory tract complications like headache with vertigo and anxiety, inflammation of the eye, nasopharyngeal congestion and irritation, nausea and vomiting with gastric derangements, diarrhea with pain, great rattling in the chest with mucus and cough, bronchitis, pneumonia, suffocative feeling with a quick throbbing pulse, shifting neuralgic pain, increasing fever, and skin complications (Goswami, 2019; Carey, 1924; Nasri et al., 2014; Mandala', 2010).
- **Magnesia Phosphoricum:** Mag Phos is a constituent of muscle tissues, nerves, bones and teeth, brain, spine, and blood corpuscles. This salt is complementary to the action of Kali Phos in its effect on the nervous system, and when used together, they provide better results. Mag Phos possess anti-spasmodic properties, and thus, is used as an anti-pain remedy. Mag Phos is effective in conditions similar to ILI or respiratory tract complications like neuralgic headache, orbital and supraorbital neuralgia, loss of sense of smell, diarrhea with nausea and vomiting, spasmodic closure of the windpipe, whooping cough with pain in the chest and shortness of breath, progressive weakness of respiratory muscles, severe fatigue, intermittent fever with body aches and pain and rashes on the skin (Goswami, 2019; Carey, 1924; Nasri et al., 2014; Mandala', 2010).
- **Natrum Muraticum:** Natrum Mur is a constituent of every solid and liquid part of the body. For the proper functioning of cells, a fine balance between Natrum and Kalium is very important. Any marked disturbance in their balance results in rapid cellular dysfunction. Even if the cellular structure does not contain Natrum or Kalium, their presence in the fluid surrounding the cells (in proper ratio) results in protective effects on the cell membrane and helps regulate cellular metabolism. This salt helps in maintaining osmotic tension. It has marked action over blood, the lymphatic system, mucus linings, the liver, and the spleen. The electrolyte balance and flow of body fluids are regulated by Natrum Mur because of its strong affinity for water. In absence of this tissue salt, normal cell division, growth, repair, and regenerative process are halted. Natrum Mur is effective in conditions similar to ILI or respiratory tract complications like congestive types of headache, inflammatory condition of the eyes, nasopharyngeal catarrh, congestion with loss of taste and smell, and diarrhea alternating with constipation. Acute inflammation of the windpipe, with watery phlegm, rattling sound in the chest with shortness of breath, inflammatory conditions of the lungs, pain at the apex of the heart worsens with deep inspiration, marked weakness and nervous exhaustion, prominent fever, and rashes on skin (Goswami, 2019; Carey, 1924; Nasri et al., 2014; Mandala', 2010).

- **Natrum Phosphoricum:** Natrum Phos is found in blood, muscle tissue, brain, nerves, and intercellular fluids. This salt helps in the formation of carbonic acid and water. It absorbs carbonic acid and carries it to the lungs where the oxygen is exchanged with carbonic acid. The oxygen is later taken up by the ferrum contained in blood corpuscles. It also acts as an acid neutralizer, and thus, effective in a wide range of diseases arising from acidic conditions of circulating blood. Natrum Phos is effective in conditions similar to ILI or respiratory tract complications like severe headache with vertigo, irritation in the eyes, inflammatory irritation of the nasopharynx, nausea with vomiting, intercurrent catarrhal conditions, soreness of intercostal muscles and the lower portion of the sternum, shortness of breath, and fever with vomiting (Goswami, 2019; Carey, 1924; Nasri et al., 2014; Mandala', 2010).
- **Natrum Sulphuricum:** Found only in intercellular fluids, Natrum Sulph regulates the fluid balance by eliminating excess water. The disturbance of the molecular motion of this salt prevents the elimination of such water from the tissues as is produced by the oxidation of organic substances. As a result of the normal biochemical process, the removal of unwanted toxic metabolic products is constantly maintained by Natrum Sulph. In the absence of this salt, toxic metabolic products are accumulated in the bloodstream leading to a state of self-poisoning. It is a chief remedy in the treatment of influenza-like conditions. Natrum Sulph is effective in conditions similar to ILI or respiratory tract complications like violent pulsating headaches with vertigo and dizziness, conjunctivitis, burning sensations and irritation of the nasopharynx, soreness of the liver, rattling of mucus and soreness in the chest, shortness of breath, anxiety and angina, and fever with extreme prostration (Goswami, 2019; Carey, 1924; Nasri et al., 2014; Mandala', 2010).
- **Silicea:** Silicea is considered a cleanser and eliminator and is found in a trace amount. It acts upon organic substances of the body involving bones, joints, glands, skin, mucus surface, spinal cord, brain, and nerves. It is known to reabsorb a bloody or serous albuminous exudate, existing within the tissues by means of lymphatics. The salt helps in eliminating non-functional organic matter from the system by promoting suppurations and thus triggering healing processes. Silicea is effective in conditions similar to ILI or respiratory tract complications like inflammatory conditions of the eyes, coryza and nasal catarrh, pneumonia, suffocative feeling with great debility, myalgia, and skin irritation (Goswami, 2019; Carey, 1924; Nasri et al., 2014; Mandala', 2010) (Table 17.1).

SELECTIVE BIOCHEMIC CELL SALTS FOR INFLUENZA-LIKE ILLNESSES AND RESPIRATORY TRACT COMPLICATIONS

Symptomatic relief means cure is a common misconception. A 100% cure is never possible with any form of treatment be it conventional, alternative, or complementary medicines, but rapid healing and restoration can be achieved with any of the forms. The drugs and treatment procedures under a conventional system provide symptomatic relief. It is to be understood that symptoms are not diseases, instead, they are the body's response to certain stress factors (see Chapter 3). Fever, dry cough, and tiredness are the most common symptoms associated with COVID-19. The less common symptoms may include loss of smell or taste, nasal congestion, diarrhea, sore throat, conjunctivitis, body ache, and skin rashes.

TABLE 17.1 KEYNOTE FEATURES OF 12 INORGANIC (BIOCHEMIC) CELL SALTS

S. No	Biochemic Cell Salt	Keynote Function
1.	Calcarea Flouricum	Provides elasticity to tissues and is an important constituent of bones and teeth.
2.	Calcarea Phosphoricum	Concerned with nutrition and crucial for blood coagulation.
3.	Calcarea Sulphuricum	Blood Purifier, eliminator, and restorer.
4.	Ferrum Phosphoricum	It is considered a biochemic first aid. Anti-inflammatory. Important for external respiration.
5.	Kalium Muraticum	It is also a blood purifier and restorer. Anti-inflammatory.
6.	Kalium Phosphoricum	It is a constituent of nerves and the nervous system.
7.	Kalium Sulphuricum	Considered as an anti-friction salt and oxygen carrier. Important for internal respiration.
8.	Magnesia Phosphoricum	It is known as an anti-spasmodic remedy. Painkiller.
9.	Natrum Muraticum	Maintains electrolyte balance.
10.	Natrum Phosphoricum	It is an acid neutralizer.
11.	Natrum Sulphuricum	Regulates the density of the intercellular fluids by eliminating excess water.
12.	Silicea	This salt is categorized as a cleanser and eliminator.

Persistent heaviness and pain in the chest, shortness of breath, loss of appetite, and confusion. Irritability, impaired consciousness, depression-associated disorders, sleep disorders, stroke, brain inflammation, delirium, and nerve damage have also been reported as the less common symptoms associated with COVID-19 (WHO, 2020a, b; CDC, 2020). ILIs are non-specific respiratory illnesses (synonym: acute respiratory illness [ARI]) that have a clinical presentation like classical influenza. The major signs and symptoms include fever, cough and sore throat, runny or stuffy nose, muscle or body aches, fatigue (tiredness), loss of taste, loss of appetite, diarrhea or vomiting, and fast breathing with shortness of breath (in moderate to severe cases). If observed carefully, we will find that the signs and symptoms of COVID-19 and ILIs are the same, thus COVID-19 may be categorized as a type of ILI. Biochemic medicine shows a promising effect in preventing and treating ILIs or respiratory infections in the initial stages. Biochemic cell salts can be administered individually or in combination form. In general, combination forms are most common as diseases are always linked to a deficiency of multiple nutritional substances. The combination of biochemic cell salts based on signs and symptoms is presented in Table 17.2.

The FDA has approved the use of several experimental drugs like hydroxychloroquine, remdesivir, favipiravir, and lopinavir-ritonavir (all of which eventually failed to show any beneficial effect on COVID-19 patients) under emergency use authorization (EUA) (WHO, 2020c). EUA was given to these unproven drugs based on their ability to deal with diseases similar to ILIs, for example, malaria, HIV infection, Ebola, influenza, severe acute respiratory infections, and so on. Based on the same ideology, biochemic medicines may also be implemented according to their ability to deal with similar ILIs. Table 17.3 provides biocombinations used for treating various common influenza-like diseases.

TABLE 17.2 POSSIBLE COMBINATIONS OF INORGANIC (BIOCHEMIC) CELL SALTS

S. No	Signs and Symptoms	Indicated Biochemic Cell Salts
1.	Coryza – acute inflammation of the mucous membrane of the nose, with discharge of mucus.	1. Ferrum Phosphoricum 2. Kalium Muraticum 3. Natrum Muraticum 4. Calcarea Phosphoricum 5. Kalium Sulphuricum 6. Calcarea Flouricum 7. Kalium Phosphoricum 8. Natrum Sulphuricum
2.	Cough – expel air from the lungs with a sudden sharp sound.	1. Magnesia Phosphoricum 2. Natrum Muraticum 3. Natrum Sulphuricum
3.	Sore throat – pain or irritation in the throat that can occur with or without swallowing.	1. Ferrum Phosphoricum 2. Natrum Muraticum 3. Kalium Muraticum
4.	Bronchitis – inflammation of the lining of bronchial tubes, which carry air to and from the lungs.	1. Natrum Muraticum 2. Calcarea Sulphurica 3. Ferrum Phosphoricum 4. Kalium Muraticum 5. Silicea
5.	Pneumonia – an infection that inflames air sacs in one or both lungs, which may fill with fluid.	1. Ferrum Phosphoricum 2. Kalium Muraticum 3. Natrum Muraticum 4. Kalium Sulphuricum 5. Calcarea Sulphuricum
6.	Asthma – a condition in which your airways narrow and swell and may produce extra mucus. This can make breathing difficult and trigger coughing, a whistling sound (wheezing) when you breathe out, and shortness of breath.	1. Kalium Phosphoricum 2. Kalium Muraticum 3. Natrum Muraticum 4. Kalium Sulphuricum 5. Calcarea Phosphoricum 6. Natrum Sulphuricum
7.	Pulmonary edema – a condition caused by excess fluid in the lungs.	1. Ferrum Phosphoricum 2. Kalium Phosphoricum 3. Kalium Muraticum 4. Natrum Muraticum 5. Calcarea Flouricum
8.	Headache – a continuous pain in the head.	1. Ferrum Phosphoricum 2. Kalium Muraticum 3. Kalium Phosphoricum 4. Natrum Muraticum
9.	Aches and pain – pain in a muscle or group of muscles.	1. Magnesia Phosphoricum 2. Calcarea Phosphoricum 3. Kalium Phosphoricum

(*Continued*)

TABLE 17.2 (CONTINUED) POSSIBLE COMBINATIONS OF INORGANIC (BIOCHEMIC) CELL SALTS

S. No	Signs and Symptoms	Indicated Biochemic Cell Salts
10.	Fatigue – an overall feeling of tiredness or lack of energy.	1. Calcarea Phosphoricum 2. Ferrum Phosphoricum 3. Kalium Phosphoricum 4. Magnesia Phosphoricum 5. Natrum Muraticum
11.	Dysgeusia – loss of taste.	1. Calcarea Phosphoricum 2. Kalium Muraticum 3. Natrum Muraticum 4. Natrum Sulphuricum
12.	Anosmia – loss of smell.	1. Calcarea Phosphoricum 2. Kalium Phosphoricum 3. Calcarea Sulphuricum 4. Natrum Muraticum
13.	Diarrhea – loose, watery stools that occur more frequently than usual.	1. Calcarea Phosphoricum 2. Kalium Phosphoricum 3. Natrum Sulphuricum 4. Kalium Muraticum 5. Natrum Phosphoricum
14.	Skin complication.	1. Calcarea Flouricum 2. Calcarea Sulphuricum 3. Kalium Sulphuricum 4. Natrum Muraticum 5. Natrum Sulphuricum
15.	Eye irritation.	1. Ferrum Phosphoricum 2. Kalium Muraticum
16.	Fever.	1. Ferrum Phosphoricum 2. Kalium Muraticum 3. Kalium Sulphuricum 4. Natrum Muraticum 5. Natrum Sulphuricum
17.	Thrombosis – the formation of a blood clot, known as a thrombus, within a blood vessel.	1. Magnesia Phosphoricum 2. Ferrum Phosphoricum 3. Calcarea Flouricum

Note: Based on the signs and symptoms associated with influenza-like illnesses (ILI) and respiratory tract complications (COVID-19).

CHALLENGES AND FUTURE RESEARCH POSSIBILITIES

The major challenge with the biochemic system of medicine is the lack of trained professionals in this domain who can take on the education, research, and treatment further. Those who exist possess faulty understanding based on homoeopathic perspectives. Proper education, research, development, and documentation are required in an evidence-based manner from the

TABLE 17.3 POSSIBLE COMBINATIONS OF INORGANIC (BIOCHEMIC) CELL SALTS

S. No	Disease Name	Indicated Biochemic Cell Salts
1.	Influenza	1. Ferrum Phosphoricum 2. Kalium Sulphuricum 3. Kalium Muraticum 4. Natrum Sulphuricum 5. Kalium Phosphoricum 6. Magnesia Phosphoricum
2.	Chickenpox	1. Ferrum Phosphoricum 2. Kalium Muraticum 3. Natrum Muraticum 4. Calcarea Sulphuricum 5. Kalium Sulphuricum
3.	Malaria	1. Natrum Sulphuricum 2. Ferrum Phosphoricum 3. Kalium Muraticum 4. Kalium Sulphuricum 5. Natrum Muraticum
4.	Dengue	1. Ferrum Phosphoricum 2. Natrum Sulphuricum 3. Kalium Phosphoricum 4. Kalium Sulphuricum 5. Kalium Muraticum
5.	Measles	1. Ferrum Phosphoricum 2. Kalium Muraticum 3. Kalium Sulphuricum 4. Natrum Muraticum

Note: Cell salts used for treating various diseases have some degree of similarity with COVID-19, based on treatment data available on similar disease conditions.

perspective of nutraceutical and functional food sciences. This system holds the potential to be established as an advanced domain of complementary immunonutrition therapy. If unapproved experimental drugs like hydroxychloroquine, remdesivir, favipiravir, and lopinavir-ritonavir, having previously recorded incidents of adverse drug reactions and iatrogenic disorders, can receive FDA-EUA, then the alternatives like complementary and alternative systems of medicine should receive equal rights under EUA because the risk of iatrogenic effects are negligible, especially in situations where conventional medicines are failing one after the other. The mainstream research community needs to come forward and take on evidence-based research initiatives on this promising mode of complementary treatment, that is, the biochemic system of medicine.

REFERENCES

Carey, G. W. (1924). *The biochemic system of medicine: Comprising the theory, pathological action, therapeutical application, materia medica, and repertory of Schuessler's twelve tissue remedies.* (22nd ed.). St. Louis: Luyties Pharmacal.

CDC. (2020, March 28). *COVID data tracker.* Centers for Disease Control and Prevention. Retrieved June 12, 2021, from https://covid.cdc.gov/covid-data-tracker/#global-variant-report-map

Goswami, S. (2019). Biochemic system of medicine: Oldest form of nutraceutical therapy. In *Nutraceutical and functional foods in disease prevention* (1st ed., pp. 403–431). IGI Global. https://doi.org/10.4018/978-1-5225-3267-5.ch014

Mandala' (2010, December). *Nutraceuticals: What they are and how they work.* European Society of Cardiology. Retrieved November 27, 2021, from https://www.escardio.org/Journals/E-Journal-of-Cardiology-Practice/Volume-9/Nutraceuticals-what-they-are-and-how-they-work

Nasri, H., Baradaran, A., Shirzad, H., & Rafieian-Kopaei, M. (2014). New concepts in nutraceuticals as alternative for pharmaceuticals. *International Journal of Preventive Medicine, 5*(12), 1487–1499.

World Health Organization. (2020a, January 30). *Pneumonia of unknown cause: China.* Retrieved May 27, 2021, from https://www.who.int/csr/don/05-january-2020-pneumonia-of-unkown-cause-china/en/

World Health Organization. (2020b, March 12). *What is a pandemic?* Retrieved May 27, 2021, from https://www.who.int/csr/disease/swineflu/frequently_asked_questions/pandemic/en/

World Health Organization. (2020c, July 4). *WHO discontinues hydroxychloroquine and lopinavir/ritonavir treatment arms for COVID-19.* World Health Organization. Retrieved November 24, 2021, from https://www.who.int/news/item/04-07-2020-who-discontinues-hydroxychloroquine-and-lopinavir-ritonavir-treatment-arms-for-covid-19

Index

C

D

E

N

O

P

R

W

Y

Z